diagnosis
and
evaluation
in
speech pathology

diagnosis
and
evaluation
in
speech pathology

LON L. EMERICK
Northern Michigan University

JOHN T. HATTEN
University of Minnesota–Duluth

prentice-hall, inc., englewood cliffs, new jersey

Library of Congress Cataloging in Publication Data

EMERICK, LON L.
    Diagnosis and evaluation in speech pathology.

    Includes bibliographies.
    1. Speech, Disorders of—Diagnosis. I. Hatten,
John T., joint author. II. Title.
[DNLM: 1. Speech disorders—Diagnosis. WM475 E52d
1974]
RC423. E58   616.8'55'075   73–16372
ISBN 0-13-208470-8

© 1974 by Prentice-Hall, Inc., Englewood Cliffs, New Jersey

10 9 8 7 6 5 4

Printed in the United States of America

PRENTICE-HALL INTERNATIONAL, INC., LONDON
PRENTICE-HALL OF AUSTRALIA, PTY. LTD., SYDNEY
PRENTICE-HALL OF CANADA, LTD., TORONTO
PRENTICE-HALL OF INDIA PRIVATE LIMITED, NEW DELHI
PRENTICE-HALL OF JAPAN, Inc., TOKYO

FOR LYNN AND PEQUETTI

contents

preface

In this volume we invite the reader to look over the shoulder of the speech clinician as he goes about his appointed diagnostic rounds. It is not a scholarly tome written in academic jargon, nor does it contain a formidable compendium of testing devices or erudite reviews of the literature to impress our professional colleagues. Rather, by focusing on case examples we hoped to provide a play-by-play account of what the clinician *does* when he evaluates individuals presenting speech or language problems.

We have purposely avoided parochial affiliations with any particular theoretical orientation. Eclecticism, in our view, is still the most fruitful way to remind ourselves that we are concerned with *people,* not speech defects.

Charles Van Riper, teacher, mentor, and colleague, first proposed the idea for the text and has followed its painful parturition with patient perspicacity. Our wives, far better diagnosticians than we, carefully monitored us for signs of information overload, while providing enormous amounts of empathy, positive regard, and constructive criticism garnished with good humor. They also typed the entire manuscript in its many drafts with their usual efficiency and attention to detail.

L. L. E.

J. T. H.

diagnosis
and
evaluation
in
speech pathology

1

introduction

Anyone who must don as many hats each working day as the speech clinician will invariably find that some are a bit snug, others flop over the ears, and only a precious few fit precisely. The tasks are not easily enumerated, since the profession is by no means static. Each active clinician also finds himself working as case selector, case evaluator, diagnostician, interviewer, parent counselor, teacher, coordinator, record keeper, researcher, and student. The boundaries between these various professional duties are not clearly defined; each clinician must be able to move freely from one area to another.

Diagnosis is among the most comprehensive and difficult tasks of the clinician. The demands for clinical skill are as great as in any other undertaking. Since speech is a function of the entire organism, the canny diagnostician must take all relevant aspects of behavior into account. The student soon learns that he is not working with speech sounds or the sounds of speech but rather with changing people in a changing environment. The mature diagnostician does not look at objective scores of articulatory skill, point scales of vocal-quality disorders, or language age as ends in themselves but rather as aspects of an individual's communication ability—we diagnose communicators, not communication! That revelation is a major factor in the transition from technician to professional.

DIAGNOSIS DEFINED

We intend to broaden the traditional concepts of diagnosis in order to present an encompassing working philosophy for performing this most important facet of a clinician's professional duties. There are essentially three aspects to diagnosis; they are by no means mutually exclusive—they are interrelated and overlap a great deal. Diagnosis is performed to

1. Determine the reality of the problem,
2. Determine the etiology of the problem, and ($Cause$)
3. Provide therapy focus.

1 diagnosis to determine the reality of the problem

The first task of diagnosis is to determine whether the presenting speech pattern does indeed constitute a handicap. Schultz (1972) has developed a model of clinical decision-making precisely directed at this question. The reader will be interested in comparing Schultz's "decision axis" concept with the present discussion. Before this is possible, however, it is necessary to have in mind a clear definition of what constitutes a speech disorder.

Van Riper's (1963: 16) definition of a speech impairment is widely quoted: "Speech is defective when it deviates so far from the speech of other people that it calls attention to itself, interferes with communication, or causes its possessor to be maladjusted." Inextricably incorporated into this definition is the concept that the speech clinician must take it upon himself to protect and preserve some predetermined and universally accepted standard of quality in the spoken signal. Unfortunately, there is no exemplary /s/ phoneme registered in the Bureau of Standards; thus, each diagnostician develops his own frame of reference.

We propose another way of identifying communication impairments. Although our criteria of defective speech are obviously related to more classical definitions, we suggest a distinct shift in emphasis. There are three aspects of the communicative act that are important in defining defective speech: the acoustic characteristics of the individual's speech signal; the influence of the acoustic signal on the intelligibility of the message; and, finally, the handicapping condition that results from the first two aspects.

The speech signal. The physical characteristics of the speech signal are subject to quantification through recording, measurement, and observation. Speech spectrographs, pitch-meters, and other instruments are available to help the diagnostician obtain an objective measure of the acoustic nature of the individual's speech. Such data are of little value, however, if no interpretation is made of the impact of the speech behavior. We must look at the physical characteristics of the speech signal and judge the *quality*. The state of the art has not progressed to the point where we can simply take the quantified data, compare it with established numerical norms, and determine the correctness of the speech sample. The physician is able to scrutinize data from a laboratory test and make an immediate diagnosis regarding the normalcy of an individual's blood count, but this kind of reference information is not yet available to the speech clinician. The question of whether the presenting speech difference is different enough to be of concern thus becomes a matter of human judgment. This judgment involves filtering incoming data through many synaptic junctions whose thresholds may have worn thin by bias and experience. An inordinately critical acoustic system is a hazard with far-reaching implications.

Each clinician must find some way to realistically judge adequate speech production under the eyes of his profession and his society. Pronovost (1966: 179) asks, "Do we consider ourselves self-appointed enforcers of society's standards of speech?" Even more perplexing is the question of whether we should appoint ourselves *determiners* of that standard. Should we protect some absolute standard of speech production? Is that the function of our profession or the function of society? If the speech difference we hear appears to have no impact upon the speaker or his environment, should the speech clinician consider it a problem and set out to correct it?

Studies of the incidence of speech disorders provide a great deal of information about the researchers as well as the subjects. One has only to compare the often-quoted figure (7 to 10 percent) of the incidence of speech disorders as provided in speech pathology literature with the 0.65 percent figure which was obtained in a Public Health Service report cited by Newman (1961). Although the Public Health Service data no doubt is open to some criticism, it was obtained from a house-to-house interview study and may more accurately reflect the general population's concept of defective speech. Incidence figures are notoriously self-fulfilling prophesies; they are also reports about someone *by someone*. If you expect that 10 percent of all grade-school children will have speech disorders, the probability that you will find just that percentage is greatly enhanced.

Johnson (1946) has emphasized the concept of the "participants of a problem," implying that in the final analysis the diagnostician becomes a part of the defect by identifying and labeling it. The widely varying estimates of the percentage of children in the schools with speech defects underscore the point that speech disorders are sometimes born in the ear of the listener as well as in the mouth of the speaker. Van Riper (1966) in his admonishing and thought-provoking article emphasizes the importance of the client's self-image in rehabilitative efforts. If our diagnosis fixates a self-image and perpetuates the error rather than helping to eradicate it, then our selection criteria must be broadened to include more than simply the acoustic nature of the speech. We are charged with the responsibility to prevent or reduce abnormality, not cause it.

What constitutes normal behavior? There are several definitions available (Johnson *et al.*, 1963), but we will discuss only two diverging philosophies with which each clinician must contend in establishing his own concept. The first theory we shall call the concept of *cultural norms*. The assumption is that there are behaviors that society considers aberrant in terms of *group* characteristics. Each bit of behavior can be judged, according to this model, against a real or theoretical standard, the nature of which is independent of the individual's personal idiosyncrasies. The second theory we shall call the concept of *individual norms*. Advocates of this model assume that each individual has made his unique adjustment to life based upon his own previous experiences, his physical limitations, and his environment's reactions to him. Any judgment as to the normalcy of a bit of behavior must be contingent upon individual characteristics such as age, intelligence, and experience.

Taken to the extreme, of course, this model would assert that each person is normal no matter what he does, since his behavior is the end product of all that plays upon his being. To this extent the concept of individual norms loses meaning, but a case example may help to clarify and give perspective. The audiologist who examines the hearing of a seventy-five-year-old individual and obtains the "typical" presbycusic audiometric curve could make a case for the judgment that this person has "normal" hearing. According to personal norms, this is average or normal behavior for a person of seventy-five; but according to cultural norms, the individual's hearing level is below the average for the total population. Follow-up procedures would be based, then, partially upon the practical matter of getting a more efficient communication system for the individual and also upon providing counseling so that the person will understand the nature of his hearing. Therefore, both cultural and personal norms play a part in diagnostic judgments and rehabilitative programs.

A severely retarded ten-year-old with a frontal lisp may not be judged to have defective speech, whereas an eight-year-old presenting a similar speech pattern, but a different intellectual potential, may be enrolled for therapy. Such judgments have implications for case selection, and the clinician must reconcile the variances between the physical differences in the sounds involved and individual variables in conjunction with what is normal for the population as a whole. Each clinician must continually use both concepts of normalcy in his diagnostic work. Every five-year-old "lisper" who leaves the kindergarten classroom for his semiweekly speech therapy session is most probably a victim of a one-dimensional definition of normal.

Far too many clinicians view diagnosis simply as a labeling process, but the actual labeling, or categorizing, is only a small part of the total assessment process. Classification systems within our profession are poor at best, and high-level abstractions (for example, lisping) tend to emphasize the similarities within a population rather than the individual differences. The keen diagnostician looks upon classifications as communication conveniences to be viewed with suspicion; he is continually alert for "hardening of the categories." Of course, the convenience factor is important, and each clinician making a determination of the reality of the problem must be willing to label it. This must of necessity, however, follow an orderly description of the characteristics of the disorder so that it can be clear what route the diagnostician took in arriving at the final classification. A diagnosis that only describes the characteristics of the problem, without judging its type or class, is a dead end. The opposite path is also dangerous; however, the diagnostician who is willing to begin his evaluation by labeling the problem has reversed the orderly sequence of acquiring knowledge and often effectively closes his mind to factors that may later point away from his premature "diagnosis."

Intelligibility of the message. The first variable in our definition of defective speech, then, concerns the physical acoustics of the speech signal. *Impact* is the crux of the problem; the clinician must be able to judge the effect of the speech difference upon the transmission of the message from speaker to listener. Objective data is of little value if they do not help us to estimate the importance of the difference for the communication of information. We have, in the main, been content with clinical insight and intuitive estimates when we judge the impact of speech differences upon intelligibility. Only a few research investigations have been concerned with this important problem (Garwood, 1952, and others). No research has so far clearly quantified the effect of a lateral lisp, for example, and yet each working day practicing clinicians must decide on the importance of such acoustic characteristics. What is needed is a massive study of how each type of speech disorder influences the transmission of information to the listener. The speech clinician is able to count the phoneme errors, quantify the number of repetitions per sentence, and establish a type-token ratio, but as yet he is unable, with any degree of reliability, to assess the intelligibility of the transmitted message.

Handicapping condition. The acoustic is one aspect of every speech difficulty, and the impact of that signal upon communication is the second. The third aspect of our definition is the resultant *handicapping condition.* The speech clinician is ultimately concerned with behavior. He does not simply identify the error and assess its influence upon the intelligibility of the message; he must also prepare a description of the person and the ways in which the particular speech symptoms shape the individual's adjusting characteristics.

Speech and speaker do not exist in social vacuums. They function in an environmental field that is extremely important. The environment is composed of an almost infinite number of factors that are affected by, and in turn have an effect upon, the speech behavior of the individual. The impact of the speech signal upon the environment is related to its impact upon the speaker, which in turn is related to its impact upon the environment.

> Tim, an adolescent with a painfully high postpubescent falsetto voice, spoke to his father only on the rarest of occasions. Tim's father later reported that he sensed his son's feeling of failure in developing a masculine voice but found himself with feelings of guilt, hostility, and frustration that he did not wish to convey to his son. These reactions became self-perpetuating, and both father and son shied away from conversation until preparations for a hunting trip brought a tearful culmination. Within a few days both father and son were visiting our office. Tim was reacting to his own reactions to his speech. The father was reacting to his son's speech, his son's reactions to the voice, and most probably his own reactions.

This third aspect of our definition of a communication impairment, then, concerns the influence of speech differences upon the adapting characteristics of the individual. In the school setting this becomes a most important factor as we look at the behaviors exhibited by the child and attempt to judge their facilitative or inhibitory potential for the child's learning. In the final analysis this third aspect justifies the existence of our profession. If the speech difference has no discernible impact on the child's behavior, and ultimately on his adjusting abilities and learning potential, there is little justification for concern on the part of the speech clinician.

Determining whether a *speech difference* does in fact constitute a *handicap* calls for careful testing, comparing the results with established norms, and a whole host of evaluative procedures that must culminate in a clinical judgment:

> Mrs. N. brought her four-year-old son into our office ostensibly for evaluation of his speech. Initial testing revealed an inconsistent frontal lisp which was easily stimulable to correction. Our first inclination was to simply inform Mrs. N. that her child's speech was within normal limits and conclude the session, but better judgment prevailed. It was noted earlier in the interview that Mrs. N. was firmly convinced of the existence of the problem and considered it quite severe. Several sessions were required before we could explain that there was no problem.

This instance of exaggerated parental reaction vividly illustrates that we must be concerned with more than just the speech signal. Total environmental diagnosis may be the only valid measure of a speech handicap.

diagnosis to determine the etiology of the problem

"Cause" has different meanings depending on its distance from the problem. As you look at a client in a diagnostic session, you search for reasons for his presenting behaviors. In fact many of these reasons may be buried in the past and can only be revealed by painstaking effort. Not only must we search through the client's past experience in order to uncover events that may help us alter current behaviors, but we must also guard against looking for causes in only one dimension of behavior. Johnny's brain damage, once identified, is probably not the only etiological factor, because speech is a complicated human function. Social, learning, motivation, and many other factors enter into the total process.

Classically, etiology has been defined in terms of *predisposing, precipitating,* and *perpetuating* factors. Agents that dispose or incline an individual toward communication impairment are designated as predisposing causes. Precipitating factors actually bring about the onset of the problem, while maintaining, or perpetuating, variables are responsible for the persistance of the abnormality.

Predisposing factors are generally thought to be important because of their potential link with a third agent. A classic example of predisposing factors is the higher than normal incidence of left-handedness among stutterers. The left-handedness itself is of little consequence, but the implication of basic underlying neurological differences has perplexed researchers for decades. The wary diagnostician must watch for factors that occur with high regularity in association with certain communication disorders. Such data could ultimately be instrumental in uncovering some basic information regarding the nature of the disorder.

Precipitating factors are generally, but not always, no longer operating and, as such, may or may not be identifiable. There is a philosophical question of whether we need to search for precipitating factors if they are not still operating, and the point is well taken. Each moment, however, there is created a new set of precipitating factors which, acting as characteristics of the past, perpetuate behaviors of the present. Speech disorders generally are not static entities developed at a given point and perpetuated without modification through time; rather they are ever-changing characteristics that are constantly influenced by intrinsic and extrinsic factors. Precipitating factors are best considered to be those agents that brought the disorder to its present state.

The perpetuating factors are those variables which are currently at work on the individual. Almost without exception, habit strength is a prime maintaining factor in developmental speech disorders. Other factors are also crucial, however, and it is the diagnostician's task to uncover the environmental and physical factors that are reinforcing and thus perpetuating the disorder.

Mrs. M. was an alert, intense person with an extremely high energy level. The referring physician's report described her as "hyper," and the description was apt indeed. Although such people do not always develop vocal nodules, they certainly seem predisposed to them. Mrs. M.'s vocal nodules had been surgically removed but were beginning to show signs of recurrence when we first saw her. In the initial interview several facts became apparent. First, it was evident that

Mrs. M. was overwhelmed by the pressures of motherhood (five children under seven years of age) and the routine and often unfulfilling chores of the daily household. She had, over the past five years, developed a method of control over the children which could best be described as the "holler and hit" technique. Unfortunately for Mrs. M.'s vocal folds, she resorted to too much hollering and too little hitting.

Mrs. M.'s case illustrates the importance of all three types of etiological factors. The personality characteristics clearly predisposed her to the resulting disorder; the intrusion of children into her life precipitated the vocal disorder by raising her anxiety and greatly increasing her vocal output; and the perpetuating influence of habit strength and the continuation of the original "irritants" were currently evident.

3 diagnosis to provide therapy focus

Labeling the speech disorder is often seen as the sole purpose of diagnosis. Similarly, some clinicians view the determination of the *cause* of a speech problem to be an end in itself. We contend, however, that if diagnosis is to be of utmost benefit it must be goal-oriented. Diagnosis without purpose is of little value to the clinician. Every classroom teacher has experienced the frustration of receiving a report from a school psychometrist stating that the child she referred because of behavioral problems does, indeed, have behavioral problems. Such a diagnosis fails to provide the crucial final link: recommendations for remedial procedures. Diagnosis is an empty exercise in test administration, data collection, and client evaluation if it fails to provide logical suggestions for therapy.

There are several major diagnostic philosophies that the speech clinician must be aware of in order to formulate his own logical and professionally comfortable personal model.

The *medical,* or *disease, model* of diagnosis appears to be based upon a few solidly entrenched tenets. First, this concept implies that a diagnosis must be completed *before* treatment. The assumption is that curative procedures are much more efficient if the etiological factors are known. Symptomatic medicine is considered tantamount to quackery. This model holds that diagnosis and treatment are two discernibly different tasks. Seldom is it possible for a physician to engage in a procedure which serves both diagnostic and therapeutic functions.

Another assumption of the medical model is that physical disturbances are generally related to organic causes. If the temperature is high, there is a structural explanation to be pursued within the soma. Identification of the site of the lesion is thus paramount in determining the cause-effect relationship. Classifications generally pertain to the site of the lesion, and it is generally assumed that the lesion is within the client. The application of this model to speech and language has been criticized because it restricts the scope of the investigation.

Medical diagnosis is generally concluded in an absolute manner. Hy-

potheses regarding etiology, nature of the problem, and prognosis are generally presented to other professionals and to the client as facts. This most useful
technique serves to build confidence and may actually hasten the recovery
process. Few of us would return to a physician who vacillated regarding the
diagnosis of our ailment. The therapeutic value of an omniscient clinical demeanor is a lesson well learned by most physicians. Absolutism is indeed a
luxury, but at times a very useful one.

The *learning,* or *education, model* of diagnosis is in a very fluid state at
present. This model is based upon traditional theories of learning and stresses
the identification of cognitive activities intervening between a cue and a
response. Classification systems are more likely to emphasize the area of behavior involved rather than the site of the breakdown. Educational writings
are beginning to emphasize the nature of the behavioral disability rather than
the causative factors.

The *psychiatric model* of diagnosis has several aspects of importance to
the speech clinician. Foremost is the concept that the state of the psyche is
capable of either interference with or facilitation of adaptive behavior. Implied therein is the idea that human behavior is related to or partially dependent upon both conscious and subconscious factors that in turn have primarily
experiential components of development. Psychiatric diagnosis, in some
schools of this currently very fractionated profession, is concerned with dis-
covering the hidden factors of the psyche that propel action.

The newest model of diagnosis, the *operant,* or *behavioral, paradigm,*
offers several applicable concepts which speech clinicians are beginning to
incorporate into their working philosophies (Sloane and MacAulay, 1968).
Typically, the operant model disavows interest in the factors that intervene
between stimulus and response, since such factors are at best only hypothetical. Probably the primary characteristic of the model is the belief that discriminative stimuli and resultant behaviors are observable, measurable, and
quantifiable, and that the establishment of "baseline," or presenting, behaviors is paramount to future therapeutic measures. The second major undertaking is to determine what reinforcers exist for the person. In other words,
the diagnostician must determine what systematic relationship exists between
behaviors and the variables that control those behaviors. Detailed examination of the subject, his environment, and his current behavioral repertoire
should lead the diagnostician to some conclusion regarding the terminal behaviors desired. This task is of vital importance in operant theory and,
strangely, has been neglected in much of the speech therapy literature. Once
goal behavior has been described, it will be necessary to delineate the exact
progression of steps necessary to achieve the goal. Precision recording is necessary in order for the diagnostician to guide the clinician's work toward the
proper level of difficulty and appropriateness.

Clearly, this presentation of classical models of diagnosis is far from complete; the points put forth are considered representative and should give the

speech clinician some basis for developing his own philosophy of diagnosis. There is no speech therapy model of diagnosis, and this is probably as it should be. Our concerns cut across many disciplines; thus, speech clinicians have typically been rather pragmatic and have adopted an eclectic approach to each new problem.

DIAGNOSIS—SCIENCE AND ART

Diagnosis demands a unique blending of science and art. The scientific method is applicable to our work as diagnosticians, both in guiding our procedures and in focusing our attitude of operation. The scientific method directs the diagnostician to observe "all" of the available factors, formulate testable hypotheses using clearly stated and answerable questions, test those hypotheses to determine their validity, and formulate conclusions based upon the tested hypotheses. The method demands rigorous adherence to standardized procedures and has as its favorable characteristics objectivity, quantifiability, and structure. The "scientific" diagnostician tends to rely upon tests, test data, and other procedures that lend themselves to quantification.

As an attitude of operation the scientific method implies that the diagnostician has not predetermined his test findings and that he is not eager to seek the proof or disproof of his hypotheses. The diagnostician sees his hypotheses as something to be tested rather than something to be defended. Many things are implied in this attitude. We have all experienced the biased clinician who finds what he expects to find in each diagnosis. The self-fulfilling prophecy is a lethal but almost universal human characteristic; it must be counterbalanced by a scientific approach to testing. The writers are familiar with one youngster who had traveled all over the country in search of a diagnostic explanation for his delay in language development that would be compatible with his parents' precepts. When we saw the child, his father brought with him a case file thick with reports from various noted authorities (the "fat folder" syndrome). Each report revealed more about the examiner than the child as it cited facts in support of a theory of etiology congruent with the diagnostician's particular specialty. Such youngsters—or diagnostic vagabonds, as we might call them—are victims of misguided, but persistent parents and nonscientific diagnosticians.

The beginning student must also guard against the "recent article" syndrome to which we all fall prey upon occasion. Typically, the behavioral pattern goes something like this: you read an article that depicts a particular syndrome and explains the distinctive characteristics of a disorder; for a few weeks thereafter every child you see appears to fall into the pattern described in the publication.

In nearly all matters the human mind has a strong tendency to judge in the light of its own experience, knowledge, and prejudices rather than on the evidence presented. Thus new ideas are judged in the light of prevailing beliefs (Beveridge, 1951: 103).

The way to overcome the "recent article" syndrome, of course, is to be aware that it exists and, incidentally, to have a thorough understanding of the nature of human perception.

The strict adherence to fact that is demanded by the pure scientific method is often a bit confining. That, in part, may explain why we all practice the "art" of diagnosis at times. The artistic approach has several specific characteristics. The "artist" is less dependent upon specific observations for the formation of hypotheses than upon his casual and nonstructured scrutiny. This type of clinician is perfectly willing to disregard formal test results or standard testing procedures in favor of what appears obvious to him on the basis of his clinical expertise. The hunch, or clinical intuition, plays a significant part in such evaluations. The diagnostician will contend that facts can be approached from several directions and that he is capable of assessing the same kinds of behaviors that are measured by formal tests. Such contentions are disconcerting to the test-bound person who has come to expect that the only valid way to gain information is through standardized procedures.

It is obvious that, in the extreme, there are weaknesses in both approaches. The scientist may tend to become so dependent upon his objective methods of measurement that he fails to see the client through the maze of percentile scores and age norms. The whole is greater than the sum of its parts, and every diagnostician must guard against simply measuring the isolated characteristics without getting a full picture of the individual. The client is often made to fit the test results even when circumstances clearly contraindicate such a conclusion. We recently received a report from a therapist who claimed great frustration with a particular child because "his ITPA results are not consonant with his classroom performance. He is not as low in psycholinguistic abilities as his test performance would indicate." This therapist believed that the child had poorer abilities than his classroom performance indicated and that there must have been something invalid about his daily behavior. Could it not be that the test results do not tell us as much as the child's everyday performance? Test data become an artifact of the child's total behavior and should be so judged, while the daily behavior may hold much more meaning for the future remedial program. Don't build altars to any testing device; every objective instrument was once only a hunch in someone's mind.

The other end of the science-art continuum is just as precarious, if not more so. The possibility of a diagnostician projecting more than a modest amount of himself into his evaluation is greater when he is less scientific in his approach. Clinical intuitions are often simply clinical biases, and it is very easy to make new evidence fit old categories. The diagnostician must find the proper admixture of each philosophy in establishing his own diagnostic procedures.

the diagnostician as a factor

Ultimately, however, the most important diagnostic tool is the diagnostician himself. The children we assess have seldom read the test manual, and the rigid structures of the testing situation may not be compatible with the child's fluid and nonstructured style of behavior. Tests are abstractions of behavior, and as such they represent only a fraction of the child's total repertoire of responses to his environment. What better measure of an individual's behavior than that behavior itself? Thus, the diagnostician becomes an important aspect of the evaluating situation as he selects, interacts, responds, and assembles information.

What skills are necessary to develop in order to become an effective, nontest-bound diagnostician? How do you develop them? There are no easy answers to these questions. Experience in the diagnostic process is an absolute necessity, but experience in terms of number of children seen is not enough; there is little value in one diagnostic experience reduplicated 1,000 times. The diagnostician must be able to gain from new experiences, and this demands *flexibility*. The stereotyped and stagnant diagnostician learns little from increased exposure to people and new situations, but those who use their experience as a pattern to be compared against, rather than as a mold into which all new experiences must fit, will continue to grow and learn.

The diagnostician must be flexible enough within the testing situation to shift from predetermined plans to new modes of evaluation as the client presents unpredicted behaviors. The examiner who steadfastly plods through a series of tests even though a child has not interacted in any significant degree may well have lost the opportunity to gain information by other means. It is not atypical for beginning speech clinicians to panic in the face of an unexpected performance and become intransigent in their application of a series of formal tests. In this regard, continued experience in diagnosis may provide the flexibility needed to move freely to other avenues of information.

A graduate student was recently observed attempting to administer a comprehensive language inventory to Mr. D., a sixty-three-year-old aphasic. Despite the student's determined attempts to complete the formal testing, Mr. D. continued commenting on the test room, the diagnostician, and other subjects irrelevant to the test. His most persistent topic was his altered life circumstances and his frustrations. The diagnostic session ended with two unfulfilled participants. The student could not understand why Mr. D. would not cooperate and came away with none of the data he desired regarding the client's language ability. Indeed, upon later discussion it became evident that the student even failed to gain much insight into the patient's current concerns because he worried only about completing predetermined procedures. Mr. D., on the other hand, left the session feeling that the diagnostician lacked any understanding of his problem, thereby adding to his feelings of futility.

Practicing clinicians often eagerly accept new and novel techniques as they become available. We have noted a generation gap within the field of speech pathology in the past few years. As the profession moves into new and uncharted areas of concern, many new materials, tests, and techniques have become available. The old guard tends to scoff at something new, and the young clinicians bristle with frustration at the inflexibility of the veteran therapists. New techniques must not be accepted or rejected carte blanche but rather must be scrutinized for their merit. Techniques grossly foreign to experience tend to threaten and bewilder the inflexible diagnostician because he perceives them as attacks upon his trusted and time-proven methods. Is it possible that training programs which emphasize testing and therapy techniques and materials are more likely to produce an inflexible therapist than those programs which emphasize theory, problem-solving ability, and creativity?

A clinician must possess many important personal attributes. Rogers (1942) speaks of empathy, congruency, and unconditional positive regard as necessary characteristics of the clinician, and they most certainly apply to the diagnostic process as well. Generally these qualities must be nurtured through consistent effort and proper guidance. Video- and audio-tape equipment now allows the developing clinician to observe his own behaviors in the testing situation in order to more fully understand his own performance. Equally important in developing these important characteristics is skillful guidance from a master diagnostician.

If the term *sensitivity* may be defined as a keenness of sense or a heightened awareness of incoming sensory data, then this much-maligned term has meaning for the diagnostician. He must be able to detect subtle physical, psychological, or interactional changes in a client's behavior; and these small changes have the most significant meaning in the diagnostic process.

Insight into the meaning of behaviors must be developed from a thorough grounding in the basic processes requisite for the speech act. Each diagnostician must become so familiar with the normal process of language acquisition and normal speech functioning that he has a built-in set of standards upon which to base judgment. The insightful clinician is the knowledgeable professional who is capable of quickly comparing the client's behavior with the norm.

The development of an *evaluative attitude* is often a rather difficult task for the beginning clinician. We are, to a large extent, slaves to our experience; each clinician tends to bring the "social attitude" into the testing setting. Rather than looking upon the client's performance as having meaning for the evaluative process, we consult our own responses and formulate our own points of view in the give-and-take of the conversation. The critical, questioning attitude must be developed so that the clinician looks upon the behaviors in terms of their meaning rather than in terms of the response expected of him. Social interaction lends itself to superficiality, whereas the flow of the diagnostic interaction must, by design, lend itself to uncovering the meaning of the incorporated behavior. Effective diagnosticians tend to question the surface validity of behaviors and search for motivations, explanations, and interpretations that are not readily apparent.

Closely allied with the concept of the evaluative attitude is the idea of *persistent curiosity*. The diagnostician must develop an inquisitiveness that will make him persistent in his search for explanations. Answers are seldom apparent at first, and continuous effort is imperative. The directors of training institutions foster weakness in this area when they assign clients to students and expect therapy to get underway in a "reasonable" period of time. They are so bound to the rigid university timetables that therapy is often discontinuous. In an attempt to give each student a variety of clinical experiences, they often tend to sever clinical undertakings with a client at each semester's end, knowing full well that the diagnostic or therapeutic process is not best served in this way. The student may not always understand this, however, and may develop the notion that diagnosis is a temporary therapy-initiating exercise to be completed in an hour or two. The curious and persistent clinician, however, continues to place the client in situations that will permit additional scrutiny.

Objectivity comes from practicing the art of controlled involvement. The diagnostician must cultivate objectivity because he is subject to human errors. He must be warm, understanding, and accepting on the one hand and objective, evaluative, and detached on the other. Without some degree of balance between the two extremes the diagnostician may so severely distort the interaction between himself and the client that he obtains little of value. Objectivity demands more than simply guarding against undue emotional involvement. The examiner must be objective about *himself*, his skills, knowledge, and personal characteristics. He must, in other words, know himself to a sufficient degree that he can judge his own successes and failures and continue to grow in professional skill.

Rapport may be defined as the establishment of a working relationship, based upon mutual respect, trust, and confidence, which encourages optimum performance on the part of both client and clinician. Rapport is developed over a period of time and is not easily established in a single session or during a few minutes at the initiation of one therapeutic encounter. Rapport must not only be developed, it must be maintained and this calls for continued effort. The list of characteristics that enhance rapport is endless, but the factor which we have found to be universally important is the *ability to maintain a nonthreatened posture throughout the testing session*. The student or clinician who is easily threatened in interpersonal interaction tends to have greater difficulty establishing rapport than one who can work with people and experience little threat from unpredictable or hostile reactions. The link between this characteristic and egostrength is probably quite strong and should be seriously contemplated by the beginning diagnostician.

Although much standardization is possible through strict adherence to test routines, the lowest common denominator in diagnostic evaluations is the examiner himself. Test results are the product of the subject, examiner, test, and test circumstance, each of which has certain influence. A baseball player's batting average is judged against many factors, including how many "at bats" he had (was this a continuing performance?) and the league he played in (who administered the tests?) to name but a few. Examinations are clearly selected as a result of the experiences and biases of the examiner. Just as the answers we receive to questions are in part a function of the questions we ask and how we ask them, the diagnostic findings we obtain are in part a function of the tests we administer and the way they are administered. A "defective speech pattern" may be partially due to a defective testing pattern or a defective tester.

diagnostic observation

How can the clinician receive the kinds of data that he needs except by formally administering tests? That question should be foremost in the mind of every examiner because it forces him to look to the test itself and ask what behaviors this test is measuring and the pertinence of those behaviors to speech and language functioning. Among the most crucial methods of obtaining information is *observation.* Observational skills are the product of many hours of hard work. There is no shortcut to developing these skills, and each student must practice by testing his skills against established measures of subject performance. There are five aspects to observation which are necessary for the orderly acquisition of useful information: focus, depth, description, interpretation, and implication.

Focus. Probably the most difficult aspect of observation for the beginning student is focusing on the pertinent aspects of behavior. It is important for the student to remind himself that *no behavior has meaning unto itself,* and thus not only must he look at the presenting conduct of the client, but he must also determine what aspects of the environment serve as stimuli or antecedent events to that behavior and what aspects serve as perpetuators. Quantification of behaviors forces the observer to become objective and he should carefully analyze the effect of the action on the environment. If the behavior is of high incidence, the events which succeed it must be suspect as maintainers and as such are of prime importance. The casual and untrained observer usually cannot focus on the descriptive level. He tends to categorize behavior as good or bad, normal or abnormal, cooperative or uncooperative, shy or outgoing, and so forth. The first step in observation, then, is to focus on a very descriptive level so that the examiner can present the actual behaviors the client exhibited rather than generalizations regarding the meaning of those actions. In order to underscore the importance of focusing attention in the observational task, we often ask students to observe some single aspect of behavior in a therapy session and report on that one characteristic. Recently five students were assigned to observe one of the following aspects of a given therapy session: (1) how much of the session was consumed by the clinician talking; (2) the amount of eye contact between child and clinician; (3) the percentage of the total therapy session in which goal directed behaviors were exhibited by both the clinician and child; (4) the mother's facial expressions and remarks as the session progressed; and (5) the entire therapy process. The interesting result of this experiment was that each of the first four students later came up with suggestions which were pertinent to the therapy process, while the last student could only add general suggestions. These microscopic observations must eventually enable the student to make general conclusions from the total situation; our experience has led us to believe that it is best to start with such a finite focal point.

Depth. The depth of the observation is determined to a large degree by circumstance, but the diagnostician must find ways to observe the client interacting with many different people and stimuli. The diagnostician cannot expect to gain a great deal of information from fleeting observations; he must be willing to spend the time and energy necessary to observe a significant amount of behavior.

Observation of the child in many and varied settings must have a reference point and that point must be normal behavior. Never let an exception to a general state go unnoticed! The unexpected may take any one of several forms. It may be bizarre and out of place with no observable precipitant, it may be the lack of response where one is naturally expected, or it may be expected in terms of the stimuli presented but bizarre in some other aspect such as intensity, frequency, or length of response.

Description. Simply selecting the proper focus and observing ample and varied behavior is not going to lead to a productive session; the diagnostician must attempt to put those observations into words. The translation from observation to description is often a much more difficult step than the novice suspects. In the early stages the diagnostician must train himself to describe behavior in writing as objectively, explicitly, and completely as possible. During these first attempts to communicate the findings of the observation, the clinician must withstand the temptation to jump to conclusions. He must stick to what he observes and what he can describe. The authors recently assigned several students to the same diagnostic session and asked them to record their observations; here are two samples of their reports:

Student A. Timmy entered the testing room and was very shy and unhappy. He was afraid of the examiner and wanted his mother. He continued to act in this spoiled manner until his mother was brought into the room. Once Mrs. H. was in the room, Timmy began to behave himself, and the testing could be undertaken.

Student B. Timmy stood in the doorway, held his head down, and refused to move into the room for three or four minutes until the clinician physically picked him up and closed the door. Timmy stood by the door and cried, while the clinician attempted to engage him in such play activities as card games, lotto, and ball. Timmy continued to cry for approximately fifteen minutes throughout all of these attempts until the clinician went out and brought Mrs. H. into the room. Timmy immediately crawled up on his mother's lap, and the clinician gave the articulation testing cards to the mother to show to Timmy. After five minutes of encouragement by the mother, Timmy began to name the pictures.

Careful examination of these two accounts shows that one student was willing to make judgments, classify behavior, and generally draw conclusions without clearly specifying just what behavior was observed; the other student made a valiant effort to report the observables. Either approach can be taken to an extreme and thus interfere with the orderly transmission of information, but we strongly recommend that the beginning clinician make every attempt to keep the early accounts of his observations descriptive.

Interpretation. Once all pertinent behaviors have been described, it is incumbent upon the observer to make *interpretations*. Without moving to this level, the observations are of little value (unless the worker is willing to allow someone else to make an interpretation based upon his descriptive data). At this point the observer makes inferences regarding the meaning of behaviors; he attempts to generalize and classify behaviors and draw conclusions as to the meaning of what he observed. All of this can only be done, however, after sufficient purely descriptive information has been compiled. Interpretations drawn from objective quantified data are much more easily checked against reality than are interpretations made from desultory observations.

We recently examined a four-year-old girl who was referred to us because "she does not talk clearly." When the traditional articulation analysis was administered using pictures to elicit single-word responses, it became evident that she was having difficulty with all of the consonant sounds. If we had stopped at this point and made no interpretation of the findings, we would have found the test results to be only of limited assistance in directing the ensuing therapy. Further interpretation was made, however, when the articulation pattern was analyzed in terms of underlying linguistic rules. It was discovered that she had not incorporated into her language system the rules of either place or manner of articulation. We recommended that the child receive therapy directed toward helping her identify the distinctive features by which sounds are differentiated prior to starting work with any given sound.

Implications. Finally, the observer is expected to explain the *implications* of the observed behavior. Implications may be found by evaluating the consistency of the disorder in various settings, the degree of intelligibility in contextual speech, and so on. Information on the etiology of the problem may also be available through observation, and such interpretations as are warranted must be ventured. Similarly, the observed behavior can be assigned a meaning in order to direct the therapeutic effort.

It should be evident to the reader that we have attempted to apply the "abstraction process" to the task of observation (Weinberg, 1959). The diagnostician moves from the nonverbal level of sensing and observing to the verbal levels of describing, labeling, and interpreting; and finally he draws conclusions and states some implications. Leaving out the middle verbal steps of description would be undisciplined because it allows too much distorting subjectivity and projection on the part of the observer. Strict adherence to the logical order of observation leads to accurate and more defensible conclusions.

Our rather extended discussion of the various skills and abilities necessary for efficient diagnosis is designed to impress upon the reader the necessity of mediating between the scientific and artistic elements of diagnosis. We are neither computers coldly collecting and collating data, nor are we just friends sitting down for a social chat. The diagnostician must possess warmth and compassion as well as observational skill and a scientific attitude.

PUTTING THE DIAGNOSIS TO WORK

Almost every training program in speech pathology conducts an active outpatient diagnostic clinic in which patients are seen for short periods of time and a "diagnostic evaluation" is conducted, complete with parent interview, test administration, and concluding interview. We contend that such practices contribute to the "ninety-minute wonder" syndrome to which many young clinicians succumb in their early years of practice. They believe that it is possible to complete the diagnostic process in a few hours.

Every client responds somewhat differently to novel and challenging situations. For example, some youngsters excel under such circumstances and perform at or near the top of their ability level; others withdraw and protect themselves from failure by putting forth only a minimum of effort. It is quite possible, therefore, that one child's performance on a single measure may be far above his actual daily performance, while another youngster, with a much lower test score, may perform well in daily adjustment. The single measure as a method of diagnosis is thus suspect and should be so considered by every diagnostician. Our knowledge of the inherent unreliability of any single measure of performance must inevitably guide us to a philosophy of continuous diagnosis.

Diagnostic therapy allows the clinician to retain the diagnostic frame of reference while conducting treatment. Simply stated, the process involves continually subjecting the patient to systematically varying therapy techniques while keeping careful record of his progress and responses to the various approaches. Through this technique it is possible, for example, to evaluate the efficacy of the auditory modality in comparison with the efficacy of a different modality. Diagnostic therapy is not simply the application of a series of formal tests over a period of time. The astute clinician will elicit in therapy many of the behaviors necessary for efficient functioning in life, and thereby provide some useful data on the general adjusting level of the subject.

> Rex, a particularly perplexing college student with a functionally based harsh voice, presented his student clinician with a diagnostician's nightmare. The first therapy procedures were aimed at altering the method of glottal attack. Although six weeks of this therapy did appear to have some positive effect, the transition was not dramatic, and a second was initiated including a slight lowering of the pitch level. However, this adjustment was extremely difficult and had no impact on the vocal quality. The enterprising therapist therefore attempted relaxation exercises with eager enthusiasm knowing full well the inherent dangers involved when female therapists attempt such procedures with male clients. These sessions, though well prepared and presented, were awkward at times as Rex showed real signs of unrest and inner conflict. Casual conversations led to therapy sessions filled with discussions of Rex's frustrations with college, women, society, and life in general. The pouring forth reached a breaking point, and the next step in this trial therapy sequence was referral to the counseling center where Rex received much-needed help. Within a few months therapy was reestablished, with emphasis once again on glottal attack, since that appeared to be a fruitful area. Progress was rapid from that point on, and dismissal was possible within the next academic year.

If one believes that diagnosis is an ongoing process to be incorporated into the total therapy schema, then one may abandon the long-held belief that knowledge of etiology is a necessary prerequisite to therapy. Certainly, there may be instances where knowledge of etiology will direct remediation, but in the main it appears more important to clearly describe the behavior of the client and his current level of functioning. There is some question as to the value for therapy of knowing that a certain child is brain damaged for instance, while there is undisputed value in knowing his language functioning, adjustive techniques, classroom performance, and primary effective modalities of learning.

In order to put the diagnosis to work efficiently, it is necessary to have clearly defined goals for the evaluation. Diagnosis must serve a function to the clinician, and this is best done if the diagnostician establishes clearly stated expectations regarding the kind of information he wishes to obtain. Adopting this goal-oriented approach, let us present some broad purposes of diagnosis:

1. To determine all aspects of behavior pertinent to speech and language production.
2. To determine why this person is at his present level of functioning. This may involve historical, developmental, maintaining, and physical factors.
3. To determine what this person's speech production should be. Is his speech behavior normal, and if not, what is the expected level of functioning with and without remediation? What is the prognosis?
4. To determine how this person should get to the desired level of performance; the diagnostic process should narrow our area of concern so that we can concentrate on a particular facet of the individual's behavior. In this way diagnosis serves to direct our therapy efforts.
5. To determine what the observed behavior means for the person. What impact, if any, does the speech pattern have on this individual's life?
6. To determine what goals the client has established for this diagnostic session. What does he expect?
7. To determine what progress has been made in the correction of previously diagnosed speech disorders. Diagnosis, as an ongoing process, should continually tell us something of the progress our client is making in therapy.

PROJECTS AND QUESTIONS

1. There are several types of speech disorders which lend themselves to objective and quantitative measurement. List some, describe how they might be quantified, and relate that quantification to a determination of the normality or abnormality of the problem.
2. Write some basic working postulates of your own personal model of diagnosis.
3. Compare the traditional etiological and symptomatic systems of classification of speech disorders with the system devised by Milisen (1957). Of what value are classification systems? Could you devise one with some novel characteristics that is of value to your understanding of speech disorders?
4. What implications for diagnosis do you find in the fact that speech is essentially an overlaid function?
5. Have society's changing definitions of aberrant behavior influenced speech therapy's definitions of speech disorders? How? Is there a relationship between our definition of what constitutes defective speech and the clinical approach to public-school therapy?
6. We have all observed other professionals undertaking diagnostic evaluations. Make a descriptive analysis of those three individuals you feel were, in your experience, most proficient. What characteristics typify these persons? How would you rate them on a ten-point scale of objectivity (scientific) versus subjectivity (artistic)?
7. What are the implications of Johnson's (1961) article for our concepts of diagnosis?
8. Most speech therapy texts quote incidence figures of 5 to 10 percent of the public-school population, and yet Newman (1961: 9–10) quotes a Public Health Service report revealing only 0.65 percent of the population as being speech impaired. If these figures are accurate, what implications does this have for our definition of what constitutes defective speech?

9. Look up the canons of J. S. Mill (1872) and relate them to our discussion of causality.
10. Review carefully the chapter by Backus (1960).
11. Read Brown and Van Riper (1966). Make up a definition of speech defectiveness based upon the many functions of oral communication.
12. What is the impact of the Perkins and Curlee (1969) article on your concept of cause?

BIBLIOGRAPHY

BACKUS, O. (1960). "The Study of Psychological Processes in Speech Therapists." In *Psychological and Psychiatric Aspects of Speech and Hearing*, ed. D. Barbara. Springfield, Ill.: Charles C Thomas. Pp. 501–35.

BATEMAN, B. (1964). "Learning Disabilities—Yesterday, Today, and Tomorrow." *Exceptional Children*, 31: 167–77.

BEVERIDGE, W. (1951). *The Art of Scientific Investigation*. New York: W. W. Norton & Company, Inc.

BROWN, C. and C. VAN RIPER (1966). *Speech and Man*. Englewood Cliffs, N.J.: Prentice-Hall, Inc.

DARLEY, F. (1964). *Diagnosis and Appraisal of Communication Disorders*. Englewood Cliffs, N.J.: Prentice-Hall, Inc.

DIETZ, H. (1952). "A Study of the Understandability of Defective Speech in Relation to Errors of Articulation." Unpublished Master's thesis, University of Pittsburg.

DUFF, R. and A. HOLLINGSHEAD (1968). *Sickness and Society*. New York: Harper & Row, Publishers.

GARWOOD, V. (1952). "An Experimental Study of Certain Relationships Between Intelligibility Scores and Clinical Data of Persons with Defective Articulation." Unpublished Doctoral dissertation, University of Michigan.

GREY, S. (1963). *The Psychologist in the Schools*. New York: Holt, Rinehart & Winston, Inc.

HADLEY, J. (1958). *Clinical and Counseling Psychology*. New York: Alfred A. Knopf, Inc. Pp. 295–307.

JOHNSON, W. (1961). "Are Speech Disorders 'Superficial' or 'Basic'?" *ASHA*, 3: 233.

——— (1946). *People in Quandaries*. New York: Harper & Row, Publishers.

———, F. DARLEY, and D. SPRIESTERSBACH (1963). *Diagnostic Methods in Speech Pathology*. New York: Harper & Row, Publishers.

LOVITT, T. (1967). "Assessment of Children with Learning Disabilities." *Exceptional Children*, 34: 233–39.

MILISEN, R. (1957). "Methods of Evaluation and Diagnosis of Speech Disorders." In *Handbook of Speech Pathology,* ed. L. Travis. New York: Appleton-Century-Crofts, Inc. Pp. 267–309.

MILL, J. (1872). *A System of Logic.* London: Longmans, Green, Reader, and Dyer.

NEWMAN, P. (1961). "Speech Impaired?" *ASHA,* 3: 9–10.

PERKINS, W. and R. CURLEE (1969). "Causality in Speech Pathology." *Journal of Speech and Hearing Disorders,* 34: 231–38.

PRONOVOST, W. (1966). "Case Selection in the Schools: Articulatory Disorders." *ASHA,* 8: 179–81.

REESE, E. (1966). *The Analysis of Human Operant Behavior.* Dubuque, Iowa: Wm. C. Brown.

ROGERS, C. (1942). *Counseling and Psychotherapy.* Boston: Houghton Mifflin, Company.

SCHULTZ, M. (1972). *An Analysis of Clinical Behavior in Speech and Hearing.* Englewood Cliffs, N.J.: Prentice-Hall, Inc.

SIEGEL, G. (1966). "Evaluative Reactions and the Pathologies of Speech." *Quarterly Journal of Speech,* 52: 70–73.

SLOANE, H. and B. MACAULAY, eds. (1968). *Operant Procedures in Remedial Speech and Language Training.* Boston: Houghton Mifflin Company.

VAN RIPER, C. (1963). *Speech Correction: Principles and Methods.* Englewood Cliffs, N.J.: Prentice-Hall, Inc.

——— (1966). "Guilty?" *WMU Journal of Speech Therapy,* 2: 2–3.

WEINBERG, H. (1959). *Levels of Knowing and Existence.* New York: Harper & Row, Publishers.

2

interviewing

The prospective speech clinician must acquire an impressive array of knowledge and skills if he is to perform his role effectively. The ability to conduct professional interviews is one of the most important of these acquisitions.[1] Indeed, no other facet of the worker's role is so central and so vital to his clinical success.

THE IMPORTANCE OF INTERVIEWING

Not only are clients' problems assessed primarily by verbal interaction, they are also corrected by means of the fragile, fleeting butterfly of the spoken word. It seems rather surprising, therefore, that the subject of interviewing has been relatively neglected in the clinical and research literature.

The paradox of speech pathology is that while all professionals talk when they are on the job, none of them writes about how they talk. After exploring the issue with many clinicians, supervisors, and personnel in university training programs, we discovered several curious concepts of interviewing that seem to make it a minor academic concern. Let us briefly examine some of these notions:

[1] This chapter is based upon *The Parent Interview* by Lon L. Emerick. © by the Interstate Printers & Publishers, Inc., Danville, Illinois (1969).

1. The good clinician communicating.   If the training program is well balanced, with the proper sequence of course work and clinical experiences, and if the clinician acquires a vast storehouse of relevant information about speech disorders and their treatment, then he will be able to convey this information to his clients.

2. The magical clinician.   Interviewing is an art that some have mastered and others have not. Since it is an art and, hence, subjective, it obviously cannot be taught or exposed to any kind of scientific scrutiny. Some holders of this position are excellent clinicians who are able to secure relationships with their clients as if by some mesmerizing process, even though they rarely talk about establishing rapport and certainly never write it on their therapy plans. Indeed, there are some clinicians who decline to study their interviewing procedures because they are fearful of casting a cold eye upon their craft and dissecting the bones; they feel that, since the process is an art, such a careful appraisal will dry up the springs of "clinical creativity."

3. The inevitable clinician.   Somewhere among the memories of his supervised clinical practice, somehow by an inevitable process that grinds along slowly, the clinician will develop interviewing skills. Practice makes perfect. Alas, practice also makes permanent, and bad habits once developed are highly resistant to change, especially when they have been formed by trial and error in the agony of the initial interviewing experiences.

4. The scientific clinician.   More and more training programs are substituting engineering for empathy and Chi Squares for clinical common sense. There is little time or tolerance for the gossamer thing that is interviewing. By the time the candidate finishes his graduate program with the magical *sine qua non*—the master's degree—he has focused so long on scientific parameters that he finds it difficult to talk to parents or clients.

5. The paper clinician.   Some clinicians consider interviewing to be secondary; they use paper to replace personal interaction. An elaborate case-history form containing a plethora of questions is mailed to the parents, and they are requested to fill it out and return it before the diagnostic appointment. The rationale for this procedure is that it saves the clinician time and alerts him to problem areas he can then explore in the personal interview. Although the clinician certainly should get some idea of the problem before the diagnostic examination, he seldom needs a twelve-page questionnaire. There are several reasons for disenchantment with the paper approach: (*a*) the questions are generic—i.e., they cover *all* possible respondents—and thus are ambiguous or not applicable to many *particular* clients; a parent may not understand the relationship between the questions posed and his child's speech problem and demand, "Why does the clinician need to know *all of this* to cure Mary's speech?" (Irwin, 1965: 76); (*b*) the queries may be threatening or engender guilt, and the clinician is not present to observe these reactions or to support and assist the respondent as he searches for an answer. Does the mailed questionnaire allow time for the respondent to plan a defense? Is it more likely that we end up with a view of what the respondent wants us to see?; (*c*) the questions, if answered by the respondent in one particular way, may prevent him from developing any other possible answers. Spoken language does tend to create a reality for the individual, but writing really lends an air of permanence; (*d*) mailed case-history forms also tend to bias the diagnostician into a set of expectancies that are difficult to change:

> Recently, one of our senior students prepared for a diagnostic session by thoroughly reviewing all available information supplied on a written case-history form by the parents of the child to be evaluated. One line of the form described the child's problem as "difficulty in producing the /s/ sound." The student zeroed in on this parental diagnosis and proceeded to collect all data possible to gird herself for the interview. The mission appeared obvious to our student—convince the parents that an /s/ distortion in a five-year-old child is not a speech handicap but simply a maturational characteristic. During the initial interview the student proceeded to spell out in rather complete detail the speech and language maturational milestones; she dwelled on the point that sibilant errors in five-year-olds are very common and not a cause for alarm. As a final gesture the clinician took a look at the child and found so many articulatory and language deficiencies that he was unintelligible.

The main objection, however, is the impersonal, routine nature of the procedure.

Our work as speech clinicians is done by means of verbal (and nonverbal) interaction between ourselves and a client or his relatives. We disturb the air and light waves to find out things about the communicatively impaired in order to modify their behavior. An understanding of the nature of this interaction, of interviewing and how to go about the task, is perhaps the most important tool in the clinician's armamentarium.

THE NATURE OF INTERVIEWING

An interview is essentially a process, not an entity—a process of verbal and nonverbal intercourse between a trained professional worker and a client seeking his services. More specifically, an interview, in a clinical diagnostic sense, is a *purposeful* exchange of meanings between two persons, a directed conversation that proceeds in an orderly fashion to obtain data, to convey certain information, and to provide release and support. The professional worker, by reason of his position and clinical expertise, is expected to (and usually does) provide the direction for the verbal exchange. Thus, an interview is not just an ordinary conversation in terms of a desultory exchange of opinions and ideas, but rather a specialized pattern of verbal interaction directed toward a specific purpose and focused upon specific content. The roles of interviewer and respondent are more highly specified in a professional interview than in a conversation.

In a good diagnostic interview, the clinician and client must become coworkers, multiplying their efforts by creating a mutual feeling of cooperation.

> The interviewer and the interviewee both bring to the interview their own characteristics, their own life histories, their own personalities. What happens in an interview, however, cannot be understood merely by studying these two participants as separate entities. Rather it is essential to realize that they relate, that they interact, and that this relationship, this interaction, a product of their personalities, is what determines the outcome of the interview (Bingham and Moore, 1959: 37).

It is futile to expect straightforward answers to simple questions. A good diagnostic interview always involves more than making queries and recording answers.

Interviewing is a unique kind of conversation. Perhaps for the first time the respondent can talk freely without fear of criticism or admonishment. Now, the *clinician* knows that an interview is a unique and distinct mode of verbal exchange, but does the client need to know? Probably not. Indeed, we typically advise students to refer to an interview as a "chat" or "a chance to get together" when they contact clients or parents to request an appointment time. An "interview" sounds rather ominous and frightening—perhaps even like a summons to account for one's failings.

In summary, a diagnostic interview is a directed conversation, carried out for specific purposes such as fact-finding, informing, or altering attitudes and opinions. The clinician's efforts are directed toward the creation of mutual respect and team effort in the understanding and solution of the communication problem.

COMMON INTERVIEWING PROBLEMS

Several factors can prevent the establishment of effective communicative bonds between a speech clinician and those he interviews. Although the list could obviously be expanded, we have picked several aspects which in our experience are the most common interviewing barriers.

fears of the clinician

There are two points in a student clinician's career when his anxiety rises to very high levels: the confrontation with his first therapy case and his first diagnostic interview. It is—and should be—an awesome responsibility to undertake the professional treatment of a fellow human being. As a matter of fact, if a student does not get somewhat tense in this situation, we suspect his suitability for the profession, since either he is so dumb he knows no fear or he doesn't care enough to be afraid. We certainly are not applauding anxiety, but we should accept and recognize our fears, specify their nature, and develop effective ways to channel the nervous energy into improving our performance.

Perhaps the most common fear expressed by beginning interviewers is that clients will not accept them in a professional role because of their youth. They doubt they can bridge the age gap, especially when they deal with parents: "Who am I to be asking questions and giving suggestions to them when they are older and more experienced?" They sigh, "Won't parents consider me a pipsqueak? Won't they look down on me if I don't have children?" Most of this is pure projection on the student's part. If the interviewer indicates his deep concern for the welfare of the child, then nearly every parent will respond in a positive manner, without scrutinizing the clinician for wrinkles, grey hairs, or diaper-pail hands. The clinician, of course, should not communicate the uncertainty he may feel in the interview situation, or he will never establish his competence or inspire confidence. The worker must abandon all thoughts of himself, his doubts and fears, how well he is doing, and channel all his energy into making the client feel that he is a coworker.

Another common fear among incipient interviewers—and one that is also largely projected—is that the interviewee will become defensive or resentful during questioning. We have seen students omit a whole series of important questions when a client, especially a parent, responded curtly or showed mild annoyance. While it is not uncommon for parents to feel ashamed because they think of their child's speech disorder as an outward and visible sign of their own failure, few in our experience are resentful or defensive about the clinician's sincere efforts to determine the nature of the child's problem. The important point is, again, to make the interviewees feel that they have done the best they could do, and now, with some assistance from the clinician, they can do better.

Many beginning interviewers are leery of questions directed at them. "What do you do when the client starts asking *you* questions?" the student interviewer frequently despairs. "Will I be able to explain to them adequately what they need to know? How will I know if I have gotten it across if they just sit there and nod?"

Finally, some beginning interviewers are frightened to deal with feelings and attitudes. Since Freud drew his vivid pictures of the mental monsters that lurk beneath everyone's psyche, many workers have maintained that the beginner should not tamper with the lids of these Pandora's boxes.

Fearful of unleashing such dreadful forces, it is small wonder that many students conduct sterile, superficial interviews with their clients.

Memory failure. A common deterrent to communication in an interview is loss of memory. Clients will simply not remember things that the clinician needs to know in order to best plan a program of therapy.

Emotional barriers. Sometimes an interviewee cannot or will not give information because there are emotional blocks that prevent free communication.

Loath to find out. Physicians have reported that some patients coming for medical assistance tend to minimize or conceal their symptoms because they don't want to find out that they have something wrong. The same device can operate in diagnostic interviews.

The class barrier. Students in training are pretty much cloistered in a middle-class milieu. Rarely are they called upon to interact with persons from lower socioeconomic levels; often they are sufficiently shocked that they lose their effectiveness when dealing with these people and their unfamiliar life styles.

The language gap. The clinician must remember that laymen often have a markedly different way of talking about a speech or hearing problem. If there is a language gap—and the clinician does not take steps to close it—the interview will be unsuccessful.

The lack of specific purpose. Many beginning interviewers either have purposes that are too broad and general or interviewing goals that are too nebulous. It is important to carefully and rather explicitly write out the purposes for the interview before meeting with the client. We must know *why* we want the answers to the questions we ask. Specifying the purposes of an interview is also an effective way to reduce the interviewer's uncertainty and anxiety.

AN APPROACH TO INTERVIEWING

We now present an interviewing approach. an eclectic product of our experience in social work, speech pathology, and clinical audiology, together with an intensive study of relevant bibliographic materials. No doubt the reader will want to modify it to suit his individual setting. It is desirable that he do so, for only through critical self-evaluation and modification can any clinician acquire an interviewing procedure that is uniquely his own.

Ṯhere are three basic goals in diagnostic interviews: to obtain information, to give information, and to provide release and support. For the purpose of discussion each goal will be considered separately, a procedure rarely possible to do in an actual interview.

goal one: obtain information

Although it may seem rather obvious, it is worth restating that as clinicians we must listen before we speak. There are essentially three reasons for this: (1) it gives clients an opportunity to talk out problems, to ventilate fears and feelings, thus enabling them to better profit from the direction and advice which the speech clinician will offer; (2) it gives the clinician an idea of the nature and scope of the information the client will need; and (3) it allows the clinician to formulate hypotheses concerning the individual's communication disorder.

Setting the tone. The first important task of the clinician is to set the right tone for the interview, to get a structured conversation initiated and channeled in the proper direction. How does one go about that? Recent research by McQuire and Lorch (1968) has underscored the importance of proper structuring. Their findings indicate that the initial style of interaction may well determine the style of interaction for the entire interview. We find that defining the roles is an effective procedure for setting the tone:

> Mrs. Seelos, I'm Miss Sullivan, Terry's speech therapist. I really appreciate the opportunity to chat with you about Terry and the things we are doing in speech. First, though, you can be of great help to me since you know Terry so much better than I do. There are several things about his early development and how his speech seems to be at home that I need to understand before planning a long-range therapy program. Before you came in today, I made some notes for myself so that we could best use this half hour before my next session.

It is helpful to think of the interview as a kind of role-playing situation. The clinician defines the roles for the client and indicates the rules and responsibilities that accrue to these roles. He tells who he is, what he intends to do, and what he expects of the client. In other words, the interviewer structures the situation by explaining the purposes of the interview— why the information is wanted and what will be done with it. Initially, of course, the client accepts the respondent role because of the nature of the situation and the official sanction of the interviewer's position. Then it is up to the worker to demonstrate his empathy and clinical expertise in order to solicit further cooperation. Two problems sometimes arise here. First, some clients may be inhibited by such explicit role definitions; respondents from lower middle or lower social classes have had little experience in holding directed conversations. In this case, a clinician can prolong the small-talk phase, emphasize the nature of the interview as a chat, and gently ease into the more structured situation as the relationship develops.

The second, more difficult problem concerns the site of the interview. Although it is generally best to conduct interviews in a clinical setting, sometimes this is not possible and one has to seek out the client or his parents at home. This is rarely satisfactory not only because of the distractions inherent in the situation (children, pets, and neighbors) but also because the interview frequently becomes a social visit.

It is vital that the interviewer convey his sincere interest in the situation as the client sees it. He must demonstrate to the client that he is genuinely trying to comprehend what the problem is, and what it means to the client personally. Most important, the clinician must not manifest concern with his own needs—even such a concern as wanting to do a good job. By being relaxed himself (even if he must simulate it for a time) he will help the client to feel comfortable.

Rapport, of course, is not a separate substance that one pours into a session; it is mutual respect and trust, a feeling of confidence in the clinician, and a large measure of understanding. Empathy, warmth, and acceptance are crucial aspects; the worker must strive for the ability to sensitively and accurately understand the interviewee's situation. He should also try to be genuine, not contrived, with a professional character armor that signals "clinician on duty." As a matter of fact, it is helpful to avoid interposing a desk—a symbol of authority—between the respondent and the interviewer (Sommers, 1969). The interview is more effective without such a barrier. In addition to the words spoken, a number of forces shape the interview. Some things are conveyed by the setting and by the dress, manners, and expressions of the participants. If our office is located in a boiler room or a storage area, we have already conveyed something of our attitude toward the client and his problem by the very physical space that we use. In professional interviewing, the goal is to provide an atmosphere that fosters communication between client and clinician.

Asking the questions. Preferably, the clinician should use an interview guide rather than one of the more elaborate questionnaires—that is, instead of a formal set of questions written out to be read and answered, he should use a form that indicates areas to explore. The interview is much more spontaneous and meaningful if the speech clinician words his questions in keeping with his understanding of the individual's situation, rather than reading prepared ones. In most cases, formal questionnaires operate as another type of barrier or crutch for the insecure interviewer.

Students frequently ask what type of interviewers they should strive to be: directive, nondirective, behavioristic, psychoanalytic, neo-Freudian, and so forth. The best answer that we have been able to give—although it sounds facetious—is that he must use whatever techniques seem to be best for the job that he needs to do. Often we feel that a beginning clinician concentrates too hard on being Johnsonian or Van Riperian rather than focusing on what he must do to meet the needs of a particular client. Some writers feel that the direct interview is unpleasant, although there is no evidence to support this assumption. As a matter of fact, one research team (Richardson, Dohrenwend, and Klein, 1965) discovered that the lack of structure inherent in the pure nondirective interview produced anxiety in some respondents, especially the less educated ones. Actually, the whole matter is an academic question, because the good diagnostic interview is characterized by a shifting of styles: objective questions that ask for specifics, subjective queries that deal with feelings and attitudes, and finally the indeterminate questions like "tell me more" that keep the respondent going.

A far better question for the clinician to direct to himself is, "Why am I asking these questions?" He should have his purposes clearly in mind. Classically, the interviewer should start with the least anxiety-producing queries, mostly objective questions, and then proceed to more subjective questions as the relationship develops.

Dexter (1956) found that the interviewer can elicit greater cooperation by vividly demonstrating that he is on the respondent's side—that is, by using the client's phraseology, his style and manner, the interviewer demonstrates he is "one of the crowd." This is sometimes effective with a very anxious or reluctant client.

The presenting story. Most persons who anticipate visiting a clinic or discussing a speech problem with a public-school speech clinician will have mentally rehearsed what they intend to say. They may even, in some cases, have had a pseudoconversation with the worker. We must allow this story to be unraveled, or the respondent will be left with a sense of frustration and lack of closure. A question such as, "What seems to be the problem?" will permit the flow of conversation to begin. The clinician should remember that this is how the *client* perceives the problem—it is his unique way of looking at the situation. It may be grossly inaccurate, but the interviewer should hear him out; nothing turns a respondent off more quickly than for the interviewer to suggest by word or action that his views are silly or misguided. Sometimes the presenting story will become a motif that recurs again and again during the course of the interview.

This is generally a crucial point in an interview. The interviewee may cautiously extend a portion of himself verbally, carefully scan the interviewer's response, and then decide whether or not to tell the whole story. Sometimes a respondent may even set up a straw man to see how the interviewer deals with it:

Mrs. Dimitri, mother of Ivan, a fifth-grader who possessed a serious lateral lisp, appeared to see herself as a modern, informed parent. At our initial interview, she launched into a lengthy diatribe about the school reading program, explaining in great detail why Ivan couldn't read. We listened intently for a time and when she paused to recycle her complaints, we praised her for her concern and suggested that she bring this up at the next P.T.A. meeting and with Ivan's teacher. Apparently Mrs. Dimitri expected a debate, and she was much mollified that we had heard her out. We then proceeded to an excellent review of her insights into the child's speech problem.

This is not the proper time for the clinician to debate an issue with the client. His story can be accepted initially on the level of feeling, and later in the interview—when rapport is stronger—the point can be discussed more fully. We feel very strongly that these initial stories, these primitive theories, should be respected as the best possible answer clients have been able to come up with. This does not mean agreeing with their conclusions; it just means we accept their judgment with understanding (the classical "I can see how you might feel that way") so that we can form a basis for further communication.

Things to avoid in the interview. Beginning interviewers commit several common errors. The list that follows is not meant to be exhaustive, but does cover the most glaring mistakes.

1. It is usually best to avoid questions that may be answered by a simple yes or no. Although open-ended questions do produce longer responses in general, it is interesting to note that respondents from lower socioeconomic groups, who have less education, become more anxious as the questions become less structured. We have interviewed several clients who are confirmed yes-men. No matter what the clinician asks, no matter what comments he makes, these respondents simply nod in passive agreement. Perhaps they are fearful of exposing their ignorance and feel that it is better to remain silent and be thought a fool than to say something and make it obvious.

We find that requesting the client to rate himself on some simple scale is more effective than either-or questions. We frequently ask the client to tell us not whether something is difficult or easy but to what degree. A simple rating procedure, with low values (1 or 2) indicating relative ease and higher values (4 or 5) indicating relative difficulty may be used.

It is important, Mrs. Pickett, that we understand certain things about your husband's personality and reactions to stress before his stroke. This will help us plan a treatment program for him. Now, in terms of social life, using an imaginary scale from 1 (very outgoing) to 5 (very shy), how would you rate your husband before his stroke?

2. Avoid phrasing questions in such a way that they inhibit freedom of response. Do not say: "You don't have any difficulty with ringing in your ears, do you?" or "You don't tell Billy to stop and start over again, do you?" Such leading questions are not effective in interviewing. The beginning interviewer tends to be anxious about asking open-ended questions. He is afraid that silence will result and that this will damage his relationship with the client. So, he will ask an open-ended question and then close it. For example, "How do you feel about David's stuttering; does it bother you?" Leave it open!

Try also to avoid abrupt shifts in your line of questioning. For example, if you are exploring the client's feelings or attitudes on a particular issue (subjective questions), don't suddenly ask an objective question. Inexperienced interviewers, fearful that they are too deep in an area, tend to jump around; often they persist with objective queries and, once a pattern of response is established, the client finds it difficult to shift to more elaborate answers.

3. Avoid talking too much. This is perhaps the most common mistake of the beginning interviewer. He feels he must fill up every pause with his own verbiage. It is much better to rephrase what the respondent has said or make some comment like, "I see," "Tell me more," or "Anything else?" Sometimes a smile and an understanding nod are effective when it is felt that the client has more to say but needs some silent time to conjure it up. If there is a positive attitude—a good rapport—and the person feels comfortable in the situation, then these encouragements increase the length of the response; if the topic or situation is neutral, these comments tend to expand the message. However, if the topic is negative or the individual feels uncomfortable, the "hmmmmhmmmm" may be taken as a criticism—that is, if he *cannot* respond at length, he will feel that he is being pressured to do so. Parents with little education are perhaps the most vulnerable to this kind of pressure.

Be careful not to fall into stereotyped verbal habits. One of our students used "very good" as reinforcement so frequently with a severely aphasic patient that one day, after making a particularly effective response to a problem, the patient—who had said very little since his stroke—finished the clinician's "very" with a resounding "good," surprising them both.

4. Avoid concentrating on the physical symptoms and the etiological factors to the exclusion of the client's feelings and attitudes. There is a little bit of Dr. Kildare in all of us; we yearn to play the role of omniscient healer. This is further compounded by instructors who dwell interminably on causation in their courses dealing with speech disorders. But it is possible to track each suspicious symptom with such zeal that we fail to obtain a basis for understanding the emotional and environmental complications of a speech or hearing disability.

5. Avoid providing information too soon. There will be plenty of time to clear up misconceptions later in the interview. The surest way to cut off the flow of information is to stop a parent, for instance, after he says, "I just tell Michael to stop, take a deep breath, and start all over again," and counsel him on the proper responses to nonfluency.

6. Avoid qualifying and hemming and hawing when asking questions. Ask them in a straightforward fashion and maintain eye contact. Rather than asking, "Did you find that, well, you know, when you were, ah, shall we say . . . with child—did you experience any untoward conditions?" say, "Did anything unusual happen during your pregnancy?" Instead of inquiring, "Did you discover, hmmmm, I mean, well, after your father, ah, passed away, did your stuttering problem increase?" say, "What impact did your father's death have upon your speech?"

7. Avoid negativistic or moralistic responses—verbal or nonverbal— to the client's statements. The flow of information will stop rapidly and the relationship will be impaired severely if the individual senses that we find him or his behavior distasteful. We do not have to subscribe to a person's values or code of behavior to show compassion and understanding for his situation. In a clinical setting we must not let our values obscure our perception of the client's frame of reference.

8. When the client causes the interview to wander, avoid abrupt transitions to bring it back to the point. Most of those whom you will interview have had little experience in directed, orderly conversation. They tend to follow chance associations and wander far afield. The experienced interviewer has the ability to make smooth transitions. How does one go about getting the interview back on the track? The best way is by building a bridge to the respondent's previous statements. For example: "That's interesting, Mrs. Davis, maybe we can come back to that in a little while; now earlier you were mentioning that your child's loss of hearing occurred suddenly. . . ." The key here is to use respondent antecedents—things that the person has said earlier in the interview. If we use only the interviewer's antecedents —questions that the interviewer has asked before—the client will not feel understood and will sense that what he has said was of little consequence. The inexperienced interviewer asks lots of questions either with no antecedents or with his own antecedents. He is afraid of losing control of the interview and thus becomes preoccupied with formulating the next question.

9. Avoid allowing the interview to produce only superficial answers. We need ways to get deeper, more significant responses from our clients. There are several interviewing devices, termed *probes*, that the clinician will find helpful:

    Crosshatch, or *interlocking,* questions are useful when we need to elicit more detail about a topic that has been glossed over. Often there are discrepancies that must be resolved. Essentially, the way to go about this is to ask the same thing in different ways and at different points during the interview. For instance, the father of a young stutterer responded in a superficial manner to our query about his relationship with the child. He assured us that he had a "loving relationship" with his son and then complained at length about his working conditions. Later in the interview when we asked him to describe the sorts of things he did with the child, he was unable to mention a single one. We don't mean to imply that the clinician should attempt to catch the client lying and then demand an explanation. The clinician must check out discrepancies, however, in order to enhance his understanding of the problem, since they could have a significant effect on the mode of treatment.

Next, *pauses* can be very helpful. When there is a lull in the interview, it may mean simply that the client has exhausted his store of information, that a memory barrier has prevented further recall, or that he senses he is not being understood. It can also mean, however, that a sensitive area has been touched upon. Do not feel that pauses harm the interview. Much significant information can be forthcoming if we keep quiet and indicate with a smile or a nod that we expect more.

Another aid is to encourage *time regression* and *association*. Memories are weak. In order to pinpoint some significant data, we may have to take the person back in time to find a memory peg such as a wedding, a natural calamity, or the like, that may call forth more information. One father, a long-time air force sergeant, catalogued everything in terms of the make and model of car he was driving. Another client, an inveterate bird watcher, remembered incidents by the times he had seen the Marbled Godwit or the Prothonatary Warbler.

The *summary probe* is one of the best ways to keep the interview moving smoothly. The clinician summarizes periodically what the client has said, ending perhaps with a request for clarification or further information. Incidentally, this procedure also demonstrates to the person that the interviewer is indeed trying to understand his problem. We generally use "mini-summary probes"—echo questions—all the way through an interview:

> *Respondent*: After my husband's stroke, my whole world collapsed.
> *Interviewer*: You were overwhelmed by the sudden change in your life.
> *Respondent*: Yes, one day he was happily planning our trip to Sanibel Island . . . and then, in just a moment, he was paralyzed and couldn't talk. Now, all our plans are up in the air . . . the new car, the checking account, he took care of all that.

The *stumbling probe* is a variation of the summary probe; we have found it helpful, especially with the reticent respondent. The interviewer rephrases a portion of the respondent's communication and then, attempting to interpret or comment upon it, he pretends to halt or stumble. For example, when interviewing the mother of a child allegedly beginning to stutter, the clinician might say: "Now, you were saying that Bruce first started to repeat and hesitate after he caught his finger in the car door. Under these conditions, it would be natural for you to . . . ah. . . ." This really works. The respondent's need for closure will precipitate significant information and, perhaps more important, significant insights.

Finally, the *assuming probe*. (This stems from the old incriminating question, "Have you stopped beating your wife yet?") Such a technique should, of course, be used sparingly and only after some interviewing experience; at times, however, it is the only way to get information out in the open. If the client has avoided an important area, if he has left much unsaid regarding his speech or hearing problem and what it means to him, then it is up to the interviewer to bring this out. One adolescent boy who had been vehemently denying that his stuttering bothered him, unburdened himself when we said, "It bothers you so much that you don't want anybody to know, do you?"

10. Avoid letting the client reveal too much in one interview. You may have had similar experiences: a good friend encounters severe trouble and you come to his aid, helping him through the crisis. A curious thing often happens when your friend recovers his equilibrium. He feels obligated to you; he felt exposed to you as a raw human being during the crisis, and now he is embarrassed, somewhat resentful, and perhaps even hostile. It is as if you are now an outward and visible sign of his former debacle. Sometimes a beginning interviewer makes the mistake of trying to get everything in one sitting. The client, sensing perhaps his first really understanding listener, may want to pour out his whole sad tale of woe. Later, however, the individual will feel embarrassed and foolish, perhaps even exposed and guilty at revealing so much of himself to this comparative stranger.

> Mrs. Mistal was an attractive but rather harried mother of six children, all under nine years of age. Her four-year-old daughter, Mary, was beginning to stutter, and Mrs. Mistal came to the clinic for assistance. The longer she talked, the more she talked about herself rather than the child. Finally, she broke down and said that her problem was her religion, a faith that forbade birth control but, as she pointed out ruefully, did not assist with the child-rearing duties. She revealed that she had a college degree but felt it was of no use since all she did was wash diapers and wipe runny noses year after year. She blurted out a lot of other things about the clergy and the trap she felt she was in. We tried desperately to shut off the flow but could not. We never saw her or Mary again.

Bringing an interview to a graceful close can sometimes be more difficult than getting it started. In our experience, an interview is most effectively terminated by summarizing what has been discussed and reviewing the specific actions to be taken. It is probably best not to consider new material at this time when neither the interviewer nor the client can devote sufficient attention to it. It is always important, however, to leave the door open for future contacts.

11. Avoid trusting to memory. Record the information as the interview progresses. Tell the client that you will take some notes during the interview so that you can plan his treatment program more effectively and make recommendations for other services. Such note-taking, or even recording devices, are rarely questioned. Indeed, we have found that clients expect you to write down some of the information that they are giving you; they doubt that you would be able to remember all of their answers. You obviously would lose your relationship, however, if you scribbled furiously while the client was revealing some sensitive information. It is axiomatic that the respondent's confidence will be respected, but we have mixed feelings about mentioning this explicitly to the client. The clinician's manner should suggest that all information received is to be held strictly confidential. At times, the clinician can suggest the possibility that he might listen and tell others, and this had never entered the respondent's mind.

Put the clinical situation, procedures, observations, and recommendations in writing as soon as possible. Commit it to paper while the facial characteristics and voice inflections can still be remembered. Make the report "alive" so that others can experience most of the clinical situation just by reading about it. Watch during the interview for things that may have significance: how the client used time (was he late or early?), postures, sighs, association of ideas, word choice, retraction of statements, insights, and so forth.

goal two: provide information

The most common complaint of patients in modern hospitals and clinics is that they have not been kept informed of their condition and progress. Interviewing 214 patients, Pratt, Seligman, and Reader report (1958: 229): "Patients who were given more thorough explanations were found to participate somewhat more effectively with the physician and were more likely to accept completely the doctor's formulation than were the patients who received very little information." We have formulated a fundamental principle in this regard: *there is never too little information, there is instead misinformation.* Not one of us can stand uncertainty. All too frequently the information, if not supplied by the professional worker, will come distorted from other sources. When not correctly informed, parents become misinformed and this leads to confusion, misunderstanding, and further compounding of the problem. It is our responsibility, therefore, to provide accurate, unemotional, objective information on the status of the individual's speech and hearing problem. Simple nontechnical language that is compatible with the person's background should always be used. Avoid false surface reassurance. Most people can see through this sort of sham. Once a person begins to understand his particular speech problem, his anxiety and uncertainty will be relieved. The best antidote to fear is knowledge.

Be sure, however, to avoid iatrogenic errors. Do not use terms or suggest consequences that will precipitate more stress for the client. One parent was told his child's hearing problem was caused by atrophy of the hearing nerve. It is difficult enough to have a hard-of-hearing child without worrying about mysterious nerves atrophying, something about which the parent can do very little. Do not communicate your negative expectations regarding the outcome of therapy to the client. We are convinced that what the clinician thinks a client can do, that he shall do. In other words, after Parkinson, the client's behavior expands to fit the clinician's concept of his potential. Do we precondition our own therapeutic behavior when we make a prognosis? Is this communicated to the client and his relatives in some manner and on some level? We think it often is. Let us illustrate this with an anecdote that arose in our practice with adult aphasics in a veteran's hospital:

> An advanced graduate student, an excellent clinician, was working for the first time with an adult aphasic. We had done the original examination on the patient and had several sessions with him but wanted the student to make her own assessment of the patient's prognosis. She presented the aphasic several picture cards and requested that he name them. The patient looked at her and said something that sounded to her ears like "I know, I know," in an exasperated tone. The student responded firmly: "I know you know, Mr. Tolonen. Now try these words in a short phrase." He did so and we nearly fell off the chair. For the patient's first name was Heino (pronounced "I know"), and heretofore he had simply repeated his name to each request for verbalization!

Below are six basic principles for imparting information to clients which we have found useful:

1. Emotional confusion may, and often does, inhibit the person's ability to understand cognitively what you are trying to say. Just because you have once reviewed the steps of ear training is no reason to expect that its importance will be grasped.
2. Refrain from being didactic, do not lecture your clients.
3. Use simple language with many examples and illustrations. If you must err, err in the direction of being too simple rather than complex. And repeat, repeat, repeat the important points—rephrasing each time.
4. Try to provide something that the client—especially a parent—can *do*. Action reduces the feelings of futility and anxiety. The activity should be direct, simple, and require some kind of reporting to the clinician.
5. Say what needs to be said pleasantly—but frankly. Do not avoid saying something that must be said on the assumption that the client cannot take it or that you will be rejected. People often display an amazing reserve of courage in difficult situations.

6. Remember, however, that the one who finally communicates what the client may have been dreading to hear is often hated and maligned. If you are the first to say the feared words, you may become the focus for all the hostile, negative feelings thus aroused. As a professional worker, you will have to be strong enough to be the lightning rod for these emotions.

goal three: release and support

The clinician does not, of course, wait until the end of the interview to provide release for the frustrations and fears of the client. Most of the parts of the interview already discussed will serve this purpose. By helping the individual talk out his problems, the worker is providing an excellent escape for pent-up feelings. The interviewer needs only to say something like: "I can see how you must feel. Most of us in similar circumstances would be concerned and anxious."

More than advice is needed during interviews for the purpose of helping clients take some specific action or move in a particular direction. They need help in sorting out the confusing choices before them. To support a respondent's real strengths, we need to make it clear that we understand what the situation means to him and that we uncritically sympathize with his feelings and attitudes. We can restore the client's self-esteem and his ability to function more appropriately if we convey our interest in him as a person and our solid acceptance of his importance. If the client feels appreciated and understood, he can sometimes drop his self-protective behavior and see how the experience will eventually benefit him.

There is an unfortunate tradition of "sweetness and light" in client counseling. A person has a problem. He is sad and depressed, and we try to cheer him up. Sometimes this degenerates into a debate, with the interviewer attempting to persuade the person that he should not feel miserable. When a person feels depressed, anxious, and fearful, he does not want to count his blessings. He wants you to feel miserable, too. He wants you to share and identify with him on his own level. Thus, the interviewer is given a basis for communication with the person. We start where he is, accept it as the proper place to start, and tell him that it is a sad state of affairs that would make anyone sad and depressed. Then, using this bond of identification, which becomes a basis for communication, we can assist him in solving the problem. The main ingredient is *empathy*, the capacity to identify oneself with another's feelings and actions.

How does one handle emotional scenes? They are bound to arise at some point in your interviewing experience. Some clinicians excuse themselves from the room and allow the respondent to recover his dignity alone. Others try to change the subject to something less emotional. Both of these approaches may, with certain clients, give the impression that the clinician is rejecting their feelings. It is more effective to indicate one's understanding of the feelings that are being expressed and accept them as natural human reactions. For example: "That's okay to let it come out, Mrs. Moody; you have been holding it back too long. Sometimes it helps to get it out in the open."

Not all clients seen by the speech clinician will need or even want extensive interviewing. In some cases, the procedures discussed here would be grossly inappropriate. Visualize an interview as ranging along a continuum from affective concern such as feelings and attitudes to objective matters such as goals and advice. Some respondents simply need objective information so that they can do the job; others require considerable support and succor before they can take over and modify their behavior. The clinician's role in some interviews may consist of simply listening to and supporting a client.

IMPROVING INTERVIEWING SKILLS

Hopefully, the material in this chapter will be useful to students majoring in clinical speech pathology and to our colleagues working in various settings. However, no one ever became proficient in interviewing solely by reading about it. It took us over eleven years of constant searching and experimenting to evolve the interviewing approach presented here. And, by the indulgence of our clients and many long-suffering parents, we continue to explore for better ways.

We have included below a series of activities and projects for your own practice. Let them serve as the beginning steps in a continual learning effort toward improved interviewing. You will find that the time devoted to such training exercises is well spent. Now, consider these steps on how to improve your interviewing skills:

   1. Read widely from a variety of sources. We have included a list of selected references to get you started. Find out what people are like by reading in sociology, psychology, anthropology, and philosophy. This is, of course, a lifetime project which we feel is delightful since there is always a new frontier, an open horizon on which we can set our sails. Our profession has arisen so abruptly, grown so rapidly, and been so concerned with the urgent scientific and clinical issues, that it has ignored the important issue—the development of a philosophical basis for our work. A speech-and-hearing clinician without a rationale is like a ship without a rudder. The fundamental and mandatory basis for sound, purposeful therapy is an overall point of view, a workable theory that does not necessarily include the specific activities that will be used to carry it out. Nothing is so pathetic as the clinician who, in a willy-nilly manner, empties a bag of therapeutic homilies on the client's lap, hoping somehow that one of them will work. Only a sequential system of logically interrelated theorems will enable us to evaluate our clinical effectiveness.

2. Listen to all sorts of people, to their dreams, their rationalizations, their insights—or lack of them—and their gripes. During the carryover stages of therapy for a stuttering problem, the senior author haunted the coffee shops in small communities around Lansing, Michigan. He talked with anyone and everyone, and it was almost always possible to strike up a conversation, contrary to what Steinbeck reported in *Travels with Charley*. This was perhaps the most valuable educational experience of his undergraduate years.

3. Form small heterogeneous groups of majors in speech pathology and audiology. Following the T-group format (a self-directed group with no set rules that meets in a highly permissive atmosphere for prolonged intervals), conduct some sensitivity training, particularly as it relates to your self-concept, assets and liabilities, your responses to people, and your relationship with your own parents and other older adults. The senior author finds, as a stutterer, that each time he works with parents of children beginning to stutter, he has a distinct tendency to summon up the "ghosts of his stuttering past." He must monitor his behavior by listening to recordings and scrutinizing interviewing protocols. In order to provide assistance to others, we must know our own foibles and potential blind spots and have them under reasonable control. As Van Riper so artfully said at a recent workshop in public-school speech therapy, "You can't heal a wound with a dirty bandage."

4. Role playing is one of the best methods to prepare for interviewing. Set up several typical interview situations in front of a class and play, for example, the roles of the reluctant parent, the spouse of an aphasic patient, or the hostile father. Discuss the interaction, and replay the situations with others assuming the roles. Write out interview purposes prior to the role playing and determine, or have the class determine, how effectively the interviewer accomplished his avowed purposes. Whenever the viewers feel that the interview went wrong or the responses were ineffective, see how many different ways it could have been handled. This builds up the beginning interviewer's repertoire of adaptive responses. You can do a surprising amount of intrapersonal role playing in your spare time. While we are waiting for a class to begin, for a light to change, or for our mother-in-law to cease talking, we frequently imagine ourselves in various interviewing situations and then explore alternate statements, probes, and so forth.

5. Make recordings of your first few interviews and then analyze them carefully with your clinical supervisor or a colleague. We believe that multiple interviewers simply do not work (although seeing multiple interviewees —such as a mother and father at the same time—can be useful and productive), and hence, we would suggest that your supervisor not observe your performance in the same room, especially for your first ventures. We have found that when the supervisor stays in the room, the student has a tendency to seduce him into taking over the role of interviewer; and if he refuses to assume the mantle, he can only sit there looking at the clients as if they were

bugs in an insect collection. We have no role sanction in our social structure for the silent scrutinizer, and his presence can seriously impair the effectiveness of the interview.

Play back your interview again and again, revising statements, underscoring errors, and scanning for the good parts. Have typed protocols prepared from some of these tapes—the errors really leap out at you from the printed page—and discuss them with your instructors, fellow students, or colleagues.

Persistent errors, such as stereotyped verbal habits, can be eradicated by using negative practice. One student was required to use his substandard "this here" and "that there" in every third utterance for a month; this procedure (and an extrathick chocolate malted as a reward) succeeded in breaking him of the habit. More substantive problems can be dealt with by using role playing.

We would like to end this chapter with a challenge to the reader. We challenge you to utilize the interviewing approach delineated above, find the errors, the things that just don't work for you, and then develop your own methods. We have given you the foundation blocks; can you use them to create steppingstones?

PROJECTS AND QUESTIONS

1. A common problem in interviewing is the tendency for both the respondent and the interviewer to become lost in extraneous and incidental details. Record an interview with a classmate who arranges to get off the track. Try several ways to bring him back to the point. Listen to the recording and evaluate.

2. Find the interviewing error in this exchange and rewrite the interviewer's queries:

   Interviewer: When did you first notice that you were having difficulty with your voice, the breathy and weak quality you talked about?
   Client: Well, let's see. My mother died two months ago and it started about a week after that.
   Interviewer: How has it changed over the past two months?

3. Look up Rogers' communication test (Rogers, C., *On Becoming a Person* [Boston: Houghton Mifflin Company, 1961], Chapter 17). Use it to sharpen your listening skills.

4. Interview a person with and without a written questionnaire. Have the respondents report their reactions in both situations.

5. Make an assessment of your roommate's behavior, particularly with respect to some problem area. Attempting to be as subtle as possible, use several stumbling and assuming probes. Report his reactions.

6. Explain in detail how you would handle an emotional scene with the mother of a mentally retarded child. The mother finally comes to the realization that her child is indeed retarded after several years of denial and repeated clinical examinations.

7. What is the Greenspoon effect (Greenspoon, 1962)?
8. What dangers are there in the use of "why" questions in diagnostic interviews? (See Benjamin, 1969: 77–84.)
9. What effect does office clutter, unusual personal dress, or grooming ("mod" or casual clothing, beards, etc.) have upon an average client or parent?
10. In what manner does the sex of the interviewer or the age of the client alter the approach employed?
11. Review the article by Woolf (1971). How does verbal output in a diagnostic interview relate to informational specificity?

BIBLIOGRAPHY

BENJAMIN, A. (1969). *The Helping Interview*. Boston: Houghton Mifflin Company. B F 637 I5 B37

BENNY, M., D. RIESMAN, and S. STAR (1956). "Age and Sex in the Interview." *American Journal of Sociology*, 62: 143–52.

BERG, I. (1954). "The Clinical Interview and Case Record." In *An Introduction to Clinical Psychology*, 2nd ed., eds. L. Pennington and I. Berg. New York: Ronald Press. Pp. 91–127.

BINGHAM, WALTER and B. MOORE (1959). *How to Interview*, 4th ed. New York: Harper & Row, Publishers. 138 B61

BIRD, B. (1955). *Talking with Patients*. Philadelphia: J. B. Lippincott Co.

BUGENTAL, J. F. (1954). "Explicit Analysis: A Design for the Study and Improvement of Psychological Interviewing." *Educational and Psychological Measurement*, 14: 552–65.

CAPLOW, T. (1956). "The Dynamics of Information Interviewing." *American Journal of Sociology*, 62: 165–71.

COUCH, A. and K. KENISTEM (1960). "Yeasayers and Naysayers." *Journal of Abnormal and Social Psychology*, 60: 151–74.

DAVIS, J. (1971). *The Interview as Arena*. Stanford, Calif.: Stanford University Press. RC 480 .5 D37 no

DEUTCH, F. and W. MURPHY (1955). *The Clinical Interview*. New York: International Universities Press. 136.42 D48

DEXTER, L. (1956). "Role Relationships and Conceptions of Neutrality in Interviewing." *American Journal of Sociology*, 62: 153–57.

EMERICK, L. (1969). *The Parent Interview*. Danville, Ill.: Interstate Printers and Publishers.

FENLASON, A. (1952). *Essentials in Interviewing*. New York: Harper & Row, Publishers. B F 637 I5 F 4v

GARRETT, A. (1942). *Interviewing: Its Principles and Methods*. New York: Family Service Association. HV 41 634

R 727.3 E47 Emerick

GORDON, R. (1956). "Dimensions of the Depth Interview." *American Journal of Sociology,* 62: 158–64.

GREENSPOON, J. (1962). "Verbal Conditioning and Clinical Psychology." In *Experimental Foundations of Clinical Psychology,* ed. A. J. Bachrach. New York: Basic Books. Pp. 510–53.

HYMAN, H. *et al.* (1954). *Interviewing in Social Research.* Chicago: University of Chicago Press. *H 62 49 LB 3454 I7*

IRWIN, R. B. (1965). *Speech and Hearing Therapy.* Pittsburgh: Stanwix.

JOHNSON, W., F. DARLEY, and D. SPRIESTERSBACH (1963). *Diagnostic Methods in Speech Pathology.* New York: Harper & Row, Publishers.

KAHN, R. and C. CANNELL (1959). *The Dynamics of Interviewing.* New York: John Wiley & Sons, Inc. *138 K12*

LANGDON, G. and I. STOUT (1954). *Teacher-Parent Interviews.* Englewood Cliffs, N.J.: Prentice-Hall, Inc. *371, 103 L27L*

MCDONALD, E. (1962). *Understand Those Feelings.* Pittsburgh: Stanwix.

MCQUIRE, M. and S. LORCH (1968). "A Model for the Study of Dyadic Communication." *Journal of Nervous and Mental Disease,* 146: 221–29.

MATARAZOO, J. (1965). "The Interview." In *Handbook of Clinical Psychology,* ed. B. Wolman. New York: McGraw-Hill Book Company. Pp. 403–50.

PRATT, L., A. SELIGMAN, and G. READER (1958). "Physicians' Views on the Medical Information Among Patients." In *Patients, Physicians, and Illness,* ed. E. Jaco. New York: The Free Press.

RICHARDSON, S., B. DOHRENWEND, and D. KLEIN (1965). *Interviewing: Its Forms and Functions.* New York: Basic Books, Inc. *BF637 I5 R5*

SOMMERS, R. (1969). *Personal Space.* Englewood Cliffs, N.J.: Prentice-Hall, Inc.

SULLIVAN, H. S. (1954). *The Psychiatric Interview.* New York: W. W. Norton & Company, Inc. *RC 480.5 S8*

VAN RIPER, C. (1953). *A Casebook in Speech Therapy.* Englewood Cliffs, N.J.: Prentice-Hall, Inc. Pp. 17–23.

———— and L. GRUBER (1957). *A Casebook in Stuttering.* New York: Harper & Row, Publishers.

WILSON, D., H. GINOTT, and S. BERGER (1959). "Group Interview: Initial Parent Contact." *Journal of Speech and Hearing Disorders,* 24: 282–84.

WOOLF, G. (1971). "Informational Specificity: A Correlate of Verbal Output in Diagnostic Interview." *Journal of Speech and Hearing Disorders,* 36: 518–26.

Wolman RC 467 W6

3

the
clinical examination
and
testing procedures

The word "diagnosis" in the original Greek means to understand thoroughly. Although an obvious oversimplification, we can gain this thorough understanding of our client and his communication problem basically by two means: *asking* and *testing*. Some kinds of information can be obtained only by setting up structured tasks for the client to do and then systematically observing his performance. The overall purpose of the clinical examination, then, is to assemble sufficient data to provide a "working image" of the individual.

In Chapter 1, we listed several objectives of the total diagnostic process; here we shall simply enumerate the several related purposes that guide the clinical examination:

1. To describe the problem
2. To make an estimate of its severity
3. To identify the factors that are related to the problem
4. To estimate prospects for improvement, and
5. To derive a plan of treatment

Thus, we are concerned with the systematic collection, organization, and interpretation of information regarding an individual and his particular communication disorder. All of this activity is carried out to provide a basis for predicting the outcome of treatment and to guide the nature and scope of the therapeutic regimen.[1]

aspects of the clinical examination

There are several important aspects of the clinical examination with which the beginning clinician should be acquainted. We have selected the most salient factors for discussion; all are potential pitfalls for the unwary.

The interpersonal context. The most crucial factor in conducting a successful diagnostic session is the client-clinician relationship.[2] No matter how well prepared and rehearsed an examiner may be, if his approach to people is poor, he is bound to experience failure. All tests, all examinations, all so-called objective diagnostic procedures are mediated by person-to-person contact.

We can be seduced into grave errors by test norms, percentile scores, and standard examination procedures: man is a total functioning unit and the various tests are multiple and fragmented. The instruments we use are relatively precise, and we are often deluded into thinking that the patient is functioning with the same degree of precision in the testing situation. But human elements may disturb the validity of the tests no matter how refined the scoring procedures or how calibrated the machines.

Impersonal, test-oriented clinical examination sessions can also make treatment more difficult since there is no absolute division between diagnosis and therapy (Johnson, Darley, and Spriestersbach, 1963). The first contact with a client initiates treatment. During a diagnostic session he is forming opinions and conceptions about the clinician and the total clinical situation. Barker and his colleagues (1953: 310) have warned that "while to the medical practitioner, diagnosis and therapy are often routine technical jobs, to the patient the situation never has such limited personal meaning. To him diagnosis and therapy are a route to highly important life conditions."

Not all clients will require the full impact of this interpersonal dimension. Indeed, some individuals simply want to find out what is wrong and then rectify the situation. The point is, however, that the clinician should be able to discern what the client needs and then adjust his style appropriately.

Age factors. Although all age levels present unique diagnostic problems, three groups in particular—young children, adolescents, and to a lesser extent, older or aged clients—require special effort and expertise.

---

[1] Repeated testing during therapy will also enable the clinician to judge the efficacy of the plan of treatment. Moreover, testing may be helpful for appropriate placement in group therapy. Finally, some speech pathologists urge more extensive testing of each client in order to provide additional scientific information on the various communication impairments.

[2] The reader will want to review the components of rapport discussed in Chapter 2, pp. 13–15.

YOUNG CHILDREN. Preschool (and kindergarten) children are often difficult to test and examine. The main problem is dealing with the child's fear of the clinical situation. This apprehension may stem from one or more of the following related factors: (1) Inadequate preparation for the examination, which produces, (2) uncertainty as to what will be done to or with him by the clinician, (3) vivid memories of trauma during visits to dentists and physicians, (4) the contagious anxieties and uncertainties experienced by the parents, and (5) stress and conflicts engendered by past listener reactions to the speech impairment. Children confront the speech examination in a variety of ways, but the two most trying responses are shyness and withdrawal and, at the other extreme, aggressiveness and hyperactivity.

The shy ones are the most difficult to deal with clinically because there is no output—no speech or language to evaluate. The lack of response per se is behavior, too, however, and has meaning we must judge; the child is always telling us something even when he isn't talking. If he cannot or will not respond to our attempts to discern his capabilities, we have to employ special procedures to get him involved with the tasks. It is fascinating to witness how our students and colleagues attempt to deal with the reticent child:

> An unfortunate but common approach is to bombard the child with stimuli, to overwhelm his defenses both verbally and nonverbally. One clinician, who claims to be able to obtain all manner of information from shy children, swoops down upon a youngster, holds him on her lap, fondles him, and chatters incessantly, repeating questions over and over at close range. Emerging from these somewhat explosive sessions, she is able to detail behavioral responses that equally competent clinicians cannot confirm. We finally discovered how she does it when we videotaped her during a diagnostic session. She is simply receiving her own stimuli as reflected by the bewildered child and is mistaking these images for the youngster's responses. She is literally answering her own questions; small wonder she confirms her own predictions.

> A few clinicians embarrass all within range by adopting what they imagine is a charming, childlike demeanor. One speech pathologist of our acquaintance adopts a vocal pitch at least a half octave above his normal pitch level (the graduate students called it his "Baby Jane" voice behind his back) and correspondingly childish inflections and immature motor behavior when he works with preschoolers. It was sometimes difficult to tell who was the client, and even the children seemed annoyed, bemused, or embarrassed by this cloying cuteness.

How *do* you get a small child to talk? Questioning is a common procedure but we must agree with Van Riper:

> Questions are demands. They immediately place the child in a subservient role, with the questioner in the position of power. Even when the child responds appropriately, the resulting relationship is one which immediately puts the questioner into the same category with other authority figures who have been controllers, a relationship which often regenerates the conflicts the child has previously experienced in threatening communication. If you ask what something is called and the child cooperates, he must either think that you must be

stupid not to know its name or that you suspect he doesn't know it (which implies stupidity), or that you must want him to do a little verbal dance for your pleasure. . . . Moreover, the eliciting of speech by questions often yields very impoverished samples. At best, you'll get just a vocabulary item, not a good speech sample. Or, if you ask him a yes-no question, you'll get a yes or no answer, often the latter. Like a marriage, we do not feel that a therapeutic relationship should start with an invitation to say no. If the question is more elaborate ("What did you have for breakfast this morning?" "What did you do in school today?") the child has probably forgotten or finds it difficult to formulate, or feels that it is none of your business, anyway. Especially with children for whom the acquisition of speech has been no easy accomplishment, any question tends to pose some threat. They have been bedevilled by too many questions from too many questioners and, when they have answered, their listeners have not always understood them or have rejected them. For these children, the interrogative inflection is almost as potent a signal as the tone that makes the rat jump in expectation of shock.[3]

Eschewing questions, then, we recommend a simple play activity—a box of common farm animals or a doll house with miniature furniture is excellent—and the use of *self-* and *parallel-talk.*

How then should one begin? We suggest that you should simply greet the child, then do some simple self-talk, commenting on what you are doing, or perceiving, and with plenty of moments of comfortable silence interspersed, until you have him playing with his box of toys. And then, in the role of the adult playmate, you can play with those in your own box—silently at first. No questions. No demands. *Solo play!* Once the child is comfortable in this activity, you should begin to put some self-talk into your own solo play; first noises (those of trucks, animals, etc.), then single words, then short phrases and simple sentences. All of these refer to what you are experiencing at the moment. Usually the child will begin to follow suit. His noises and his self-talk begin to flow. Next you should shift to contact play very gradually. Let your toy truck occasionally touch his fire engine, or help him find a block, or put another one on his toppling pile, or straighten it up a bit so he can make it higher. When you feel the time is ripe in this *tangential contact play,* begin to accompany it with some noises or commentary, using *parallel talk,* telling him what he is doing, perceiving, or feeling, again making sure you have more silence than speech. From tangential play, you can often proceed rapidly to *intersecting play* in which your activity becomes a part of his. (Let your truck go over the bridge he has built or feed your doll or toy dog a piece of the play fruit he has put on the play-house table). Verbalize what you are doing. Next seek to achieve *cooperative play,* assisting him in what he is doing. (Have your truck bring him the blocks he needs to build his tower.) Usually by this time, the child is speaking very easily and often copiously, your own verbalizations primarily confined to reflecting what he has said. From this point onward, the communication can proceed fairly normally and naturally. We hope we have not given the impression that this process is too time-consuming. Often we can accomplish all the progressive interaction in a single session and build a very warm communicative

[3] Charles Van Riper, *Speech Correction: Principles and Methods,* 5th ed. © 1972, pp. 108–10. Reprinted by permission of Prentice-Hall, Inc., Englewood Cliffs, N.J.

relationship in less than an hour. There are, of course, many children for whom such a careful approach may not be vitally necessary, children who have learned that big people always seem to have to ask stupid questions, children who are willing to dance when the interrogative strings are pulled, children who relate easily. Yet even with these children this approach seems to work very well. The relationship established is less superficial, more satisfying. We do not meet with as many moments of resistance or negativism later on in therapy (Van Riper, 1972: 108–10).

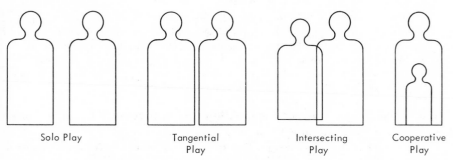

| Solo Play | Tangential Play | Intersecting Play | Cooperative Play |

FIGURE 1   Diagram of Interaction Between Clinician and Child (Van Riper, 1972: 109). Reprinted with permission.

We recently watched a colleague perform a very effective language evaluation on a particularly reticent and reluctant child:

> The clinician approached the child sitting tensely by her mother in the waiting room. Quietly introducing himself (without maudlin gestures or syrupy promises of what fun this is going to be), he extended his hand expectantly to the child and they disappeared into an examining room. We watched through a one-way mirror as the clinician explored the room with the child. He talked softly, almost in a whisper, as he itemized the objects and structures visible in the room. Still talking softly, in short, simple sentences, he opened a small box containing several plastic farm animals. Arraying the creatures on the table top, the clinician named them, purposely confusing the pig and the goat. Sara smiled slightly and shifted her chair closer. The clinician then proposed an animal parade and pranced the horse and the cow closer and closer to Sara. In a short time, the child was playing eagerly with the animals and chatting freely with the therapist.

But what do you do with the aggressive, active ones, the children who cannot or will not sit still, who demand to structure the situation in the way they desire? First, and most important, the clinician must retain control of the situation. He does this, basically, by defining the limits for the child and by a firm, but accepting manner. The child must see clearly that he cannot test the examiner, that the examiner is not threatened and has no intention of acquiescing. We do not mean a rigid intransigence, for it is often desirable to alter the testing situation to fit the child. To be sure, much of the behavior manifested by these children is for testing the limits of the situation; they want to know the rules of the game before they will cooperate. On some occasions, with a highly distractible child, we have had to reduce the stimuli in the room; we may have the child sit facing a plain wall, draw the window shade, and keep all test materials out of sight until used. We have even turned off lights in a room to force the child to focus on us. In a few instances we have found it necessary to take the child out of the testing situation and go for a walk before returning to the clinical tasks:

> Tim migrated restlessly from the window to the door of the examining room, whining belligerently. When an item was presented to him, he either threw it away or ignored it. We then took the child for a walk about the clinic; we looked into each room while carrying on a running commentary about what was going on. Then Tim was able to return to the examining room and was content to move through the various tasks we had planned.

With a few genuinely hyperkinetic children we have resorted to mild physical restraint, generally holding them close to us.[4] They seemed to need and actually like external controls on their flighty behavior that they could not control from within. Although we don't recommend the procedure, we know one highly successful clinical audiologist who, when confronted with a recalcitrant child, firmly squeezes the youngster's trapezius muscle as he guides him toward the examining booth.[5]

Second, don't plead or cajole the obstreperous child. If he ducks beneath the table and announces he will not cooperate, we go ahead with the various tasks, using self-talk. Don't reinforce crying or whining by soothing or placating. It is, however, a good practice to distract the child with some interesting task and then praise his attentiveness.

There are obviously many other considerations that could be discussed; additional suggestions will be offered in the several chapters concerning various disorders. But for the present, here are several basic precepts on the management of children in a clinical examination:

1. As a general rule, you ask less and observe more. Children usually lack the insight and cooperation necessary to analyze their problem rationally and objectively.

2. The prospective diagnostician should learn all he can about normal children in order to provide a baseline for his observations of youngsters presenting problems. He can do this by taking courses, studying relevant norms, but

---

[4] Hyperkinesis, or hyperactivity, considered a so-called soft sign of neurological impairment, has been overused. We suggest that you follow a four-year-old normal youngster for a day before you glibly use the term. The abundant activity of normal children is generally goal-directed, it has some "logical" sequence or flow to it. True hyperactivity is simply random behavior. The point is that the normal child may actually be more active, although he may not seem to be because we can see some order in his play.

[5] See Sloan and MacAulay (1968) for the use of operant control methods in managing a flighty or recalcitrant child.

most of all by extensive scrutiny of children in nursery school and other settings. He should have a good idea of the typical or modal behavior for children at various age levels. One student claimed her four-year-old client was in grave need of psychiatric appraisal and treatment. We remembered the child and were somewhat puzzled by this recommendation. We demanded a rationale. It seems that the child had an imaginary companion, a wrinkled green elephant that served as a scapegoat and alter ego. We chuckled and then sent the student scurrying to the Gesell profiles to see how common such fantasies are in four-year-olds.

3. Limit the choices you offer a child. Don't ask if he would like to go with you, do this or that, unless the alternatives do not conflict with the examiner's goals. He will invariably say "no" and you will be left with egg on your face.

4. Be flexible in your use of tests and examinations. If you cannot employ the rigid standardized format for administration, use the test to obtain all the data you can. If the child refuses to name the pictures and objects, you might be able to get a language sample from the items he has in his pockets.

5. Absolute honesty—even candor—is important in working with children. Recently the senior author was examining a nine-year-old stutterer who had a particularly disfiguring portwine stain covering a large portion of his face and neck. Inadvertently glancing at the mirror during a horrendous and agonizing block, he suddenly screamed, "Ugly, ugly, ugly!" My instinctive response was to reassure him that he was not ugly, but quietly and matter-of-factly I said, "Yes, ugly-ugly-ugly . . . right now." He looked searchingly at my face for a long moment and then, with a shy smile, he moved closer.

6. The whole assessment does not have to be done in one session.

7. You should understand that parents are people, too, not just vehicles to assist diagnosis or carry out therapy (Emerick, 1969).

ADOLESCENTS. Experienced clinicians frequently report that adolescents —the classical teenager, especially in grades 7 through 11—are often difficult to examine and resistant to therapy. The main problem seems to be getting through to the person. There is no magic formula for this, but we would like to make some suggestions that we have found helpful in guiding our work with adolescent clients:

1. Acquire an understanding of the many pressures and changes the teenager is experiencing: rapid physical growth, sexual maturity, conflicts between dependence and independence, definition of a new ego-ideal, a search for identity and life work, intense group loyalty and identification, and many more. Empathy that flows from understanding is a powerful force in establishing a working relationship.

2. There is an intense desire to be like others, not to stand out from the pack in any way that would suggest frailty. Hence the adolescent will find it extremely difficult to reveal a speech impairment, even if he does want help. He will tend to cover it up with a sullen bravado or a dense "it-doesn't-bother-me" shell. Denial is their particular forte. You can't beat this down nor can you simply dismiss the individual with a shrug. We advocate a straightforward approach: acknowledge the forces that are bearing on the individual, point up objectively the paths others have taken, provide information about the economic and social penalties that accrue to the speech-defective person

(have him talk to older clients). Basically, try to demonstrate by your demeanor and what you say that you do care about him. Personal involvement and commitment are key factors.

3. Don't try to "swing" with teenage clients; empathy is not identification. Don't abandon your professional role for that of a teenager. Not only does it weaken your effectiveness, it also looks ludicrous and invites rejection.

One public-school clinician had a painful experience in learning to maintain her role and status as adult therapist. While waiting one day for a fourth member of a therapy group to arrive, she attempted to enter a rap session with three teenage males. She wanted to know the meanings of several "in" words, but the boys demurred and looked rather curiously at her. She responded by saying, "Look, teenagers want to know all about the adult world, right? So, turnabout is fair play, why shouldn't I learn about yours?" One of the bolder adolescents suggested that they were becoming adults and thus they needed to know—but was the clinician going to be a teen?

4. Approach the adolescent with tolerance and good humor. Don't be shocked or annoyed by their overstatements and superlatives. Sometimes they will, in order to uphold their protective armor, resort to all sorts of strategies to confuse, defeat, or anger the clinician. The ability to laugh at yourself and to use humor in a gentle, needling manner is an asset.

5. Demonstrate your competence to deal with this person and his problem. We like to do this by explaining what we are about, the reasons for the various tests and examinations, how we will use the information, and the process of checking out our hypotheses. We encourage the adolescent to challenge and question what we are doing. Finally, we usually give him an idea of the route we would follow when therapy commences; we enumerate the steps and even do some trial therapy.

6. Avoid the teacher image as much as you can. Unfortunately, many of our schools are more concerned with keeping order than with learning or with human relationships. Teacher is always right in some schools. We eschew this image by our style of interaction, by keeping the person's confidences, by listening to him when he complains about a teacher or a course. We don't enter into the criticism or side with the client against the school, nor do we try to defend the institution or retreat to moralisms.

These recommendations have been distilled from our clinical experience and are not presented as magical touchstones for all diagnosticians or all clients; nor do they represent the full range of possibilities for successful interaction with teenage clients. We present them here to provoke other workers to develop clinical generalizations on the basis of their experience.[6]

---

[6] It is very easy to retreat behind the smug slogan, usually uttered with an unctuous smile, "It all depends on the individual." While it certainly is true that each client is unique as a human being, it does not follow that broader generalizations about the common ways people respond are undesirable or untrue. Clinicians must make many implicit generalizations about their professional interaction with clients. We quite agree with Williams (1968: 54): "If the questions for which the researcher seeks answers are not meaningful, then the clinician is at fault for failing to provide the basis for meaningful questions." We shall never have a scientific basis for our work if we regard each new case as a law unto himself.

OLDER OR AGED CLIENTS.   Older clients present some rather special problems for the diagnostician. The clinician should be alert to fatigue, disorientation, failing eyesight, and hearing loss. With advanced age, the person may find it more difficult to focus his attention on a task, and he generally has trouble remembering directions because of short-term memory decline. We need, therefore, to explain each step of our clinical procedures at greater length and repeat instructions several times to insure understanding. Our pace should be geared down, if necessary, to the client's slower level. Since many older clients tend to feel useless and discarded in our youth-oriented culture, and resentful that their bodies are betraying them, we may find it important to spend some time listening to their memories of past achievements.

As with children and adolescents, the diagnostician should know as much as possible about aging (some training programs are pretty much child-oriented in course work and practicum). Further, the clinician should recognize and have under control his own ambivalence toward growing old. Finally, it is absolutely imperative that a multiprofessional approach be employed in rendering services to older clients (Leutenegger and Stovall, 1971).

The factor of sex.   In what manner does the sex of the diagnostician influence the clinical examination and testing situation? Do young children relate better to female clinicians? Do adolescent boys feel more comfortable, and hence more able to reveal information about themselves, with male diagnosticians? We know of no scientific basis on which we can answer these questions, and no doubt it is often a highly individual matter. However, in our own practice, in the supervision of student clinicians and extensive consultation with colleagues working in various settings, we have observed several principles at work:

1. Female clients of all ages, with the possible exception of female adolescents, seem to experience little difficulty with a male diagnostician. This might be the product of countless experiences with male dentists and physicians.

2. Adolescent females, girls in the process of becoming women physically and psychologically, seem to be more comfortable and open with a female clinician; likewise male adolescents seem to work better with male clinicians.

3. Female clinicians of college age sometimes find it difficult to maintain a clinical context when performing diagnostic examinations on men of the same age level. College-level male clinicians may experience some of the same difficulties in diagnosis with female students.

Obviously, the factors of age and sex are interrelated in a complex manner in the clinical relationship. We do know that the interpersonal context does influence the *kinds* of responses clients will give to various tasks; it also may influence the *amount* and *style* of response. Men talking together assume a rather distinct verbal style (the "locker room" set) as do women (the "bridge club" set). Since the clinician can do little about his or her sex at this point, he should inspect his value systems to see that this particular facet does not become obtrusive in the clinical setting.

The work setting. Ideally the speech clinician performs his professional role as he has been trained to do, regardless of where he works. However, diagnosticians working in schools often report several difficulties: (1) The speech clinician is identified in the child's mind with the teachers, some of whom may be penalizing or disturbing listeners. In addition, the clinician may find himself identified with authority figures, and this hampers the development of a clinical relationship. (2) The type of diagnostic regimen best suited for the client may be difficult to implement within the school. (3) The child usually has no choice about entering the examining situation; he is brought for diagnosis by his parents, referred by a teacher, or is "screened out" by the speech clinician. (4) It seems more difficult to secure active parental participation when children are seen in school. Some parents are suspicious of the authority which a school represents; they may harbor resentment for alleged bad treatment when they attended school. Inherent in this is the natural resistance manifested by many persons toward official institutions of government. The clinician may find that he has been tarred by the same brush, and may be unable to obtain the cooperation of some parents.

Some clinicians, however, give up too easily; with a resigned shrug, they suggest that it is impossible to do careful, thorough diagnostics in the schools with the heavy caseload requirements. But *the nature of the child's problem, not the characteristics of the work setting,* dictates the nature of the clinician's responsibility. The needs of the client, not the arbitrary and often antiquated state codes or educational policies of the school, should and must determine the scope of the speech clinician's professional activities. To be accorded professional treatment, one must behave as a professional. The hallmark of professionalism is doing what needs to be done for the good of the client. A clinician's responsibilities do not end when the last school bell rings.

We have attempted to show how three factors—age, sex, and work setting—influence the clinical examination. There no doubt are many other conditions which also impinge: the timing of the diagnostic examination should coincide with the individual's readiness for help; the manner of referral; and idiosyncratic aspects such as the motives and fantasies of some clients. Additional comments will be presented in the discussion below dealing with test selection.

THE SELECTION OF TESTS

There are many diagnostic instruments to assess all aspects of a client and his communication abilities. Thus, it becomes a matter of critical selection among the diverse tests available. What factors are employed in making a selection? In addition to the rather obvious criteria such as the nature of the client's problem (you would generally not give a dysarthric client a test measuring attitude toward stuttering), the client's age (high school seniors take umbrage at picture-naming tests of articulation), and the diagnostician's training ("that's the way we did it at dear old Mossy Rock"), the following additional factors should be considered:

1. Does the test provide information that cannot be obtained by interviewing or observation? All diagnostic instruments cause a certain amount of stress to the client; if it is feasible within reasonable time limits to obtain data by indirect means, then the clinician should be wary of using the test. When desirable, however, test information might be a very valuable check on hypothetical constructs emerging from the interview and observation.

2. Is it possible to convey the instructions without lengthy and complicated explanations?

3. Is the test relatively easy to administer and score? The complexity of a diagnostic tool does not necessarily correlate with its precision or validity.

4. Is the test economical in terms of the client's time and energy? How much time does it consume relative to the quality and quantity of data obtained?

5. Are the theoretical constructs upon which the test is constructed congruent with the examiner's beliefs?

6. Does the test permit objective scoring? Although the important decisions, clinically as well as scientifically, are judgmental, the basis for making the judgments is sounder to the degree that human bias is at least identified and, hopefully, limited. Is the test standardized—are the procedures and materials fixed so that, regardless of where or by whom a client is evaluated, the same methodology can be employed?

7. Will the test actually make a difference in solving the person's problem? Is it practical in the sense that the results lead logically to a program of treatment?

8. Does the test suggest to the client that he might have additional problems? A diagnostic procedure should not be iatrogenic. Related to this is the inadequacy of some attitude and personality inventory scales in which the respondent can recognize the acceptable and the nonacceptable answers.

9. Does the test violate the client's integrity? We have already alluded to the painfully obvious error of using a picture test of articulation with older clients; some violations are less obvious.

10. Does the diagnostic instrument permit the development of clearly defined and reportable concepts regarding the patient and his communication disability?

11. Is the instrument reliable? Does it give consistent measures when administered repeatedly to the same client? Do separate examiners arrive at the same conclusions from this instrument when making independent judgments?

12. Is the test valid? Does it test what it says it does? Obviously, an instrument must be reliable—you must evoke the same "something" each time—before it can be valid; for example, if every time we said "corn" a client responded "tree," he would be reliable but consistently wrong. There are several types of validity: content validity (how well does the test *sample*—all tests obtain only a sample, not a parameter or whole—the particular aspect in which we

are interested?); predictive validity (how well does the test predict performance?); concurrent validity (how well does the test data we have check
with other evidence available?); and construct validity (how well does the
test show or reflect some trait, quality, or construct presumed to underlie
performance on the test?).

— 13. In what manner was the test standardized? What types of norms are set
forth and on what population are they based? Is it "fair" to give a measure
of verbal intelligence, based on suburban, middle-class vocabulary, to an
Ojibway Indian child?

14. - any risk to the child? (HEW regulations)

We will delineate later some possible dangers involved in testing. At
this point we would like to suggest that a common danger is dependence upon
formalized instruments and atrophy of observational skills.

observation

We have discussed the clinical examination as if it consisted solely of
formal testing. However, every test was once a system for looking at clients
that existed in one man's mind. In Chapter 1 we pointed out the critical importance of observation and described the process in terms of *focus, depth,
description, interpretation,* and *implications.* In this section we remind the
reader of two common difficulties encountered when beginning clinicians set
out to observe clients: first, instead of observing, they simply look at global
behavior; and secondly, there is a distinct tendency to rush into interpretation

before the description phase has had sufficient attention.

Beginning students, unless they are guided closely, simply watch clients
without observing specific items of behavior. In order to train themselves in
critical observation, incipient diagnosticians must select one or two facets of
the individual's behavior (*focus*) that they wish to scrutinize or prepare detailed *descriptions* of ongoing activity according to a rigorous time schedule
(*depth*). Here is an example from a student report:

> We noted that Dave [a ten-year-old with several articulation errors, including a
> pronounced lateral thrust of his lower jaw on /sh/ and /ch/] had a facial tic—
> he blinks his right eye—which may be related to the lateral jaw thrust. So we set
> up an observation schedule: for five two-minute periods during his last therapy
> session, we counted each occurrence of the tic and related it to the therapy ac-
> tivity he was doing and to the mandible thrust.

They found that the tic was an antecedent of the jaw thrust, and the clinician
altered his therapy to include the management of the eyeblink. Sometimes we
insist that the student record everything a given child does, also on a time
schedule. This is especially useful in assessing the behavior of children presenting severe language disorders as well as other types of impairments. From
these masses of data, inferences (*interpretations*) can then be made and *implications* drawn.

We find that observation of ongoing behavior affords us a better idea of a child's *typical* behavior (what he usually does) than many formal tests that assess abilities (what he can do in maximum performance). It must be stressed, however, that both observations and test information are hypothetical constructs and only samples of the client's total repertoire. We must not place too much credence in only one isolated observation or test score:

> Nonverbal behavior is a case in point. Although very useful as an adjunct to interviewing and testing, no one item has universal meaning. If a parent leaves her coat on during an interview, for example, it may mean that she feels vulnerable and the garment provides protective armor. It may also mean that she has a spot on her dress where the baby spilled Similac that morning as she rushed to make the appointment, or that all the hangers in the waiting room were taken again by forgetful students. The issue here is not to make any one item of behavior the sole basis for interpretation. All observations should be compared with others to see if patterns emerge.

DANGERS IN TESTING

At some point in the future, the speech-and-hearing clinician might have a massive diagnostic computer system for rapidly assessing speech and language disorders. Into the maw of this marvelous machine, the diagnostician will feed certain key signs, and error-free diagnosis, with suggestions for remediation, will emerge following a short wait. But, alas, this is a mythical beast, at least for the present.[7] We must rely on the fragile magic of human perception.

It is axiomatic that no testing device or examination procedure is any better than the person who administers it. Tests, after all, are mere tools and can be used wisely or foolishly. In this section, we focus on some of the dangers involved in using tests: overtesting, undertesting, and other assorted dangers.

overtesting

Many clinicians employ a shotgun approach to diagnosis. They administer several tests and collect a plethora of data on the assumption that quantity is the key issue—the more information they have, the more likely they are to have something relevant. This type of procedure is especially evident in some training programs where the unfortunate client is poked and prodded in the interest of clinical experience.

The worst aspect of overtesting is the tendency to fragment the patient into a series of clinical artifacts and, in the process of sorting out the scores and profiles, to lose his unique wholeness. *We miss the person for the percentiles.*

---

[7] But see the exciting novel by Michael Crichton, *The Andromeda Strain* (1969).

We recently participated in the staffing of a pretty little blond ten-year old girl with a slightly nasal voice. The child, who had Perthe's disease and wore a large, cumbersome brace on her left leg, was referred by a local speech clinician for a voice, language, and hearing examination. The two advanced graduate students assigned to the case diligently administered a lengthy language inventory, a verbal intelligence measure, a comprehensive audiometric evaluation, and an extensive voice analysis. Two hours later when all these data were arrayed, it showed that Penny was within normal limits in most dimensions and slightly below normal on the remaining. By this time, however, the child was lost in the welter of profiles and percentiles. Straining mightily at the gnats of information, three faculty members and the two bewildered students attempted to come up with some meaningful recommendations. The fact that Penny was doing fairly well as a person despite the obvious physical deformity, the fact that she was communicating intelligibly and openly with only mild hypernasality, was obscured by the barrage of information from the "routine test battery."

Overdependence on the process of testing and test scores may prevent us from seeing important clues about the person and his life situation. By placing too much emphasis on the formal diagnostic instruments we can ignore how the client and his family see the problem.

Another danger, also a form of overtesting, is delaying treatment. The structure afforded by the administration of various diagnostic instruments does provide a sense of security to the clinician.

Finally, since diagnosis and treatment are part of the same continuous process, we should carefully consider how tests may structure relationships in an undesirable way. Extensive test batteries may lead the client to suspect that his problem will be handled in a detached and authoritative manner.

undertesting

Grave errors may also be committed by not having sufficient information on a given client. Many clinicians who work in schools operate as if they have made a diagnosis when they state that a child has a frontal lisp; this is a description—and a superficial one at that—not a diagnosis. It is certainly not the basis for a therapeutic program.

Consider the child who was enrolled in speech therapy year after year for a "simple" functional disorder of articulation. More extensive assessments revealed sensory problems, mild motor impairments, psychological conflicts, and other learning disabilities—all hiding behind the "simple lisp" label. The ubiquitous diagnosis of "functional articulation problem" may result from insufficient scrutiny of the client. Obviously, then, a very real danger in undertesting is the fact that you may well overlook something serious if you do not investigate beneath the obvious. Also, you will not have enough information to convey in reports to experts in the field when you want to refer a client; perhaps you may not even know when there is a need for referral.

Finally, certain tests, when judiciously used, can prevent us from creating speech defects where none exists (Van Riper, 1966):

> Many first-grade children have "maturational speech differences" which, in most cases, will clear up by the end of the school year. Some, of course, will not. There is no need to include all first graders with lisps in speech therapy, to catch the few who will not mature into better speech. By using a screening test to identify those in need of help, we not only conserve our efforts but also prevent the development of a self-concept that includes "I have trouble with /s/."

 assorted dangers

In addition to the polar dangers of over- and undertesting, there are several other possible risks involved in the use of tests. They are all interrelated:

The client's participation. No diagnostic procedure is a one-way street; if the client cannot or does not participate in the testing to the level required —because of attitudes, moods, his personal background—the results may be spurious. We are, in a very real sense, at the mercy of the respondent's co-operation.

> We tested Ruth during the initial stages of therapy for stuttering, with a popular test of verbal intelligence. Although a college sophomore, she received the astoundingly low IQ score of 81. On the basis of our prior interaction with her, we suspected the validity of the measure. On a later retest, using a different form of the examination, she obtained a score of 120. In talking with her about her performance, it was revealed that, on the day before the first test, she had been notified that she, as a candidate for Homecoming Queen, had not been chosen, nor was she even selected for the Queen's Court. Her performance becomes explicable in light of the antecedent event.

The competence of the examiner. The prospective diagnostician should be thoroughly familiar with a diagnostic instrument before he attempts to administer it. The test manual should be carefully studied and several trial attempts with normal-speaking individuals completed before assessing a client.

The magic of tests. Some clients feel that a test will do something for them; once the test has been administered, someone will be able to figure out the exact cause of their problem and pinpoint a solution. Tests, thus, often raise false hopes.

The mean scores. Most diagnostic instruments have tables for interpreting given scores obtained; these norms are generally based upon the average performance of a large number of subjects. Hence, their application to a given individual is problematical.

The presumption of the test. Some tests are contraindicated because they presume normal speech and hearing. Their application to clients with communication problems is suspect:

> Our favorite aphasic client, perhaps our all-time favorite client, was Charles S. Hanford. Following a thrombotic stroke, with resultant auditory aphasia, his employer demanded a psychological appraisal, fearful of the possibility of brain damage. Mr. Hanford was taken by his wife to a local clinical psychologist, who gave him a comprehensive intelligence measure. The psychologist, although noting the aphasia, did not modify the test instrument. He made recommendations on the basis of the test results, including an IQ score of 54, which was remarkable in terms of Mr. Hanford's degree of auditory aphasia at the time. The client's wife was told that "he had suffered extensive brain damage, would be unable to work or drive again [he had no paralysis] and would not be able to make judgments with regard to the family finances, etc." When Mr. Hanford eventually learned of this, he was furious. In retribution for the psychologist's actions, he paid the twenty-five-dollar fee in quarters and other small change over an interval of eighteen months, always demanding a receipt and always indicating that if the psychologist left town he would immediately pay his bill in full.

Looking where the light is. The joke about the drunken man looking for his lost watch under the bright illumination of a street light rather than in the darkened alley where it was lost applies to the way some clinicians use tests. They have a pet instrument which they apply willy-nilly to each client without regard to his particular needs.

Following the fads. It is very difficult to identify the beginning and end of a particular fad or intellectual *Zeitgeist* when you are in the middle of it. There are some workers who make a total commitment to one way of assessing and talking about a particular communication impairment and cannot change to meet the needs of a client who does not fit the mold of the test in vogue.

Hardening of the categories. Following the fads can easily lead to that dread clinical disorder, "hardening of the categories." This involves being able to see behavior only through well-worn perceptual grooves with regard to identification and classification of clients and their responses.

With all these possible pitfalls it is easy to see why some impressionistic diagnosticians, the artisans described in Chapter 1, eschew formal tests. Many of these individuals feel that tests tend to traumatize clients. There is little hard evidence that this has to be true. Indeed, Schuell, Jenkins, and Jimenez-Pabon (1964: 159–76) observe that when the tasks are presented in the spirit of mutual exploration, they can be factors in correcting misapprehensions and misinformation. This is to say that a diagnostic session can be therapeutic; the client explores himself and the dimensions of his problem with the objective support of the clinician. The unknown begins to take on limits and definition; the client is no longer faced with a global failure. Testing can and should reveal the client's strengths as well as weaknesses.

PROGNOSIS

Prognosis may be defined as a prediction of the outcome of a proposed course of treatment for a given client: how effective therapy will be, how far we can expect the client to progress, and perhaps, how long it will take. Since diagnosis is a continuing process, prognosis should, like therapy planning, have both long-range and immediate facets. Immediate prognosis covers what the person can do now, what steps in therapy are possible, what is the best route to take. Prognosis for specific communication disorders will be discussed in subsequent chapters; in this section we will present some generic purposes and a possible danger involved in predicting a client's response to therapy.

Prognosis also provides direction for treatment; we must know where we are going so that we will know when we have arrived. Some predictive factors are specific to a particular speech or language disability and will be discussed in the appropriate chapters. There are, however, a number of general factors that the clinician must consider when making predictions: the client's age, habit-strength, the existence of other problems, the type and intensity of reactions from significant persons in the client's environment, the client's motivation, and secondary gains the client may derive from the problem.

Accurate prognoses can help establish our credibility with other professions. The ability to predict with reasonable precision is perhaps the highest form of scientific achievement. Needless to say, however, these predictions should be based on something more than clinical intuition. Impressionistic conclusions, especially when made by experienced workers, can often be startlingly accurate, but they should always be labeled as impressionistic: a prognosis should be supported by a substantial amount of information.

In what sense might a prognosis be dangerous? We have become suspicious of what these predictions can do to our therapeutic interaction with the client; we are becoming increasingly convinced that the clinician's expectations regarding the case's potential influences the treatment program. It is certainly possible that our negative prognoses can be communicated to a client and affect the course of therapy.

SOME TESTS AND EXAMINATION PROCEDURES
COMMON TO MANY DIAGNOSTIC UNDERTAKINGS

A number of tests and examination procedures are clinically useful regardless of the client's particular communication impairment. In order to avoid repetition in the chapters that follow, these commonly utilized assessment techniques are discussed here; in the chapters dealing with the various disorders, we shall present diagnostic procedures that are pertinent to the specific speech problem.

the oral peripheral examination

It is a common practice to inspect a client's oral structures to determine their structural and functional adequacy for speech.[8]

To provide an example of typical data gathered during an oral peripheral examination, we have included notes hastily scribbled during an evaluation of a nine-year-old boy with a hoarse voice and several articulation errors:

> Lips look okay. No asymmetry of face. Slight open bite; poor dental hygiene (lots of cavities and tartar buildup). Tongue has good mobility, no paralysis or sluggishness; can protrude, wiggle from side to side swiftly, and touch the alveolar ridge; can even curl and groove. Hard palate seems OK, no scars. Soft palate has good tissue supply; elevates fine, no asymmetry. Palatine tonsils are *really* enlarged, filling the whole isthmus between the fauces. Pharynx looks inflamed (possible postnasal drip?). Good gag reflex. Wonder why he has mandible thrust to left side on /*sh*/ and /*ch*/?

Note the systematic nature of the inspection. Although the period of observation was relatively brief—an oral examination is generally completed in less than two minutes—the clinician has a sound basis for making a referral to a laryngologist. Now we shall present a rather detailed procedure for conducting an oral examination.

Tools you will need. You will need a light source; a small flashlight is good (we avoid the head mirror because it makes us look like a physician). Next, obtain a supply of plain applicator sticks. We dislike tongue depressors because of their association with doctors; in addition they are so blunt they do not permit evaluation of point-to-point sensitivity in the oral area. If you do use tongue depressors, the individually wrapped ones are best for sanitary purposes (it is curious that no one has yet invented a flavored tongue blade). Finally, your kit might include several pads of cotton gauze (for holding onto tongues), a few candy suckers, and a mirror.

How to get into a small child's mouth. Most older children and adults will open their mouths on request. Small children, however, are sometimes rather reluctant to let the clinician examine their tongue and teeth:

> Jimmy cooperated, cautiously but willingly, in all the diagnostic tasks until the clinician brought out a tongue depressor. He clamped his little jaw shut in bulldog fashion and tears began to form in the corners of his huge brown eyes. The

---

[8] Beginning students often perform an oral peripheral examination in a rather mechanical fashion, almost as if they are simply following a ritual. Observation is of little use if one is not competent to learn something from what one is looking at. If you don't know anything about the range of normalcy in oral anatomy and physiology, then there is little you can discover by idly looking around in a buccal cavity. See Project 2 at the end of this chapter.

clinician unwrapped the wooden blade and produced a small pen light, chatting amiably all the time. "Let me see, here is my mirror. I wonder if that little black dot is still on the back of my tongue. Hmmmm. Only three boys have ever seen it. . . ." (The clinician opened his mouth and looked intently with light and mirror.) Then, turning to Jimmy, the clinician requested, "Say, can you help me find that black dot? It's way on the back of my tongue. That's right, here's the flashlight." Jimmy, curious now, looked cautiously into the clinician's mouth. The clinician giggled and suggested he look further back. "I taw it, I taw it," Jimmy said triumphantly. "Hmmmm. You did? Say, I wonder if . . . no, I bet you don't . . . but maybe you do, maybe you have a black dot, too?" suggested the clinician. The child handed the light to the clinician and opened his mouth, erasing a small grin.

There is another method we have used which, although slightly indelicate, is more universally effective:

Children are engrossed with magic and guessing games. We make a wager—some small token will do—that he cannot guess what we had for breakfast (or lunch). Then, after he scrutinizes our oral cavity and makes a guess, we agree, with shocked surprise at his wizardry. Now we ponder aloud what he might have had for the most recent meal. Generally, their mouths pop open like baby starlings. Our first guess is usually something outlandish (like sardines and Bermuda onions) which provokes much mirth and a chance to look and guess again.

With some especially shy children or those for whom the oral examination conjures up vivid memories of past trauma, we have used another technique. It may take more time, but children almost always like to play follow-the-leader games. Using a large mirror so that we can see each other, we go through a series of comical movements of our arms, legs, and torso. Gradually we shift the focus of movement to our head, using our eyes and lips. Finally, we open our mouths and make weird movements with our tongue. The children usually follow in this "play," and we end up peering into each other's mouth before the glass.

What to look for.   It is important to be *systematic* and *swift* when conducting an oral examination. This demands considerable practice. Use every opportunity to scrutinize normal-speaking persons, not only to perfect your technique and observational skills, but also to establish a frame of reference on the range of structural and functional variation. The following outline is presented as a guide for conducting oral peripheral examinations:[9]

1. Lips and lip movement: inspect the lips first for relative size, symmetry, and scars. Can the client pucker his lips and retract them? Can he close his lips

[9] Laryngoscopic examination is the professional responsibility of the physician. While the speech pathologist usually describes breathing patterns, and examines the external musculature of the larynx for tension, an assessment of the vocal folds must be undertaken by a laryngologist.

tightly for the sounds /p/, /b/, and /m/? Can he utter the nonsense syllable "puh" at least once per second?

→ 2. Jaws: scrutinize the client's jaws in a state of rest; observe for symmetry. Can he open and close his mandible at least once per second?

→ 3. Teeth: inspect the client's bite during a state of rest. A normal dental bite is characterized by the upper incisors overlapping the lower incisors by not more than one half of their vertical dimension. Is there an open, under-, or overbite? Does the client have cavities, jumbled teeth, gaps between teeth or more than the normal complement of teeth?

One of the senior author's first clients was a college girl with supernumerary teeth. The presenting problem was lalling, severe distortion of the /l/ and /r/. When we looked in her mouth we were astounded to find an extra set of upper incisors directly behind the normally positioned set. She apparently had learned to make the two semivowels with the blade of her tongue in order to avoid the sharp serrated edges of the extra teeth.

→ 4. The tongue: note the size of the tongue relative to the oral cavity. Observe for symmetry in structure and during movement. Is there scarring, atrophy, or fasiculations? Can the client protrude and retract his tongue, wiggle it from side to side, and touch the alveolar ridge without random movement or extraordinary effort? Inspect the tip of tongue and the frenulum for any evidence of tongue tie.[10]

Can he trill his tongue when the mandible is stabilized? Test for diadochokinesis by having him utter "tuh"; can he say one per second? Is there any evidence of tongue thrust? (An open bite might alert you to this possibility.) When he swallows does he have an exaggerated lip seal? Does his tongue protrude beyond the incisors? Is there no apparent bunching in the masseter? If the answers to these last three queries are positive, then the client may be a tongue-thruster.

→ 5. Hard palate: note the shape (is it flat? high and arched?) and width of the hard palate. Are there any scars present? Can the client produce /r/ and /l/? One public-school clinician noted that three of his cases with persistent /r/ defects had rather high and arched hard palates. He experimented with several materials (bubble gum and peanut butter were consumed too swiftly) to reduce the palatal height; finally, in cooperation with a local dentist, he made prosthetic devices of denture material. All three children began to make the elusive /r/ with their devices. The dentist gradually shaved off the structures. The cases' tongues were thus coaxed higher and higher until they were making the /r/ on their own hard palates.

→ 6. Soft palate and velopharyngeal closure: inspect the velum for size, scars, and symmetry. Does the soft palate move back and up toward the posterior pharyngeal wall? Can you visualize lateral movement?[11]

---

[10] Some children, especially those presenting neuromuscular problems, may find it difficult to elevate the tip of their tongue to the alveolar ridge on command. We use a sucker, placing the moistened candy behind the upper incisors and encouraging the child to go after it. A spot of peanut butter or a tiny paper wedged high between the central incisors can also be used.

[11] Individuals presenting nasal vocal quality or nasal emission will require more extensive evaluation of their velopharyngeal competency. See Chapter 8 and Project 2 at the end of this chapter.

→7. Fauces: inspect the pillars for scars, the status of the palatine tonsils, and the width of the isthmus. Check the general condition of the oropharynx.

→8. Others: observe the client's breathing during speech and at rest. Is there tension apparent when phonation is initiated? Is the client a mouth-breather?

For further information regarding the oral peripheral examination, consult the work of Van Riper (1963: 472–90) and others (Johnson, Darley, and Spriestersbach, 1963: 111–32; Darley, 1964: 91–105). Remember, one swallow does not make a summer, and one deviancy in the oral area does not necessarily cause disordered speech:

> Laymen have a distinct tendency to blame speech defects on even minor oral abnormalities. One university student, who had a particularly vivid lateral lisp, insisted that his deviant /s/ was caused by a moderate gap between his upper central incisors. Even when we plugged the space and the lisp persisted, the adamant collegian continued to insist that the gap was the cause of his problem.

 motor abilities

During the oral examination the diagnostician may observe disturbances in the client's gross and fine motor abilities that suggest possible neurological dysfunction. While the diagnostic appraisal of motor dysfunction is the responsibility of the neurologist, the speech clinician should have a basis for making intelligent referrals. This can be accomplished by comparing various facets of the client's motor performance with norms corresponding to his age level.

A public-school clinician referred Steve Munroe to us with the following note:

> "Steve is almost unintelligible. . . . His whole pattern of articulation seems uncontrolled and bizarre. Although he is nearly thirteen, he is only in the sixth grade and that's where the problem lies. Unless we can show, somehow, that he belongs in the orthopedically handicapped room—where he could stay through high school—they will put him in a junior high class for the trainable retarded. Why? Solely on the basis of his score on the Wechsler; although he obtained an IQ of 62, I don't think he is retarded. His articulation is so bad I'm sure he failed the verbal items because the psychometrician could not understand him; and I think his incoordination shot him down on the motor tasks. Anyway, I need help. The physician at the public medical clinic refuses to refer him for a neurological examination; he claims that Steve is clearly retarded and belongs in the trainable room."

We decided to examine Steve in two sessions. We first wanted a global impression of his motor abilities, following the format presented by Wood (1964: 64–71). Here are our notes:

1. General body description. Steve is thin and wiry, has a slightly stooped posture. He appears on the small end of normal in height and weight.

2. Locomotor. His gait is characterized by a slight shuffle, and he seems to drag

his right foot slightly. His stance is not broad-based (not wider than his shoulders). Speed and range (distance or extent of excursion) seem restricted and "jerky"; they lack synergy.

3. Balance. He can stand for three seconds on one foot (left) with both arms extended and his eyes closed; he refused to attempt the task with his right foot. He tried to walk forward with one foot directly ahead of another but failed after three steps and refused to try again.

4. Manual dexterity. His copying and drawing attempts are jerky, and he must exert great effort to control a slight intentional tremor in his right arm and hand. He picked up eleven small buttons and put them in a box in seventeen seconds, using his left hand for the task after fumbling for a few seconds with his right.

5. Psychomotor. The tremor in Steve's right hand was more noticeable when we asked him to place a knitting needle through a small plastic loop suspended on a string. There was overflow of movement in the shoulder and upper chest area while he attempted this task. His speech efforts are often grotesque when he attempts to produce certain phonemes, particularly /r/ and /l/; some drooling was observed.

At the end of our first session we tape-recorded Steve reading a standard passage ("My Grandfather"). Later, using the procedures detailed in recent articles by Darley, Aronson, and Brown (1969a; 1969b), we rated the speech sample on the several dimensions provided by the authors. Our clinical hunch was confirmed; the ratings showed that Steve's performance was startlingly identical to the several clusters associated with pseudobulbar palsy (Darley, Aronson, and Brown, 1969b: 483). We were now certain that we had sufficient ammunition to insist upon a neurological referral but, knowing we had to work through the obdurate institutional physician, we wanted our case to be overwhelming. Well aware that medical practitioners are impressed by percentiles and normative comparisons, we administered the Oseretsky Test (Doll, 1947) during our second diagnostic session with Steve. This instrument evaluates motor proficiency by means of age-graded tasks and yields six measures. Here are the results we obtained:

1. General static coordination. Steve failed at the seven-year-old level (he could not balance on tiptoe, bending forward from the hips for ten seconds).

2. Dynamic coordination. He performed at the eight-year level. (This test requires the subject to touch all the finger tips of one hand successively with the thumb of the same hand, beginning with the little finger; it took him five seconds with his left hand and nine seconds with his right.)

3. General dynamic coordination. Steve passed all the items up to the ten-year level on this subtest. (Ten-year test task: given three trials to jump and clap his hands three times while in the air, Steve was successful on his third attempt.)

4. Motor speed. Steve also passed all the age-graded tasks up to the ten-year level. (He was required to make four piles with forty matchsticks in thirty-five seconds for the right hand, and in forty-five seconds for the left.) He took almost two minutes to complete the task with his right hand but finished in less than forty-five seconds with the left.

5. Simultaneous voluntary movements. Steve had trouble with this subtest, a task that requires simultaneous movements with both limbs. He got up to the eight-year level (tapping the floor rhythmically with his feet, alternating

right and left, while at the same time tapping the table with his fingers in the same rhythm.) He became upset and confused, pounded on the table in anger, and refused to continue.

6. Synkinesis. This subtest requires the subject to perform muscle movements without overflow such as wrinkling the forehead without any other movements at the eight-year level. Steve was tired and refused to do any of the tasks.

We held a formal conference with the physician, reviewed our findings and suggested politely but strongly that, since Steve had never been evaluated by a neurologist, we were sure that the doctor would certainly want conclusive evidence beyond a reasonable doubt before relegating the child to the irreversible category of "trainable." Somewhat defensive at first, the physician eventually concurred and expedited the referral; he even went one step further and enlisted the professional counsel of a physiatrist to direct the planning for a comprehensive, long-range program of rehabilitation for Steve.

Obviously not all of our clients will require such extensive investigation of their motor abilities. The point is, however, that the clinician must be capable of supporting his convictions with data. An emotional appeal—which the public-school therapist had tried unsuccessfully in the case of Steve—without carefully prepared evidence serves only to create a rather unprofessional image.

For further information concerning the evaluation of motor abilities, see the work of Berry (1969: 205–7, 219–70) and Van Riper (1963: 481–82). Grinker and Sahs (1966: 3–137) and Chusid and McDonald (1967: 158–278) present extended discussions of the neurological examinations.

estimates of development

Experienced clinicians recognize that in order to understand handicapped children, it is absolutely essential to have a thorough working knowledge of normal patterns of growth and behavior. What is typical or modal behavior for a four-year-old? What should he be able to do at this age level? It is possible, of course, to answer these questions in an impressionistic manner *if* the diagnostician has a clear idea of what is normal for various age levels. However, standardized scales devised on the basis of extensive observation of many children provide greater reliability and objectivity.

Ilg and Bates (1955) have prepared a very useful guide for comparing behavior patterns at various age levels based upon the exhaustive research of the Gesell Institute for Child Behavior. When preparing for a diagnostic session with a child, we review the descriptions of characteristic behavior for that particular age level.

Several checklists and interviewing guides have been devised from the data gathered at the Gesell Institute and from other research dealing with child development. Many clinicians find the Vineland Social Maturity Scale

(Doll, 1946) a useful device for assembling information on a child's maturity; the diagnostician does not observe the child directly but rather queries the parents on the youngster's ability to dress and feed himself, his social inter-action, and daily activities. The items on the scale are arranged in age cate-gories. For example, here are the six items at the three- to four-year-old level:

1. Walks down stairs one step per tread
2. Plays cooperatively at the kindergarten level
3. Buttons coat or dress
4. Helps at little household tasks
5. "Performs" for others
6. Washes hands unaided.

Although it is possible to derive a social age and social quotient on the basis of the information obtained in an interview, we often prefer to use the Vine-land as a screening device, which affords a way to compare the child's develop-ment—at least as perceived by his parents—against normative expectations.

There are distinct advantages to directly observing the child's performance instead of relying solely upon an informer. At the present time there are three tests (actually checklists for recording behavior that allow comparison with established norms) that permit the clinician to chart the development of a child in age-graded tasks. Both the Communicative Evaluation Chart (Ander-son, Miles, and Matheny, 1963) and the Utah Test of Language Development (Mecham, Jex, and Jones, 1967) concentrate on assessing language develop-ment; they are easy to use and do provide the clinician with an objective means of evaluating expressive and receptive verbal language skills. The Com-municative Evaluation Chart also includes items that assess physical well-being, motor coordination, normal growth and development, and visuomotor perception.

For a practical, clinically useful tool to help detect children with serious developmental delay, we prefer the Denver Developmental Screening Test (Frankenburg and Dodds, 1969). The Denver instrument is very simple to ad-minister, takes less than twenty minutes to finish, and in its published version, comes complete with all the forms and materials needed. It permits evaluation of the following aspects of a child's functioning: gross motor abilities, fine mo-tor coordination, language development, and personal-social maturation (the ability to perform tasks of self-care and relate to others). Here is a portion of a report we submitted to a family physician regarding Robbie O'Neill, a three-year-old child tentatively diagnosed as autistic:

> The vertical line drawn through the four dimensions represents the child's chronological age (see Figure 2). We administered the items through which this line passes in each dimension. On those items Robbie passed, we placed a large letter "P" on the horizontal bar at the midpoint; "F" indicates a failure and an

"R" stands for refused. In order to assist you in interpreting the scale, we quote from the Manual (Frankenburg and Dodds, 1969: 7): "Each of the test items is designated by a bar which is so located under the age scale as to indicate clearly the ages at which 25%, 50%, 75%, and 90% of the standardization population could perform the particular test item. The left end of the bar designates the age at which 25% of the standardization population could perform the item; the hatch mark at the top of the bar 50%; the left end of the shaded area 75%; and the right end of the bar the age at which 90% of the standardization population could perform the item. Normal children will generally show a fair amount of scattered successes and failures on items within one area and between the four areas. A *delay* is defined as any failure by a child on an item if he is older than the age at which 90% of the children pass that item. In other words, his vertical chronological age line is to the right of the right end of the bar representating the items he fails."

Robbie appears to be well coordinated in gross motor functioning; even though he refused most of the fine motor tasks, we noted a great degree of manual dexterity (he played almost continually with baby food jars filled with small nails, transferring the nails from one container to another). Note that he does not use language in a meaningful way; his parents report only "compulsive" laughter, but no speech per se. Consider also Robbie's responses on the personal-social dimension: he refuses to associate with others and is operating in a very delayed fashion.

Although the speech pathologist is concerned with developmental milestones and patterns of maturation, we quite agree with Berelson and Steiner (1964: 55): "Maturation, by definition, is always a *necessary* condition, but it is not always (strictly speaking, never) a *sufficient* condition; no child can do anything he is not biologically equipped to do, but no child can do everything he *is* biologically capable of."

intelligence and educational performance

Since the development of speech and language is dependent, in part, upon a child's capacity to learn, the speech pathologist is interested in his client's intelligence; many disorders of oral communication stem from low intelligence or inability to utilize an existing level of intelligence. A client's intelligence is also an important consideration in planning therapy.

We like to obtain a general impression of a client's intelligence and, if further testing is indicated, we refer him to a qualified psychometrician. The two most comprehensive measures of intelligence are the Stanford-Binet Intelligence Scale (Terman and Merrill, 1960) and the Wechsler scales for children (1949) and adults (1955). These instruments provide a multidimensional profile of an individual's intellectual abilities. Unless the clinician is qualified to administer these tests, he will generally rely on some screening device such as the Goodenough Draw-A-Man Test (1926), the Ammons Full Range Picture Vocabulary Test (Ammons and Ammons, 1948), or the Peabody Picture Vocabulary Test (Dunn, 1958). We prefer the latter test because of its ease

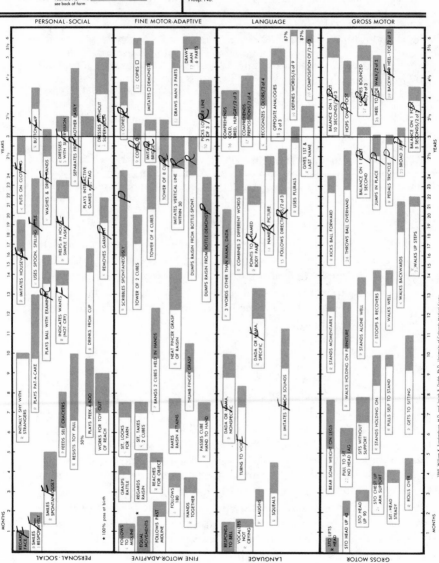

FIGURE 2 Score Sheet for Denver Developmental Screening Test. (W. Frankenburg and J. Dodds, *Denver Developmental Screening Test.* © 1969, reprinted with permission.)

70

of scoring and interpretation and the modern stimulus pictures provided. (However, see precautions noted in Chapter 4.) The Peabody Test is really a measure of recognition vocabulary, but it correlates highly with the more comprehensive instruments cited above (Taylor, 1963).

We do not generally report an IQ score or percentile if the client's performance is within normal limits. If a client's performance is not within normal limits, we usually cite the age level at which he responds:

> Conrad's recognition vocabulary was evaluated with the Peabody Picture Vocabulary Test (Form A). His performance on this scale was characteristic of children two years younger; in terms of auditory word recognition, then, Conrad appears to be functioning at a level of six years, or two years below his chronological age.

The Peabody Test is also useful because it allows the examiner to observe the client's behavior on a structured task and to get a feel for how he uses language. We can scrutinize his style of responding, how long he takes to complete the items (latency of response), and how he reacts to failure. Many children comment about the pictures, and the task thus provides another sample of their language output.

We should not give undue importance to one measure of intelligence. This is especially important in dealing with youngsters, since the younger the child, the less reliable is any intellectual assessment. We have also seen wide fluctuations in the tested intelligence of older children that seemed to stem from environmental events. Finally, IQ scores, like all test data, should be related to other sources of information, such as case histories, interviews, direct observation, and, when possible, school performance.

A child's school folder can be a rich source of information regarding his ability to learn and adjust. What scores did he obtain on various achievement tests? How does he go about learning? What are his attitudes toward success and failure in school? What about his abilities in problem-solving, reasoning, and identifying relationships? How does he perform in the language skills— spelling and reading in particular? What kinds of things does he perceive as worth working for in the classroom?

motivation

Motivation is a critical variable in speech therapy, particularly at the outset of treatment and again during the carryover phase of therapy. The assessment of a client's motivation, by means of testing or impressionistic observation, is then a very useful clinical procedure.

> What is motivation? A motive may be defined as: . . . an inner state that energizes, activates, or moves (hence, "motivation"), and that directs or channels behavior toward goals (Berelson and Steiner, 1964: 240).

Motives may be classified as primary (hunger, thirst, sleep) or secondary (need for social stimulation or recognition). Speech clinicians are generally interested in the relative strength of various secondary or social motives. Low motivation is commonly regarded as a poor prognostic sign; however, if the individual is highly aroused, if he manifests very high motivation, he may not be able to concentrate on the sequence of treatment.

One widely used means of assessing a client's motivation is to measure his level of aspiration:

Bill said he wanted to work on his lateral lisp, but his laconic nature and scholastic underachievement belied the fact. In order to assist him in gaining insight and provide us with some examples of his typical goal-setting behavior, we administered the Cassell Test (1957). This instrument measures goal-setting behavior by means of a graphomotor task: the client draws squares around circles as swiftly as he can. A four-page booklet consisting of eight units with three rows of twenty small squares each is provided. Within a specified time limit—thirty seconds—Bill attempted to draw the squares. Prior to each trial, he was requested to estimate or predict the number of squares he felt he could complete in thirty seconds. The Cassell Test yields a "D" score, which is the average of the difference between performance and subsequent estimate for all test trials. When a client consistently bids higher than his previous performance, his "D" score is positive. When he bids lower than his previous performance, his "D" score is negative. Here are Bill's scores:

Prediction	Performance
10	12
11	14
12	16
12	16
13	16

"D" score = −3.2. Divide 5 (the number of trials) into 16 (the total discrepancy between prediction and performance).

Normally, individuals tend to have slightly positive discrepancy scores because they balance their idealistic aspirations against realistic expectations of attainment. As a group, handicapped persons, as well as persons with a long history of failure, manifest "D" scores that are lower than those obtained by normal groups. We have also noted that some handicapped individuals react to failure with very high shifts in their goal-settings; by so doing, they put the attainment of their goal out of reach and thus insulate themselves from failure. For another means of measuring level of aspiration, see Rotter (1954).

There are other ways of assessing a client's motivation. McClelland (1955, 1961) has devised an intriguing system for determining the strength of an individual's "achievement motive" by analyzing thematic content in stories they write and scrutinizing their doodling.

We have also used an informal "test" of motivation in our work with young stutterers. It is based upon the observation that highly driven persons tend to feel uncomfortable if they are interrupted while completing a task and will tend to return to it as soon as they are permitted. We have used various activities— arithmetic problems, classifying and sorting objects, puzzles; when the young- ster is well into the task, we interrupt him and then record the time elapsed un- til he resumes the activity. Although lacking sufficient data to present norms, we have found that children with high motivation—those who strive for success— tend to return to the task more swiftly than those with low motivation—those who avoid the threat of failure. The former also do better in treatment. Per- sistence is essential to success in therapy as well as in life.

In a recent publication, McDaniels (1969: 139) presents a provocative formula for analyzing the potential motivation of a handicapped individual:

$$\text{MOTIVATION} = \frac{P(Os) \times U}{C}$$

Where:
$P(Os)$ = the probability of a *successful outcome* of treatment (based on the client's and clinician's judgment).
U = the meaning or value (*utility*) the client places upon the particular performance to be acquired.
C = the expense (*cost*) in money, and the physical and mental effort re- quired.

For extended discussions of motivation, consult the work of Raph (1960) and others (Berelson and Steiner, 1964: 239–96; Atkinson and Feather, 1966; McDaniels, 1969: 133–64).

audiometric evaluation

Because of the close relationship between auditory acuity and speech and language development, we generally perform an audiometric assessment on each client. We often do this simply by combining informal, nonaudio- metric testing with an audiometric screening procedure. Individuals manifest- ing abnormality on these tests should receive more complete audiological evaluation. For a discussion of hearing loss and assessment, consult the work of Emerick (1971) and others (Newby, 1964; Darley, 1961; Glorig, 1965; O'Neill and Oyer, 1966; Sataloff, 1966; Davis and Silverman, 1970).

socioeconomic status

Speech clinicians do not routinely obtain a measure of socioeconomic status on each client. However, social class may have a bearing on the assess- ment and management of an individual's communication problem in one or more of the following ways: (1) parental attitudes toward clinical assistance may differ between classes (lower-class parents are more distrustful of authority; (2) child-rearing practices—including the amount and type of speech stimulation—seem to differ between lower and middle classes; (3) the economic position of the parents will influence the recommendations made; and (4) some types of speech differences, rather than being regarded as speech defects, may more appropriately be designated as subculture dialects.

There are several measures of social class; the scales devised by Hollingshead and Redlich (1958: 387–97) and Warner, Meeker, and Ells (1960: 139–42) are representative, and we have found them useful for conducting research or for an extensive study of a particular child:

> Social class alone may not be as important clinically as the identification of discrepancies between the elements (occupation, source of income, place of residence, amount of income) used in ranking. When there are gaps between these elements—for example, high-prestige occupation but low salary—it can provoke intense striving behavior and subsequent pressure upon children. Social mobility can produce stresses and strains that the clinician may wish to identify.

The occupation of the head of the household is the most reliable index of social status, and many clinicians find, the Minnesota Scale for Parental Occupations (1950) a useful tool for ranking various jobs. We prefer, however, the North-Hatt Scale of Occupations (Reissman, 1959: 401–4); the authors present an alphabetical listing of various occupations and, on the basis of empirical research, assign a prestige or ranking score to each job.

personality

Although the evidence suggests no systematic causal relationship between personality disturbances and speech defectiveness, clinicians recognize that many clients present varying degrees of emotional reaction to their impaired communication (Van Riper, 1963: 40–73). Speech is perhaps man's most human attribute, and when a person cannot talk well, it affects him in a most profound way. However, a few speech impairments are a direct result of psychological conflict:

> Hugh did not seem like other stutterers we had seen: he was so calm, so relaxed, with a perpetual bittersweet smile on his face as he discussed his problem. His stuttering had started suddenly in his junior year at a religious college where he was studying to be a minister. His blocks were long, silent vigils during which he assumed a posture startlingly like one being crucified. He talked at great length, revealing sadly that now he could obviously not be a clergyman. Stuttering, he said, was a sign from the Almighty, a cross to bear. For Hugh, it seemed to us, stuttering, rather than *being* a problem, was a *solution* to a problem. The psychiatrist to whom we referred him confirmed our hunch: Hugh had made a dramatic emotional commitment during a religious revival meeting when he was an impressionable teenager. His decision had been vividly reinforced by his relatives who scrimped and saved to send him to college to be a minister. As he proceeded through school he began to realize that the church

was not "his thing" but could find no face-saving way out of his commitment—until he began to stutter.

A speech clinician should not play psychologist unless he is qualified by virtue of training and experience to administer and interpret psychodiagnostic tests.[12] Obvious psychopathology is not difficult to identify, and appropriate referral should be made. It is important that, when we first set out to examine a client, we let him know that it may be necessary to look at his problem from many aspects, including psychological. We should not pop out of a box at the end of a diagnostic session and recommend that the client see a psychiatrist. Nor, in our judgment, is it clinically wise to make a psychological referral (without prior indication that a referral may be necessary) when the client is not responding to therapy. Such a referral is basically assaultive: we are saying, in effect, that if you don't respond to our treatment you must "have your head examined."

One of the most useful procedures in clinical work is the information contained in Hahn's (1961) classic article on direct, nondirect, and indirect methods in speech correction.

> We made a grave mistake with Ricky: we assumed that he could profit from the same kind of direct therapy the other children were receiving. From the start he tried to show us that he needed something different; despite our best efforts he persisted in his misarticulations. Recalling Hahn's article we decided to make a change. We assigned a senior student to work with Ricky, a student who by his appearance and manner was childlike and "simple." His job was simply to do things *with* Ricky such as making airplanes, taking him for cokes, and so on. After they had done this for a time, the senior author entered the scene and accused the student therapist, in front of Ricky, of wasting time and goofing off. The child did more work in the remaining six weeks of the school year than he had ever done; he had to achieve to protect the student, his friend.

For discussions of psychodiagnosis, see the work of Anderson and Anderson (1951) and others (Pennington and Berg, 1954; Stern, Stein, and Bloom, 1963; Sunberg and Tyler, 1962).

PRECEPTS REGARDING THE CLINICAL EXAMINATION

In this chapter we have presented rather explicit methods for conducting the clinical examination. We dislike diagnostic formulae, and our purpose has not been to give out recipes, but rather to describe some way of approaching various problems without going too far astray. By way of summary, we now

---

[12] Since the advent of behavior therapy, however, some psychologists have no compunctions about playing speech clinician. It does not matter what the presenting problem is, baselines are established, reinforcement schedules devised, and subjects "run."

present a list of interrelated and overlapping precepts regarding the clinical examination.

1. We examine persons, not speech defects or speech defectives. Our primary concern is with communicators, not communication.

2. The clinical examination is conducted interpersonally; the catalyst of a diagnostic session is the person-to-person relationship between therapist and client.

3. There is an element of magic in every transaction between people. A diagnostic session can, in some instances, meliorate a problem situation by engendering hope or be deeply disappointing to a client who hopes that a test or examination will resolve his difficulty.

4. A most important requisite for conducting a clinical examination is a thorough understanding of normalcy.

5. Diagnosis is the initial phase of treatment. The very first contact with a client—the manner in which he is treated during a clinical examination—is a crucial determining factor in his response to therapy.

6. The clinical examination, or more broadly, diagnosis, is not necessarily confined to a single session.

7. Treatment is often diagnostic; we often discover the nature of a client's problem during therapy.

8. The clinical examination is performed to provide a working image of the individual; it is accomplished by interviewing, examining, and testing.

9. An important aspect in acquiring a working image of an individual is determining how he perceives himself and his situation.

10. An individual makes certain adjustments to his problem; his attempts to solve his difficulty—which may include a protective cover of defenses—may be a part of the problem but must not be confused with it.

11. Behavior is a function of the individual and the situation. We should be aware that our test results reflect not just the client's abilities but also his performance *in* the diagnostic setting.

12. Our diagnostic activities should include an assessment of a client's larger social context; the younger the individual, the more important this aspect of the evaluation becomes.

13. Tests are only tools to provide a systematic guide for our observations. They enable the clinician to scrutinize a client in a structured manner.

14. Although for the examiner the testing situation may be very familiar and routine, for the client it is a novel experience.

15. Examination and testing can be iatrogenic. It can suggest problems to the client that he had not considered.

It is remarkable that those who live around the social sciences have so quickly become comfortable in using the term deviant, as if those to whom the term is applied have enough in common that significant things can be said about them as a whole. Just as there are iatrogenic disorders caused by the work that physicians do (which gives them still more work to do), so there are categories of persons who are created by students of society and then studied by them (Goffman, 1963: 140). Do we create problem children by labelling them "tongue-thrusters," "culturally deprived," "learning disabled"?

16. Simply because a testing device is made up of a series of precisely defined tasks, administered and scored in a rigidly structured manner, this does not mean that a client's responses are similarly precise.

17. It is as important to observe *how* the client responds during a testing procedure as it is to obtain a score.

18. There is a distinct tendency for students to be caught up in diagnostic fads —the "recent article" syndrome.

19. It is very easy to reify a particular testing instrument, to endow a scale or diagnostic concept with a special form of reality independent of its creator. Some clinicians embrace a diagnostic device with militant enthusiasm and attack all intellectual queries or criticism with apostolic zeal.

20. An intellectual awareness of the nature of his problem, or the factors causing it, will not guarantee insight, acceptance, or remission by the client.

21. Impressions formed on the basis of the first careful evaluation of a client are generally accurate. There is a distinct tendency to discount or deny our findings especially, for example, if they suggest a child is mentally retarded or that an adult aphasic is not capable of further improvement.

22. A professional works when and where he is needed. The needs of the client, not the setting in which the clinician works, determine the scope of his professional activities.

PROJECTS AND QUESTIONS

1. When conducting a speech evaluation with children, which technique works more effectively: to take the child away from the mother or to take the mother away from the child? That is, is it better to lead the child away from the parent into the examining room with you or should both mother and child be ushered in together and then, when the child is occupied, have the mother take her leave unobtrusively? Research this issue with at least twenty nursery-school children who do not have speech defects.

2. The oral peripheral examination:

a. Look up the following terms: angle, neutroclusion, distoclusion, mesioclusion, edentulous, prognathic, cineflurography, cicatrix, deciduous teeth, palatography, uvula, bruxism.

b. Draw a diagram of normal dentition in children and adults. Consult a standard textbook in anatomy and inspect the norms provided by Johnson, Darley, and Spriestersbach (1963: 126).

c. Consider the three major malocclusions: employing your knowledge of motor phonetics, identify the phonemes most likely to be troublesome in each type of abnormal bite.

d. Write an abstract of B. Weinberg, "A Cephalometric Study of Normal and Defective /s/ Articulation and Variations in Incisor Dentition," *Journal of Speech and Hearing Research,* 11 (1968): 288–300.

e. Review S. Fletcher and J. Meldrum, "Lingual Function and Relative Length of the Lingual Frenulum," *Journal of Speech and Hearing Research,* 11 (1968): 382–90. What conclusions can you reach about the reported low incidence of tongue tie?

f. What do the following articles have to say about tongue-thrusting?

HOFFMAN, J. and R. HOFFMAN. "Tongue-thrust and Deglutition: Some Anatomical, Physiological, and Neurological Considerations." *Journal of Speech and Hearing Disorders,* 30 (1965): 103–20.

LEWIS, J. and R. COUNIHAN. "Tongue-thrust in Infancy." *Journal of Speech and Hearing Disorders,* 30 (1965): 280–82.

RONSON, I. "Incidence of Visceral Swallow Among Lispers." *Journal of Speech and Hearing Disorders,* 30 (1965): 318–24.

WOOD, J. "Tongue Thrusting: Some Clinical Observations." *Journal of Speech and Hearing Disorders,* 36 (1971): 82–89.

g. What does McDonald say about testing for oral diadochokinesis?: E. McDonald, *Articulation Testing and Treatment: A Sensory Motor Approach* (Pittsburgh: Stanwix, 1964), p. 183.

h. An assessment of oral stereognosis is not routinely done during a clinical examination. However, when we study children who persist in their articulation errors (after one year of therapy), we find that many have disturbances in oral-tactile kinesthesia. Study the following articles for methods of evaluating oral sensitivity:

DELLOW, P. G. *et al.* "Oral Assessment of Object Size." *Journal of Speech and Hearing Research,* 13 (1970): 526–36.

FUCCI, D. "Oral Vibrotactile Sensation: An Evaluation of Normal and Defective Speakers." *Journal of Speech and Hearing Research,* 15 (1972): 179–84.

McCALL, G. "The Assessment of Lingual Tactile Sensation and Perception." *Journal of Speech and Hearing Disorders,* 34 (1969): 151–56.

RINGEL, R. "Oral Sensation and Perception: A Selected Review." In *Speech and the Dentofacial Complex: The State of the Art. ASHA Report No. 5* (1970), pp. 188–206.

────── *et al.* "Some Relations Between Orosensory Discrimination and Articulatory Aspects of Speech Production." *Journal of Speech and Hearing Disorders,* 35 (1970): 3–11.

RINGEL, R., J. SAXMAN, and A. BROOKS. "Oral Perception: II. Mandibular Kinesthesion." *Journal of Speech and Hearing Research,* 10 (1967): 637–41.

RINGEL, R. and S. EWANOWSKI. "Oral Perception: I. Two-point Discrimination." *Journal of Speech and Hearing Research,* 8 (1965): 389–98.

RINGEL, R. and H. FLETCHER. "Oral Perception: III. Texture Discrimination." *Journal of Speech and Hearing Research,* 10 (1967): 642–49.

i. Write out in detail how you would introduce the oral peripheral examination to: (1) a kindergarten child, (2) an adolescent male, and (3) an elderly person with aphasia.

3. Devise a flow chart depicting the diagnostic process. Here is an example:

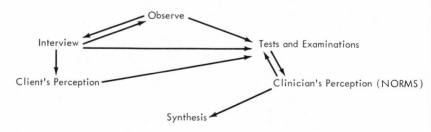

See also N. Sunberg and L. Tyler, *Clinical Psychology* (New York: Appleton-Century-Crofts, 1962), p. 87, for another example of a diagnostic flow chart.

4. Is there an appropriate *order* in which the various tests and examination procedures should be administered? In the interview we suggested moving from less to more threatening questions as the rapport develops. Work out a pattern for conducting a comprehensive examination on a child or an adult.

5. Select one of the tests described in the present chapter or a diagnostic instrument already known to you, and analyze it using the format presented by Sunberg and Tyler (1962: 141–42).

6. Research the concept of nonverbal communication; the following books will give you a start:

BIRDWHISTELL, R. *Introduction to Kinesics.* Philadelphia: University of Pennsylvania Press, 1970.

DAVITZ, J. *et al. The Communication of Emotional Meaning.* New York: Holt, Rinehart & Winston, Inc., 1964.

FAST, J. *Body Language.* New York: Evans and Co., 1970.

GOFFMAN, E. *Interaction Ritual.* Garden City, N.Y.: Doubleday Anchor Books, 1967.

HALL, E. *Proxemics.* New York: International University Press, 1963.

———. *The Silent Language.* New York: Doubleday & Company, Inc., 1959.

SOMMER, R. *Personal Space.* Englewood Cliffs, N.J.: Prentice-Hall, Inc., 1969.

BIBLIOGRAPHY

AMMONS, R. B. and H. AMMONS (1948). *Ammons Full Range Picture Vocabulary Test.* Missoula, Mont.: Psychological Test Specialists.

ANDERSON, H. and G. ANDERSON (1951). *Projective Techniques.* Englewood Cliffs, N.J.: Prentice-Hall, Inc.

ANDERSON, R., M. MILES, and P. MATHENY (1963). *Communicative Evaluation Chart.* Golden, Colo.: Business Forms, Inc.

ATKINSON, J. and N. FEATHER (1966). *A Theory of Achievement Motivation.* New York: John Wiley & Sons, Inc.

BARKER, R. *et al.* (1953). *Adjustment to Physical Handicap and Illness: A Survey of the Social Psychology of Physique and Disability.* New York: Social Science Research Council, Bulletin 55.

BERELSON, B. and G. STEINER (1964). *Human Behavior.* New York: Harcourt, Brace & World, Inc.

BERRY, M. (1969). *Language Disorders of Children.* New York: Appleton-Century-Crofts.

CASSEL, R. (1957). *The Cassel Group Level of Aspiration Test.* Beverly Hills, Calif.: Western Psychological Services.

CHUSID, J. and J. McDONALD (1967). *Correlative Neuroanatomy and Functional Neurology,* 13th ed. Los Altos, Calif.: Lange Medical Publications.

CRICHTON, M. (1969). *The Andromeda Strain*. New York: Dell Publishing Company.

DARLEY, F. (1964). *Diagnosis and Appraisal of Communication Disorders*. Englewood Cliffs, N.J.: Prentice-Hall, Inc.

————, ed. (1961). *Identification Audiometry*. JSHD Monograph Supplement No. 9.

————, A ARONSON, and J. BROWN (1969a). "Differential Diagnostic Patterns of Dysarthria." *Journal of Speech and Hearing Research*, 12: 246–69.

———— (1969b). "Clusters of Deviant Speech Dimensions in the Dysarthrias." *Journal of Speech and Hearing Research*, 12: 462–96.

DAVIS, H. and S. SILVERMAN (1970). *Hearing and Deafness*, 3rd ed. New York: Holt, Rinehart & Winston, Inc.

DOLL, E. (1946). *The Vineland Social Maturity Scale*. Philadelphia: Educational Test Bureau.

————, ed. (1947). *The Oseretsky Test of Motor Proficiency*. Minneapolis: Educational Publishers.

DUNN, L. (1958). *Peabody Picture Vocabulary Test*. Minneapolis: American Guidance Service.

EMERICK, L. (1971). *A Workbook in Clinical Audiometry*. Springfield, Ill.: Charles C Thomas.

——— (1969). *The Parent Interview*. Danville, Ill.: Interstate Printers and Publishers.

FRANKENBURG, W. and J. DODDS (1967). *Denver Developmental Screening Test*. Denver: University of Colorado Medical Center.

GLORIG, A., ed. (1965). *Audiometry: Principles and Practices*. Baltimore: Williams and Wilkins.

GOFFMAN, E. (1963). *Stigma: Notes on the Management of Spoiled Identity*. Englewood Cliffs, N.J.: Prentice-Hall, Inc.

GOODENOUGH, F. L. (1926). *Measurement of Intelligence by Drawings*. Yonkers, N.Y.: World Book Company.

GRINKER, R. and A. SAHS (1966). *Neurology*, 6th ed. Springfield, Ill.: Charles C Thomas.

HAHN, E. (1961). "Indicators for Direct, Nondirect, and Indirect Methods in Speech Correction." *Journal Speech and Hearing Disorders*, 26: 230–36.

HOLLINGSHEAD, A. and F. REDLICH (1958). *Social Class and Mental Illness*. New York: John Wiley & Sons, Inc.

ILG, F. and L. BATES (1955). *Child Behavior*. New York: Dell Publishing Company.

JOHNSON, W., F. DARLEY, and D. SPRIESTERSBACH (1963). *Diagnostic Principles and Methods*. New York: Harper & Row, Publishers.

LEUTENEGGER, R. and J. STOVALL (1971). "A Pilot Graduate Seminar Concerning Speech and Hearing Problems of the Chronically Ill Aged." *Journal of the American Speech and Hearing Association,* 13: 61–66.

McCLELLAND, D. (1961). *The Achieving Society.* Princeton, N.J.: D. Van Nostrand Co., Inc.

——— et al. (1955). *Studies in Motivation.* New York: Appleton-Century-Crofts.

McDANIELS, J. (1969). *Physical Disability and Human Behavior.* New York: Pergamon Press.

MECHAM, M., J. JEX, and J. JONES (1967). *The Utah Test of Language Development.* Salt Lake City: Communication Research Associates.

Minnesota Scale for Parental Occupations (1950). Minneapolis: Institute of Child Welfare, University of Minnesota.

NEWBY, H. (1964). *Audiology,* 2nd ed. New York: Appleton-Century-Crofts.

O'NEILL, J. and H. OYER (1966). *Applied Audiometry.* New York: Dodd, Mead & Co.

PENNINGTON, L. and I. BERG (1954). *An Introduction to Clinical Psychology.* New York: Ronald Press.

RAPH, J. (1960). "Determinates of Motivation in Speech Therapy." *Journal of Speech and Hearing Disorders,* 25: 13–17.

REISSMAN, L. (1959). *Class in American Society.* New York: The Free Press.

ROSENZWEIG, S., E. FLEMING, and H. CLARK (1947). "Revised Scoring Manual for the Rosenzweig Picture-Frustration Study." *Journal of Psychology,* 24: 165–208.

ROTTER, J. (1954). *Social Learning and Clinical Psychology.* Englewood Cliffs, N.J.: Prentice-Hall, Inc.

SATALOFF, J. (1966). *Hearing Loss.* Philadelphia: J. B. Lippincott Co.

SCHUELL, H., J. JENKINS, and E. JIMENEZ-PABON (1964). *Aphasia in Adults.* New York: Harper & Row, Publishers.

SLOANE, H. and B. MACAULAY, eds. (1968). *Operant Procedures in Remedial Speech and Language Training.* Boston: Houghton Mifflin Company.

STERN, G., M. STEIN, and B. BLOOM (1963). *Methods in Personality Assessment.* New York: The Free Press.

SUNBERG, N. and L. TYLER (1962). *Clinical Psychology.* New York: Appleton-Century-Crofts.

TAYLOR, J. (1963). "Screening Intelligence." *Journal of Speech and Hearing Disorders,* 28: 90–91.

TERMAN, L. and M. MERRILL (1960). *Stanford-Binet Intelligence Scale: Manual for the Third Revision* (Form L-M). Boston: Houghton Mifflin Company.

VAN RIPER, C. (1966). "Guilty." *Western Michigan Journal of Speech Therapy,* 2: 1–2.

————— (1963). *Speech Correction: Principles and Methods,* 4th ed. Englewood Cliffs, N.J.: Prentice-Hall, Inc.

————— (1972). *Speech Correction: Principles and Methods,* 5th ed. Englewood Cliffs, N.J.: Prentice-Hall, Inc.

WARNER, W., M. MEEKER, and K. ELLS (1960). *Social Class in America.* New York: Harper & Row, Publishers.

WECHSLER, P. (1955). *Manual for the Wechsler Adult Intelligence Scale.* New York: Psychological Corporation.

————— (1949). *Manual for the Wechsler Intelligence Scale for Children.* New York: Psychological Corporation.

WILLIAMS, D. (1968). "Stuttering Therapy: An Overview." In *Learning Theory and Stuttering Therapy,* ed. H. Gregory. Evanston, Ill.: Northwestern University Press.

WOOD, N (1964). *Delayed Speech and Language Development.* Englewood Cliffs, N.J.: Prentice-Hall, Inc.

4

diagnosis
of language disorders
in children

This chapter can be only an introductory statement to a very complex area of human behavior. The information explosion in this subject will no doubt date much of what presently is being written, and contradictory or conflicting points of view should be considered healthy and encouraging rather than demoralizing and frustrating. The vastness of the language areas is a challenge—not a threat—and should be met with interest and enthusiasm. The student should set small attainable goals, systematize his study, and work for an understanding of the rationale of diagnosis and therapy as well as the technique.

We trust this chapter will not mislead its readers into supposing that by reading it they will become expert diagnosticians of language disorders overnight; nor that they will be saved the trouble or stimulation of reading widely themselves.

THEORETICAL FRAMEWORK

In order to understand language, judge its normalcy, evaluate its parameters, and provide adequate therapeutic measures, it is essential that the clinician understand the theory upon which the behavior is based. We shall not try to discuss fully the various perspectives on language; rather we shall simply indicate the major trends and encourage the reader to pursue each as completely as is practical and beneficial. The task is formidable, but the reward in terms of understanding and insightful professional behavior should make the labor worthwhile.

An appreciation of the various theoretical explanations of language should assist the reader in his scouting of the literature in three basic ways. First, the developmental nature of language acquisition will be more meaningful if it is placed in some unified context. The knowledgeable student of language is able to measure individual development based upon the factors that influence the child, the child's typical stages of language learning, and the general characteristics of the normal process. Second, the nature of language as a symbol system is only truly put into perspective from a theoretical base; without some background in theory the student is helpless to interpret conflicting information and points of view. Third, the theoretical foundations must be familiar to anyone who wishes to investigate and manipulate abnormal language behavior. An understanding of the abnormal most logically stems from a thorough appreciation of the normal.

We have selected four areas of knowledge that we feel each student should pursue to gain a full understanding of the language process. These are: learning theory, linguistic theory, communication theory, and neurophysiology data. No doubt much of the information in the last area is also theoretical —so in fact we have four areas of "theory" that warrant investigation.

learning theory

Almost unchallenged, learning theory has held the limelight as the primary source of authoritative information about language for many years. Speech pathology has drawn heavily upon learning theory both for its understanding of normal behavior and as a therapeutic rationale. Wingate (1971) aptly describes the dependency relationship developed between speech pathology and psychology in stuttering theory and therapy, and the same case could be made for our understanding of language. At the foundation of all learning theory is the understanding that language, as a form of human behavior, is basically learned.

Several scholars have pointed out that no single learning analysis can fully explain the complexities of language—i.e. reception and expression, denotation and connotation, and so on. Staats (1968) has formalized a theory that borrows aspects from both classical and operant theories. He is convincing in his attempt to defend the idea that learning analyses are possible of such complex behaviors as language. Staats makes an interesting rebuttal to the adversaries of his approach when he states:

> Because a learning analysis of various complex human behaviors has been lacking should not increase the credibility of a biological explanation of the development of human behavior. Only the direct evidence of biological determinants should do that. We cannot infer biological or maturational causes when all we have observed is the behavior itself (1968: 386).

linguistic theory

Psychology and linguistics are, of course, parallel disciplines and rarely converged until recently. This unfortunate hiatus has produced quite different views of language behavior. The currently most popular and seminal linguistic theory is probably the generative grammar theory attributed to Chomsky (1957) and his associates. Although there have been several variations and major modifications since its inception, one central theme appears paramount. Perkins (1971: 108) states it clearly:

> Human infants apparently begin life as cryptographers innately equipped biologically to "crack" society's communication code within a few years. No other hypothesis offered so far comes close to explaining a baby's extraordinary capacity to decipher speech.

The biological orientation of Lenneberg (1967), the "sentence-centerism" of McNeill (1970), and the "transformational" postulates of Chomsky all appear to rely heavily on the assumption that language facility is a basic part of human nature.

The classic battle is clearly in focus: Is language a learned behavior that requires just the right amount of motivation, stimulation, and reinforcement? Or is it an innate characteristic of the human species, in which case a child has all of the language potential at birth and only needs maturation and progressive refinement of potential to fit into his own language system? The awesome impact of this conflict has yet to be felt in any real, applicable way in the rehabilitation fields. In fact, it is curious to note that although the theories differ significantly, there have been only minimal attempts to synthesize the linguistic postulates into some practical therapeutic application. The unfortunate consequence has been that speech pathologists have followed the shifting winds of psychological theory for the past fifty years. Since linguists have displayed (until recently) little interest in clinical applications of their formulations, it is understandable that speech clinicians have relied more upon applicable psychological theory.

> When we accept that a human behavior is biologically determined, then we attribute problems of that human behavior to the personal defects of the individuals involved. If language or cognitive development comes from biological determinants, then the child who does not develop normal language, or what have you, is biologically inferior (Staats, 1968: 387).

communication theory

Shannon and Weaver (1949) published papers describing a mathematical theory of communication which had far-reaching impact upon several disciplines, including language research. Communication theory attempts to formalize the nature of communication and its potential for transmitting information by engendering models that explain communication situations. This has forced speech pathologists to organize their thinking regarding language and its place in the entire process of communication; of paramount importance have been the many applications of the feedback model proposed by Fairbanks (1954), Mysak (1959), Van Riper and Irwin (1958), and others.

neurophysiological data

The biological and neurological requisites that underlie language behavior are very complex subjects. In a review of the current knowledge on this topic, Berry (1969) makes the cogent observation that knowledge of the neurological and biological systems creates a basis for more critical evaluation of other models of language behavior.

GUIDING PRINCIPLES

We now present five interrelated principles which we feel will aid the clinician in conducting a more revealing and productive diagnosis of language disorders in children. In the ensuing discussion we shall try to be consistent with these principles; however, it is the student's responsibility to put each principle into practice.

1. Language is a broad and all-encompassing category of human behavior: *Know your competency areas and remain within them.* Speaking, listening, writing, reading, thinking, problem-solving, discriminating, perceiving, recalling—all directly involve language. No one can be expected to be knowledgeable in *all* of the areas of language, but an understanding of the breadth of the language system creates a reverence for its impact upon human behavior. The well-informed diagnostician is aware that the area he is assessing has far-reaching implications.

2. Our knowledge of language, both normal and abnormal, is fragmented and incomplete: *Accept this state of affairs not as a source of frustration but as a source of motivation to learn more and add to the body of knowledge.* The student of language disorders is often demoralized by the apparently overwhelming amount of information available and the inconclusive nature of so many vital issues. No final chapters have been written on any aspect of language disorders and diagnosis.

3. No single measure (or session) is adequate to totally evaluate and understand a child's language ability: *Make your diagnosis an ongoing rather than a static undertaking.* There are two major arguments in favor of this point of view. First, a child's language behavior is continually changing, and no single measure can predict or describe the course of the change. In fact, the course of language development may be as important to diagnosis as the presenting problem. Second, the language process is so complex that it de-

mands more than one method of diagnosis. Diagnosis must tell us where the child is, how he got there, where he should be, and how to initiate work with him to move him from where he is to where he should be. Diagnosis must reflect the progress made and point out the progress not made. It must serve as a continuing source of information to be monitored. Although we are continually seeking knowledge, we must not fall prey to the common human inclination to find only what we seek.

4. Diagnosis of language facility should be made *in situ*—rather than through some abstracted process—as much as possible: *Know the normal process of language development.* The importance of this point of view cannot be overestimated. Language diagnosticians have for too long been satisfied with test results which, in reality, only measured some small portion of a child's total language performance in an artificial testing situation. This is not to say that test data are of no importance; on the contrary, most of the remainder of this chapter will be devoted to a discussion of the practical application of standardized tests. We simply wish to encourage the diagnostician to look carefully at the child's total language behavior as he uses it for everyday functioning. This demands a great deal of knowledge and familiarity with the normal language-development process, because the information gained through observation of this behavior will have to be measured against some criterion of adequacy. This can only be done accurately when the observer has a clear and correct conception of the normal process. A language-development scale similar to those provided by Berry (1969) may prove helpful. These observation scales are intended, however, as general guides rather than specific checklists and have the greatest value to those who have assimilated the knowledge and can make judgments rapidly and accurately. The continuous use of such scales should help the student to commit much of the information to memory; however, because the information does not lend itself to easy memorization without continual practical application, the student should study the checklists with reference to a specific child, rather than in the abstract. There are no armchair (or textbook) experts on language disorders. The only valid route to knowledge is through continuous, frequent, and varied clinical experience. Isolated bits of information, or "facts," about a child are not really meaningful; it is only when the student has synthesized these facts into a working gestalt that the data are of value.

5. Language diagnoses can take many shapes and forms depending upon the type of data requested: *Know the purpose of your diagnosis.* Knowing the purpose of the diagnosis gives direction to the ensuing events.

DIAGNOSIS OF ORAL LANGUAGE DISORDERS

The complexity of language diagnosis is a direct reflection of the myriad of variables that impinge on language acquisition. "A young child's success in learning to talk depends on his ability to perceive and organize his environ-ment, the language that is a part of that environment, and the relation be-tween the two" (Bloom, 1970: 1).

Language is a set of *systems* that have social, neurophysiological, psy-chological, and temporal requisites and that allow the individual to relate sound to meaning as an individualistic, internalized, representational process. We are concerned with the development of the systems that affect sound dif-ferentiation and production, syntax and grammatical acquisition, vocabulary development, conceptualization, and the transfer of these basic attributes to varying modalities through such skills as speaking, writing, reading, and understanding.

determining the existence of a problem

With the exception of traumatic cases, every eight-year-old child with deviant language behavior was once a three-year-old with *deviating* language behavior. Language, therefore, is an emerging behavior which explodes to nearly full maturity in the first three years of life and continues to be refined and developed for several years thereafter. As we look at the language of a preacademic child, we must look not only at his behavior of yesterday and today but beyond to his future potential. With a clear knowledge of what is expected of a child of a given age, it is possible to accurately identify existing or potential language difficulties in very young children; with our current understanding of the importance of these first few years, early diagnosis and therapeutic intervention are imperative.

Determining whether a child's language behavior is within normal limits is not always an easy task. Parents, teachers, physicians, and other re-ferring sources often seek assistance without having a clear concept of the exact nature of the problem:

> Jimmy was an alert two-year-old with observing eyes and a placid disposition. He understood directions and conversations appropriately for his two years but was speechless. Jimmy's mother was concerned, but not to the point of seeking help until a year later when the child passed his third birthday without (re-portedly) emitting a single meaningful word. The family physician calmly acknowledged all the information offered by Mrs. H. and then offered his pro-fessional opinion: "Jimmy will grow out of it." As the child approached his fourth birthday, he spoke his first words, his first phrase, and indeed his first sentence, all at the same time. "Mama, kitty's got a robin!" came the shriek from the backyard. Mrs. H. knew at once that the voice was that of her son and the doctor's sage advice had come true. Jimmy's expressive language was normal by his fifth birthday.

The trouble with this account is that all too often the frail hopes of matura-tional miracles turn into real nightmares as the five-year-old struggles unsuc-cessfully to compete in a verbally oriented kindergarten class.

The speech clinician cannot afford to be uncertain about the existence of a problem. He must have tools available to him which will aid in the determination, and he must have the knowledge to use those tools effectively. Father says his son is speaking well for his age, mother says her son doesn't talk right, the physician claims the child will grow out of it, and the speech clinician must resolve the dilemma. This, then, is the starting point in diagnosis. The information gained will lead the diagnostician logically into the other areas of evaluation or encourage him to terminate the diagnosis at that point.

Does the child have a language problem? In a sense this concern is more theoretical than real, since we are asking the diagnostician to keep the concept in his head during the total assessment instead of segmenting his diagnosis into artificial categories. The clinician looks at a child through the prism of any of the various measuring techniques, and he uses this focus to organize and classify the information received. Continuous refinement of technique will provide greater diagnostic information regarding not only the existence of the problem but at what level of competence the child is performing. Such information has direct implications for the therapy process when the clinician attempts to initiate work at the proper level of complexity.

Early students (Head, 1926; Myklebust, 1954) promulgated a three-part concept of the language process that employed the categories of reception, central integration, and expression. Myklebust's clinical applications of this early formulation to an assessment and therapeutic model were widely accepted, and the terms receptive, inner, and expressive language are still extensively used by practicing therapists. Even the most recent revision of the ITPA (Kirk, McCarthy, and Kirk, 1968) and similar measures rely heavily on the input-integration-output concept. Berry (1969) refutes the validity of this model on the basis of neurological as well as behavioral findings. Even though we acknowledge that reception and expression are not separate entities, but interrelated behaviors with strong neurological interdependencies (Schuell, Jenkins, Jimenez-Pabon, 1964), the convenience of the breakdown and the efficiency of the classical model are too great to ignore. Consequently, we shall employ the concepts of receptive, expressive, and receptive-expressive to present a survey of various assessment techniques for determining the existence of a language problem. Project 3 at the end of this chapter will help the student acquire a fuller understanding of the conflicting points of view.

Language is the function of the central nervous system. As such it is not indebted to specific input or output modalities. Language assessment, therefore, should most logically deal with central processing functions and not the various receptive and expressive channels. From a practical basis, however, this would lead to a restricted form of information. Clearly, language acquisition would be impossible if auditory, visual, and haptic channels were all dysfunctioning; and language competence would be of limited value if all methods of expression were peripherally interrupted. We have chosen this pragmatic solution to the theoretical issues in the hope of bridging the gap between the traditional procedures and the new psycholinguistic theory.

Receptive. The speech examiner is interested in determining if a problem exists and is not necessarily concerned with etiology of the problem or the direction of ensuing treatment. For this reason it is usually necessary to determine in only a general way the child's nonverbal (sometimes called prelinguistic) skills. The understanding of gestures, meaningful reactions to intonations, inflections, and facial expressions are all aspects of a child's language skills and are normally displayed within the first few months of life. Signs of auditory discrimination are evident before the third month of life as the child localizes sound sources and responds differentially to familiar and unfamiliar voices.

Comprehension of speech is more likely to be of prime concern at this point, however, and several formalized tests of receptive language are available to the examiner. One way to measure a child's reception of language is to determine the number of spoken words he understands. Two well-known tests are: the Peabody Picture Vocabulary Test (Dunn, 1965) and the Ammons-Ammons Full-Range Picture Vocabulary Test (1958). The PPVT consists of sets of pages with four line drawings on each page. The scoring procedure results in a language age, intelligence quotient, and percentile rank. The test does an admirable job of indicating the child's receptive vocabulary level; however, its use as a measure of intelligence, particularly when such measures are interpreted as indicating intellectual potential, may penalize children with a language delay of any given etiology. It may be best for the examiner simply to use this test to evaluate a child's ability to understand words presented singly and withhold further judgment as to intellectual level.

Since both instruments cited above use words presented with no overt or related clues (such as facial expression, context, intonation), and since children probably learn language skills from the whole (context) to the part, these assessment tools probably do not provide an accurate picture of how the child will perform in everyday speaking situations. As Berry (1969: 265) points out, ". . . they do not assess the child's ability to understand words joined in language sequences or to use them in connected speech."

> It is not uncommon to learn more about the testing process during a diagnostic session than about the child. Timmy S. taught us a great deal one morning. Following a completely fruitless testing session in which we were examining Tim's ability to understand prepositions, the child was given a chance to go out and play with the other children of the summer clinic. The test had called for the child to point to pictures that depicted the preposition spoken by the examiner. The child was unable to identify even the most elementary items, which led the examiner to conclude that he understood none of them. During the following play session, Tim demanded that he be *in front of* the line, cried when the ball went *over* the fence, told the aid that the ball was *under* the car, and urged his playmates to crawl *between* his legs during a game of leapfrog. In other words, Tim used and understood many prepositions during everyday activities but was unable to display his knowledge in a single test situation.

The Ammons Full-Range Picture Vocabulary Test taps essentially the same semantic skill as the PPVT and should in our opinion be similarly restricted in interpretation.

The Assessment of Children's Language Comprehension (ACLC) (Foster, Giddan, and Stark, 1969) currently in a research edition begins to answer some of the shortcomings of the pure vocabulary tests by adding increasing amounts of contextual elements to the task. The authors state that the purpose of this test is "to provide a more precise description of the level at which the child is unable to process lexical items" (2). The test consists of four levels of difficulty beginning with a fifty-item vocabulary test in which the child is required to identify common words. At the second level of difficulty the child is required to correctly identify the picture (from four stimuli) when the examiner indicates not only the noun but a verb or a modifier as well. As an example, the child may be asked to point to *the man sitting* when the four pictures include a man walking, a man sitting, a cat walking, and a cat sitting. At the next level of difficulty a preposition is added to the stimulus; and at the fourth level the child must understand the subject (with or without a modifying word), the verb, and the prepositional phrase. Although the examination lacks substantial normative data at this time, it is apparent that the test will prove helpful in identifying receptive language problems.

Linguistic decoding involves not only the comprehension of vocabulary but also an understanding of the grammatical systems within which the words are packaged. Careful study of a child's interaction with his parents or others should provide clues to his ability to respond to verbal commands, questions, and statements. To be valid, such studies almost always demand verbatim transcripts because they are often not standardized. In this case, however, standardization may not be of prime importance since such observations display the actual behavior we are concerned with—that is, the child's ability to perform in his environment. McNeill (1970) describes an interesting approach to the study of comprehension conducted by Slobin and Welsh (unpublished) in which the researchers used imitation to measure comprehension. As McNeill (1970: 13–14) points out, "They exploit the fact that a successful reformulation in imitation depends on a successful comprehension of the sentence imitated." The point of interest regarding comprehension is not verbatim repetition but rather preservation of meaning. In this case it is possible for the diagnostician to construct a series of sentences of varying complexity and incorporate varying types of grammatical classes. This device as currently in practice does not provide a clear indication of the need for therapy or distinguish between normal and abnormal ability levels, but standardized procedures incorporating these techniques will no doubt be forthcoming. This should provide an added dimension to the testing of comprehension.

Carrow (1968) presents a promising approach to the study and evaluation of children's auditory comprehension of language structure. Her testing technique examines the ability to comprehend the lexical and grammatical aspects of language of children aged 2–10 and 7–9 years. The author describes the test as follows:

> The instrument we designed permitted the assessment of oral language comprehension without requiring language expression from the child. The test consists of a set of plates each of which contains one or more black and white line drawings; the pictures represent referential categories and contrasts that can be signaled by form classes and function words, morphological constructions, grammatical categories, and syntactic structure (1968: 103).

Expressive. The expressive skills of a child are classically categorized into the following areas: phoneme or sound production, expressive vocabulary development, syntax development, and level of transformational sophistication.

The developmental nature of sound-production acquisition is well documented (Templin, 1957; Irwin, 1960; Poole, 1934), and a test of articulation ability should provide the examiner with a clear picture of a child's level of performance. The fact that articulation is more than a simple motor skill and indeed is an essential aspect of a child's general language development will be discussed in Chapter 5. The Fisher-Logemann Test of Articulation Competence (1971) is an example of an articulation measure which takes linguistic issues into account. The interrelationship between sound production and word and sentence production needs further exploration.

The longitudinal observational studies of children learning to speak provide some clues to the diagnostician in evaluating expressive language. McCarthy's (1930) classic work served as a reference point for many later studies of language development. McCarthy used the child's spontaneous speech as elicited through pictures and toys as a criterion for language development. Further refinement of this technique was accomplished by Day (1932), Davis (1937), Templin (1957), and Johnson, Darley, and Spriestersbach (1963). Johnson, Darley, and Spriestersbach suggest that the following measures be used to analyze speech samples: mean length of response, mean of five longest responses, number of single-word responses, and structural complexity (as measured by techniques originally devised by McCarthy); others have added such measures as standard deviation of response length and number of different words used (type-token ratio). Templin (1957) devised a structural complexity score procedure that classifies the remarks of the child and gives increasing weights (0 to 4) to increasingly complex responses. This procedure has not received a great deal of attention, since it tends to be unstable.

The linguist may evaluate a child's language production in order to develop a theoretical framework for the understanding of language acquisition, whereas the diagnostician must look at the child's language skill in order to compare it with the norm. Nonetheless, some techniques have been developed for the former purpose that may be useful in diagnosis. Careful analysis of the child's verbal behavior may reveal which grammatical classes he has incorporated and which he has not. The development of negation, plurals, question form, pronouns, auxiliary verbs is well documented in linguistic literatures, and this enables the diagnostician to establish whether or not there is a language deficit. The works of Bellugi (1964, 1967) may give the reader some insight into this aspect of language development. Berko's test of language production (1958) incorporates the study of the child's ability to pluralize nouns, give the past tense form of verbs, and some other skills.

Several authors have made direct application of linguistic theory, which aids our understanding of the language-impaired child. Menyuk (1964) compared the language development of normal and "language-delayed "children and concluded that the delayed youngsters differed from the normal group *qualitatively* as well as *quantitatively*. Menyuk classified the syntactic errors of the delayed group as substitutions, omissions, and redundancies, indicating substantive differences in the syntax structure of the language-delayed child and the normally developing child.

Lee (1966) describes syntax development in terms of successive levels of sophistication. Her "developmental sentence types" method provides the diagnostician with a frame of reference against which to compare a given child's language structure. Lee made comparisons of the language of a normal and a language-delayed child based upon sentence types and found significant differences, once again indicating that there is a qualitative difference in syntactic output between the two groups of children. Thus, children with language disorders not only have limited vocabularies, they also have a limited ability to order and arrange words.

Extending this general concept, Lee and Canter (1971) devised the Developmental Sentence Scoring (DSS) procedure, which provides a developmental scale of syntax acquisition. The procedure, as described by the authors, evaluates the child's use of grammatical rules in spontaneous speech and judges his performance against the adult standard. Fifty "complete, different, consecutive, intelligible, nonecholalic sentences" must be elicited from the child by the adult examiner for scoring (317). Many syntactical structures were not included in this test; the eight selected appear to be acquired early and have developmental characteristics. Lee and Canter provide normative data on 160 children aged from three years to six years, eleven months.

Berko's (1958) now-classic test of the child's use of morphological rules is of interest for its ingenious technique and excellent potential. Berko tested the child's ability to produce the plural and possessive forms of nouns, the third-person singular of verbs, past tense of verbs, comparative forms of adjectives, and others. The test included drawings of hypothetical creatures engaged in various activities and ordinary creatures engaged in hypothetical activities. The most often described example is a creature introduced as follows: "Here is a wug. Here are two others, there are two————." The attempt is to elicit the plural "wugs." Similar techniques could be devised for testing several grammatical skills. Berry (1969) describes an exploratory test of gram-mar for children aged five to eight years which did indeed expand on the Berko concept.

According to McNeill (1970: 157), "Every sentence, however simple, has some kind of underlying structure related to some kind of surface structure by means of certain transformations. The substance of grammar consists of making explicit these three terms." The child's level of sophistication in trans-formational skills—i.e., the ability to change an underlying thought from one sentence form to another, to produce question forms, passive sentences, or negative sentences—may be informative. McNeill reports that Brown and Olds devised a means of testing transformational level through the use of puppets. No formalized test has yet been devised to measure all of the avail-able transformational forms, but the general technique holds promise for further understanding of language acquisition and language performance.

All of the measurement techniques mentioned to this point have been arbitrarily classified as strictly receptive or expressive in nature. The reader should be aware that most of the procedures have been experimental, that they have not been extensively standardized, and that there is little data on their validity. Most of the standardized and commercially produced tests of lan-guage have combined both input and output aspects into one instrument.

The following section describes testing techniques currently available for measuring both the comprehension and expression capabilities in order to determine the existence of language deficit.

Receptive and Expressive. Until recently a single diagnostic instru-ment, the Illinois Test of Psycholinguistic Abilities, enjoyed a monopoly in the clinician's language assessment armamentarium. First published in experi-mental form in 1961, the test swiftly filled a void in the field of speech pathol-ogy and language rehabilitation. Unfortunately, the test was met by an uncritical audience eager for tangible measures useful with the children they had to deal with. There were few reference points with which to compare the ITPA, and the users displayed a startling lack of sophistication. The time has come for the ITPA to take its rightful place as only one of many measures of language ability; it has its inherent strengths and weaknesses and should be used only as a *part* of a total language evaluation.

Growing out of Osgood's (1957) three-dimensional model of language behavior, the current edition of the ITPA (Kirk, McCarthy, and Kirk, 1968) is comprised of ten subtests and two supplementary tests. The scoring pro-cedure for the test produces a profile of psycholinguistic abilities that allows comparison of receptive and expressive skills with chronological age and de-velopmental norms. The intended purpose of the ITPA was to aid in direct-ing remediation, but the test nonetheless offers some data that can be used to determine the existence of a language problem.

Bzoch and League (1971) clearly state their preference for a separation between reception and expression in their publication of the Receptive-Expressive Emergent Language Scale (REEL). This measure, primarily an interview technique, provides the examiner with a receptive quotient, expressive quotient, and composite language quotient on children from birth to three years of age. As the authors state:

> The REEL Scale is grounded on three basic premises regarding language function. Briefly stated, these are as follows:
>
> 1. The auditory modality is the primary means of acquiring language.
> 2. Language is an innate (genetically based) capacity of man.
> 3. Speech behavior and cognitive development are inseparably interconnected (16).

Although the authors indicate its usefulness for differential diagnosis, the REEL appears to have greatest value in revealing language problems and determining the level of language functioning of a given child. The interview technique has inherent shortcomings, and although the authors contend that a single brief interview is adequate to accurately score the REEL, it is better to use it in conjunction with extended observation of the child.

Similarly based on the receptive-expressive dichotomy is the Preschool Language Scale of Zimmerman, Steiner, and Evatt (1969). The test gives an auditory comprehension age and quotient as well as a verbal ability age and quotient; it is designed for children from one and one-half years of age to seven years. Unlike the REEL, this test requires the clinician to examine the child directly and provides all the necessary materials.

Lee has effectively transformed her knowledge of linguistics and language disorders into an effective screening instrument for syntactic development, the Northwestern Syntax Screening Test (Lee, 1969). Administered to children three to eight years of age, the test includes both receptive and expressive measures of syntax; tentative norms have been established.

The Parsons Language Sample (Spradlin, 1963) is comprised of seven subtests based on the Skinnerian system of language behavior. The subtests acknowledge the receptive-expressive nature of language and include tests of tacting, echoic, intraverbal (all vocal), echoic gesture, comprehension, intraverbal gesture (all nonverbal), and the test of manding which is both verbal and nonverbal. It is interesting to note that Spradlin (1967), author of the PLS, later made several criticisms of the test and similar instruments. His criticisms included the fact that the PLS, in the main, demands only single-word responses from the child, thus giving little opportunity to measure the intricacies of grammatical acquisition. Strangely, the Skinnerian model of language development has failed to generate a great deal of research in the diagnosis of language disorders. This is no doubt in part due to the fact that the behaviorists have shunned diagnosis in the traditional sense in order to concentrate more heavily on other factors.

The Michigan Picture Language Inventory (Lerea, 1958) evaluates vocabulary comprehension, vocabulary expression, language-structure comprehension, and language-structure expression. Lerea's tests of grammatical structure included the following areas: nouns (singular and plural), personal and possessive pronouns, adjectives and adverbs, demonstrative articles, prepositions, and verbs and auxiliaries. This initial edition of the MPLI is considered by the author to be experimental, but the general assessment concept holds promise. It is anticipated, however, that it will be necessary to evaluate greater amounts of language (both input and output) than one-word stimuli and responses in order to get a true picture of a child's language structure.

In conjunction with a research endeavor, Fraser, Bellugi, and Brown (1963) devised a test of imitation, comprehension, and production of language. The child's ability to differentiate between each of ten grammatical contrasts is evaluated through the use of paired pictures. Although the test was not designed as a diagnostic measure, the process may have value as an assessment procedure. The ten grammatical contrasts included are:

> mass noun/count noun
> singular/plural (inflections)
> singular/plural (is–are)
> present progressive tense/past tense
> present progressive tense/future tense
> affirmative/negative
> singular/plural of third-person possessive pronoun
> subject/object–passive voice
> subject/object–active voice
> indirect object/direct object (127).

The Verbal Language Development Scale (Mecham, 1958) is an extension of the communication portion of the Vineland Social Maturity Scale and as such provides the diagnostician with a language age-equivalent for a child through the interview technique. However, the scale fails to elicit a great deal of essential information on the nature of the child's language performance.

Crabtree (1958) developed the Houston Test for Language Development for children up to three years of age:

> An attempt was made to include at each age level, items that represented the various aspects of language, both from the broad classifications of reception, conceptualization, and expression, and the more specific categories of melody, rhythm, accent, gesture, articulation, vocabulary, grammatical usage, and dynamic content (3).

Scoring for this test results in a language age, and although no exact procedure is available, the careful examiner could extract information regarding the various language attributes. In 1963 an extension of this test to age six was constructed.

The Utah Test of Language Development (Mecham *et al.,* 1967) provides another overall measure of expressive and receptive language skills; however, there is no specific way to differentiate certain language characteristics in the scoring procedure. The authors state that this is the direct test form of the Verbal Language Development Scale (cited above), and as such it also results in a language age-equivalent.

The foregoing discussion is not intended to guide the diagnostician in determining the existence of a language problem; rather its purpose is to present various tests and testing procedures currently in practice which serve that end. The authors are well aware of the risks involved in such an overview. The uncritical reader will consider the list final; the outline of procedures above is not meant as an end, but rather a starting point in the study of diagnosis. The assessment devices we have presented are, of course, merely temporary touchstones in the continuous growth and maturation of the discipline. It is possible to be beguiled into treating the *proposition of diagnosis as the application of a series of tests.* We hope that the student will not draw this implication from the foregoing discussion.

There is one additional confounding factor in testing for language acquisition: most tests abstract only fragmented language samples and never really engage the child in the practical business of protracted speaking. However, contextual speech will ultimately make or break him in his environment, and it is this that must be judged.[1] Also, as conversational speech is produced in more complex ways, the load factor may come into play; the child may be able to handle single-sentence construction or simply give the past tense of a verb form in the test setting, but may fail that same task when the verb form is buried in a grammatically demanding sentence. Tests which meet this criticism, however, tend to be laborious, lengthy, and unstandardized, and therefore compromise measures must be found.

In a sense this diagnostic category is both theoretical and practical. The diagnostician does not apply a series of assessment procedures to determine language level without also using that information as a guide for therapy (although few language tests are precise in specifying logical starting points for therapy) and as a basis for differential diagnosis. On the other hand, there comes a time in nearly every evaluation when the diagnostician must decide whether or not the child's language deficit will benefit from treatment. The first purpose of diagnosis, of course, is to determine whether or not a problem exists, and this is often slighted by the diagnostician.

However, the matter is further complicated by the necessity of differentiating between language development that is slow but essentially normal

---

[1] Hatten and Hatten (1971) reported on their attempts at ongoing diagnosis; what comments do they have regarding observation of routine behavior in the home?

and development that is genuinely abnormal. In other words, is there a clear distinction between "delayed" language and "disordered" language? Theoretically, it is possible to quite clearly differentiate between delayed and disordered language development; however, on a practical basis the distinction is often so well hidden by intervening variables that it disappears.

Perplexing to the diagnostician is the fact that children often have acquired the various linguistic competences necessary for language functioning but do not know when to apply them. Knowing when to speak and how much to say is as much a skill to be learned as any of the language concepts. The child may have a language competence equivalent to his age but be unable to apply what is expected, appropriate, and effective in varied environments.

From the behaviorist's standpoint, assessment of a language-disordered child may terminate with this initial aspect. Three basic types of information are necessary for a behavioral diagnosis: (1) Specific information must be available on the child's performance level. This is variously termed "entering behavior" or "baseline performance level." Such information should be available from the diagnosis to determine the existence of the problem. (2) The clinician must have a specific concept of what language behavior he expects from the child. This is the "terminal" behavior and would be comprised of those language skills found within the language community of the child. (3) The clinician must be able to apply discrete, measurable steps that will logically lead the child to the desired level of performance. He should have a clear understanding of the normal process of language development and be able to apply it to the sequential steps of therapy.

This "task analysis" concept is very valuable to the clinician in devising a clinical sequence; however, there is no clear agreement among linguists, psychologists, or speech pathologists about the exact sequence of language development. Further complicating the issue is the paucity of information on the internal (CNS) manipulations that take place in language development, and whether language development in the language-disordered child should necessarily follow the normal sequence of development. Chalfant and Scheffelin (1969) present in tabular form task analyses for acquisition of auditory receptive, expressive auditory, and vocal motor language.

determining the etiology of the problem

At this point we have determined that the child under investigation has some sort of language deviation: his language-development rate is lagging and his language-development procedure is exhibiting significantly aberrant patterns. We must now determine exactly *why* this language deficit exists.

West (1957: 596) defines differential diagnosis as "a discriminating diagnosis aimed at distinguishing a given case of disorder from one or more other disorders presenting confusingly similar symptom pictures." This is essentially what we must undertake at this point. The fact that children show strikingly similar symptom patterns led the profession, at one time, to make indiscriminate use of the term "delayed speech" as a category of speech disorders. This general term offered no causal explanation and encouraged the idea that language disorders of differing etiologies do indeed result in similar speech patterns. However, the clinician must identify the differences that exist in the language patterns since these symptom differences are the key to the determination of etiology. Differing etiological classes result in differing patterns of language, and lumping them all under the heading of delayed speech or any such wastebasket term may discourage the examiner from detecting subtle, but important, nuances.

The need for information on the etiology of a language disorder is not always clearly evident; in fact, some therapy approaches make no such demands upon the examiner. We would like to submit the following reasons for the need for such diagnosis:

1. Differential diagnosis gives broad direction to the therapy effort. If a child is determined to be hard-of-hearing, the ensuing therapy should, logically, take that fact into account. Without such information it would be possible to direct therapy to specific deficit areas, but the efficacy of the entire effort would be blunted.

2. Differential diagnosis may aid in the prognosis, or prediction of the rate and range of growth of the child. Knowledge of the etiological category may provide the clinician with some information about the typical group characteristics of growth patterns and the rehabilitative growth possible. Although the clinician should not apply group norms to the individual, such general patterns may prove helpful.

3. Such diagnostic information may help eliminate any agents that may yet be active. Perpetuating etiological factors should be identified and, if possible, eradicated.

4. Differential diagnosis may help to prevent the recurrence of the syndrome of behavior in other members of the client's family. If the etiological factor is such that it may occur again to affect younger children, the family should be informed and helped in taking preventative steps.

5. Differential diagnosis serves as a therapy agent for the environment in yet another way. Parents, when seeking help for their children's problems, find comfort in knowing *why* a particular problem occurs. Such information generally lessens guilt feelings and aids in the general environmental milieu.

6. Every diagnostician should seek such information for its own sake. It will add to his basic knowledge of disorder types and help him in future diagnostic ventures.

What are the potential factors that might interfere with language acquisition? Unfortunately the answer is not as clear-cut as it was once thought to be; and, in part, we must rely on the definition of language offered earlier. If we assume that language acquisition consists of a broad spectrum of skills that include vocabulary-building, phonemic development, grammatical development, concept formation, problem-solving, and so forth, then it appears that the factors traditionally supposed to interfere with language development may indeed be active. If, however, we consider language development to be the learning of the abstract rules that govern language behavior, then the research findings are much less certain.

This sounds very much like we are making a distinction between language competence (the underlying understanding of the language system) and language performance (the actual language behavior as exhibited through speaking, and writing); in fact, this may be the case. Part of the reason that the original question of which factors influence language acquisition is so difficult to answer straightforwardly is that much of the research on language acquisition has failed to make the distinction between speech ability and underlying linguistic competence. Adding further to our dilemma is the always-present influence of bias. Those who theorize that language is primarily a learned behavior tend to find many factors that have an impact on language acquisition, whereas scholars who propose that language competence is largely an innate human skill tend to find that the traditional factors of sex, intelligence, and socioeconomic status have little impact on acquisition. Since we are looking at language acquisition as it is displayed in speech behavior, we shall discuss differential diagnosis from a rather traditional stance.

Intelligence. The correlation between *speech* behavior and intellectual level has been fairly well established: speech develops at a slower rate in retarded children. Except in extreme or severe retardation, however, intelligence appears to have little impact on language competence (Lenneberg, 1967). Although the measurement of intellectual functioning is seldom the province of the speech clinician, he is often called upon to make referrals and draw conclusions from test data. Most of the traditional measures used by psychometrists to measure intelligence are not applicable to children with language disorders. Speech performance, either from a production or reception standpoint, strongly influences the results of nearly every major measure of intelligence, and thus the language-deficient children are placed at an immediate disadvantage. Measures such as the Leiter International Performance Scale (Arthur, 1952) are free of language interference. The speech clinician has the duty to warn psychologists and educators against overinterpreting intelligence measures that deal harshly with language-deficient children.

In looking for historical and behavioral clues to substantiate or refute the diagnosis of mental retardation, the clinician should be aware of certain group characteristics. Many retarded children have certain illnesses in their medical histories which aid in the diagnosis of mental retardation. There may be retardation in the family history, but it is often found that the most severely retarded children (probably the result of agenesis or some massive cerebral insult) come from families with no history of mental retardation.

It is to be expected that the retarded child will follow a rather typical but slower growth pattern. The retarded are not currently being viewed as a homogenous group, as was popular at one time. The diagnostician must be on the lookout for signs of potential retardation, which may be reflected in inconsistent developmental patterns.

Emotional Disturbance. There is little question that the emotional stability of a child affects the quality and quantity of his verbal behavior. However, there is some question as to whether the emotional state significantly affects the child's ability to learn the language system. The net result of severe emotional disturbance is often bizarre speech behavior that ranges from mutism to complex and continuous verbiage. Once again, the task of analysis does not fall to the speech clinician; however, it is important for the diagnostician to keep in mind that how a child talks may reflect as much about his psyche as what he says.[2]

Leaving the formalized testing to the psychometrician, the speech clinician may look for the following characteristics that indicate the need for psychological evaluation.

1. Infantile language patterns that are not consistent with the overall potential of the child.
2. Language patterns that change significantly in both quality and quantity from one environment to another.
3. The persistence of echolalic and monologue speech to the exclusion of socialized speech behavior beyond the fourth year.
4. Atypical patterns of tonal quality, along with restricted or bizarre characteristics of emotional expression—generally, a lack of crying and laughing or strange patterns thereof.
5. Conversations filled with "tangential" remarks and responses. Eisenson (1963) explains tangential responses as replies which speak to an incidental aspect of a statement but disregard the meaning.
6. Speaking too much or too little in a given circumstance is a warning signal. Child-rearing practices no longer stress that children should be seen but not heard, and the mute child should be earnestly encouraged to communicate in the testing situation. If, on the other hand, a child is exceedingly verbal to the point of obsession, this too may be diagnostically significant:

Sally had been variously diagnosed as retarded, cerebral palsied, and aphasic, but whatever the diagnosis, she was, at age thirteen, still without speech and was using a language board to communicate. Upon entering the examining room with the student clinician, she began pointing to the word "Helen" on her board and then to the word "visit." Once the student commented that it was nice that Sally was going to visit Helen (her aunt), Sally pointed to the phrase "I like you" and spelled out "we are good friends." Within five minutes of the initiation of the diagnostic session, Sally had told about the new curtains in her bedroom, her father's operation for back trouble, and how much she loves her mother. Following the session the student was incensed when it was suggested that Sally had some emotional problems in conjunction with her speech and

[2] Rousey and Moriarty (1965) suggest that the psyche has a profound impact on articulatory accuracy. What implication might this have for language evaluation?

language difficulties. The idea that she said too much and volunteered too much unrequested and unimportant information never occurred to the student, who was completely taken by this "friendly" and "outgoing" child.

7. Language is an extension of the thought process, and therefore the diagnostician must look at the logic and organization displayed.
8. A disinterest in people or communication, together with a preoccupation with mechanical objects, is typical of this group.

Such lists could, of course, be endless, but they do serve as a baseline for further elaboration. A word of warning is in order about the interpretation of behavior, however. It is essential that the examiner make a careful analysis of the child's total environment before drawing conclusions about the significance of his behavior. Not only are there cultural and subcultural differences in modes of behavior, but family environments also have significant variances.

> Bert was totally confounding the student clinician with his apparent euphoria and inability to understand any questions put to him. When asked if he walked to the clinic, Bert would pose a taut, wry, little smile and nod in affirmation. Later he was asked if he got to the clinic in a car, and he gave the same kind of response. In fact, the student got a similar smile and nod to the same question substituting a train, cab, bicycle, and kitchen sink. Things clarified greatly when the mother was interviewed, and her face froze in a meaningless smile as she resisted any meaningful interaction with sterile and superficial answers.

In this day when difference is supposed to be a sign of individuality, it is sometimes difficult to judge truly aberrant behavior from the norm. It is important for the diagnostician to be in tune with the times and have a keen awareness of acceptable variations in human behavior before attempting to make judgment.

3 *Brain Damage.* The third etiological category, brain damage, presents yet another domain that falls outside of the jurisdiction of the speech clinician. This time it is primarily the physician who must make such diagnoses; however, there is much the speech clinician can do to aid the physician and to fully understand the diagnostic process.

There are so many valid arguments against the use of the term "brain damage" as an etiological category for language disturbance that it is amazing that it is still in use. It is a testimony to the early works of scholars such as Strauss and Lehtinen (1947), who were so effective in describing a syndrome of behavior, that the term became solidly accepted. We perceive and remember best those characteristics that have labels, so it is often convenient, if misleading, for the brain to group many variables into a single category. Our argument against the use of the term "brain damage" centers around three aspects: (1) impact on the environment, (2) the impurity of the diagnostic category, and (3) the lack of usefulness as an aid to therapy.

The impact of the term "brain damage" on the parent can be devastating. Feelings of guilt arise, along with the implication that some sort of actual physical damage has taken place to an otherwise normal organism. Nearly every parent can recall some severe fall or imagined trauma to his child which could have caused the problem and might have been prevented. Parents tend to hear the term as a sort of static characteristic that dooms their child to a life of inadequacy; the label has an unchanging, permanent, hopeless ring to it. Many parents also equate the term with mental retardation, since brain functioning is obviously associated with intellectual potential. The studies of Siegal and Harkins (1963) show what can happen to adult-child interaction when the adult assumes that the child is mentally retarded; the change in the quality and quantity of verbal stimulation may be significant. Lastly, there is a tangential environmental effect in the frequently prescribed medication for brain-damaged children. Not infrequently the use of medication places the onus of control of the child on some outside authority—in this case the pre-scribed medication. We have observed several instances in which both child and parent believed no control was possible without medication.

> Paul was an active four-year-old when he was diagnosed by the neurologist as brain damaged. A then-popular medication was prescribed and used for six years. When Paul was ten years old, however, his parents felt that further prob-lems were evident, and they returned him for additional testing. The diagnosis was reconfirmed and a new medication prescribed. The neurologist informed the child that the new pills were "memory pills" and must be taken every morn-ing before school. Not long thereafter, Paul returned home from school admon-ishing his mother for forgetting to give him his pill that morning. "I must have forgotten to take it, mom; I forgot all sorts of stuff today and got in lots of trou-ble," he said. The idea that the pill was all that was keeping the child function-ing was instilled in his and his parent's thinking and should serve as a stinging indictment of the misuse of medication.

The term "brain damage" is not a pure diagnostic category. Cerebral-palsied children are brain damaged, epileptic children have brain differences, some emotionally disturbed children, some deaf, and some retarded children have brain damage; the aphasoid child is brain damaged, as is the child with central dysarthria, whether or not he fits into one of the other categories. If brain damage implies brain difference, we are all "brain damaged" to some degree.

The use of the designation "brain damage" as an aid to future therapy has not been fruitful. The term is not descriptive as once thought, and no single rehabilitative technique has come forth to help this type of child. The continuing search for specific treatment methods to fit specific causes keeps alive, however, our search for the causes, and without this pursuit the answers that must ultimately come will be lost.

The ability of the central nervous system to deal with symbolic abstrac-tions is critical to language development. If the attribute is lost or diminished

due to agenesis or trauma, the resultant disorder is termed "childhood aphasia," or "aphasoid syndrome." Whatever the label, the possibility that the
child without language or speech development is aphasic should be investigated.

Differentiating the aphasic child from other etiological groups is an ex-
hausting, time-consuming, and often frustrating undertaking. Since it is inherent in the concept of aphasia that the child have some central nervous
system differences, the possibility is very real that this child may also have a
degree of retardation, hearing loss, and eventual secondary emotional reactions. Seldom, if ever, is it possible to arrive at a diagnosis of aphasia in one
session, and once again we must stress the need for ongoing diagnosis. The
eventual need for diagnostic treatment and the possibility of gaining diagnostic information from observing the results of treatment must not be over-
looked.

Since it takes the combined efforts of several disciplines to arrive at a
satisfactory diagnosis of aphasia, it may well, and often does, fall upon the
shoulders of the speech clinician to collate and integrate the various diagnostic findings and draw some conclusions from them. In light of this Wood
states:

> First, the classification of aphasia in children assumes that the major factor sepa-
> rating this disorder from all other speech and language problems is the distur-
> bance in symbolic language formulation. . . . The deaf child does not develop
> speech normally, but his lack of speech production is related directly to his in-
> ability to hear sound. Yet deaf children may have integrated symbolic language
> in all language functions that do not require sound. The mentally retarded
> child functions at a retarded symbolic level, but symbolic formulation is not the
> only area of his deficiency. Thus, the mentally retarded child is expected to de-
> velop symbolic language in proportion to his mental age. The emotionally dis-
> turbed child may reject sound and may not talk, but his problem, again, is not
> relegated to a primary disturbance in symbolic formulation. Diagnostically,
> these differentiations are of extreme importance. Second, some of the more
> overt symptoms of aphasia may resemble the symptoms of other childhood prob-
> lems, but the total problem constellations are distinctly different. . . . Third,
> the classification of aphasia cannot be used merely because all other possible di-
> agnostic classifications have been excluded (1964: 32–33).

To further complicate our task of diagnosis, most authorities differentiate between children with primarily motor, or expressive, disabilities and
children with primarily sensory, or receptive, disabilities; and although these
two subcategories overlap a great deal, there are some distinguishing patterns
of behavior. It should be noted, however, that when the disability is linked
either to a single input or output modality and does not appear to interfere
with the central language process, it is technically not aphasia but rather
apraxia, agraphia, or agnosia (Wepman *et al.,* 1960).

Since any single characteristic may well indicate more than one etiological category, it is often necessary to look for a constellation of factors that
indicate aphasia. The following may provide a starting point:

1. The case-history information may suggest possible brain cell damage—i.e., anoxia, trauma, or hemorrhage.

2. Neurological examination findings may suggest possible brain damage—i.e., EEG abnormalities, infantile reflex patterns, or motor incoordination. Landau, Goldstein, and Kleffner (1960) found that aphasic children have a higher percentage of EEG abnormalities than the normal population, but it should be remembered that the absence of abnormal EEG or any other neurological signs must not rule out aphasia.

3. Intelligence scores on verbal and nonverbal tests may vary significantly, with the nonverbal being higher.

4. Shows an interest in people and seeks to interact with them and participate in social activities. (This may diminish somewhat as the child grows older.)

5. The aphasic child is significantly behind his age group in ability to classify and group things into some sort of organized pattern. He is generally unable to see the similarities among members of a given class or category, and thus is unable to deal well in abstractions. This is admittedly an oversimplification, and the reader is warned that there is a wide spectrum of behavior to be judged.

6. The aphasic child has difficulty imitating articulatory movements and recalling sequences and patterns. This is generally typical of the motor aphasic child.

7. With great stimulation and time-consuming effort the aphasic child is able to learn and produce articulatory patterns, but appears unable to generalize this skill to new words without repeating the laborious task of drill once again.

8. After learning articulatory movements for a given word, this child may need an unusual amount of help in transferring this skill to other settings.

9. The aphasic child's comprehension of speech is poor, and it is not improved with amplification. Some authorities claim that actual decrements in understanding are typical of aphasic children under amplification. These comprehension difficulties may be manifest in poor auditory discrimination for individual speech sounds or be so extensive as to make the comprehension of speech difficult or impossible. Obviously discrimination ability is partly dependent upon reception of the speech signal, but the actual task of comparing and judging the similarities and differences is a function of the central nervous system.

10. The child shows confusion or is delayed in establishing laterality, but not always.

11. The child commonly has difficulty in establishing a flow of speech, which results in awkward grammatical constructions, numerous hesitations, false starts and repetitions, and altered timing patterns. The term "cluttering" is often used to identify this speech pattern.

12. The child usually has difficulty perceiving forms or patterns. He finds it difficult to select the significant auditory, visual, or tactile pattern from the surroundings. This "figure-ground" difficulty often appears related to a tendency to fix on some aspect of the stimulus without perceiving that aspect as a part of a gestalt.

13. Hardy (1962) speaks of the child's inability to process successive stimuli rapidly. These children tend to be able to handle fewer bits of information than normal children, and this is exhibited in poor recall ability for serially presented stimuli.

14. Hardy also discusses the capacity of the child to "track" verbal stimuli. He defines tracking as "a matter of being able to process an indefinite variety of incoming information, employing all the attributes of the sensorium, and to relate this to previous and presently pertinent experience" (42). The ability to use what is remembered of past experiences by recalling them and applying them to present stimuli is sometimes deficient in these children.

Many workers disagree with the use of the term "congenital aphasia" as an etiological category. Lenneberg (1964) articulates the argument clearly, citing evidence that the cortex has a large degree of functional equipotentiality during the first three years of life. He states further:

> Whatever function becomes localized in adult life can become established in early childhood in spite of the presence of fixed cortical and subcortical lesions, and it seems immaterial where these lesions are located. The entire left hemisphere may be incapacitated during the first two years and remain so thereafter without interfering with the establishment of language at the usual age. However, a similar lesion would result in irreversible language loss if it occurred during or after the middle of the second decade. Neither trauma nor surgical lesions, nor focal infections, nor agenesis (including the corpus callosum) regardless of cortical locality will prevent acquisition of language as long as the insult occurs at early enough an age, is confined to a single hemisphere, and does not reduce the individual to a state of idiocy. . . . Thus there is clearly no justification for speaking of congenital motor aphasia (168–69).

Neuromotor coordination. In order for articulate speech to be produced, it is imperative that the brain be capable of organizing neural impulses before sending them to the speech structure, that the neural pathways be capable of transmitting these organized impulses to the musculature, and that the musculature itself be capable of receiving the stimuli and responding appropriately. If the child is unable to produce such coordinated action, articulate speech will suffer. This implies, however, that such circumstances will probably result only in an expressive language deficit. This is probably not the case. As Berry (1969) points out, we perceive speech-sound sequences only after the neuromusculature patterns of articulation have been established. If this is indeed true, then the child's receptive and internal language skills are no doubt linked to his production skills and will suffer some sort of limitation if the organized production of speech is deficient.

In addition to this alleged association between motor speech and language acquisition, there is another relationship which must be mentioned. Several workers, Kephart (1960), for example, have postulated a hierarchical relationship between lower-level functions, i.e., perceptual-motor behavior, and higher cognitive functions. If this hierarchy of development does exist, motor coordination takes on even greater significance for language acquisition. Lenneberg (1964), on the other hand, speaks of the congenitally inarticulate child as a youngster who has an excellent comprehension of language and a fully developed language system, but who cannot control the speech musculature to produce articulate speech patterns.

Sensory-motor control. The control of the speech musculature is, in part, a function of nerve-muscle patterns that lead from the brain; it is also a function of the nerve-brain–nerve-muscle patterns. That is to say, coordinated muscle control is indebted to the feedback of information from the tactile, kinesthetic, proprioceptive sensors informing the brain where the structures are and where they are going.[3] In certain types of expressive language impairments, it may be necessary to differentiate between neuromotor and sensory-motor breakdowns. Liberman gives priority to the kinesthetic feedback information over the auditory in the control and comprehension of language. He states:

> We believe that a speaker (and listener) learns to connect speech sounds with their appropriate articulations and that the sensory feedback from these movements (or, more likely, the corresponding neurological processes) comes to mediate between the acoustic stimulus and its perception (1957: 117–23).

Environment. Environmental factors, such as quantity and quality of language stimulation, motivation to speak, number of siblings, and order of birth, have long been cited as critical to the development of language in the child. These, and all other so-called environmental factors, do not, however, appear to be related to *language deficits* as much as they are to *delays* and *distortions in the learning of speech.* A child apparently is capable of learning the basic systems of his language under, or perhaps, in spite of, the most adverse learning conditions. However, he will probably show the effects of his experience in his vocabulary, grammar, and articulation.

Sally is a prime example of a child whose speech pattern has been adversely affected by environmental conditions. We first saw Sally when she was five years old. She was brought to the clinic by her third set of parents. Sally was taken away from her real parents by the welfare office, which made the following claims: Sally had been confined to her crib for essentially every minute of her first year of life. She displayed continuous diaper rash from infrequent changing and improper cleansing. Both parents worked, and Sally was cared for by her five older brothers and sisters, the eldest of whom was twelve. At six months of age she was able to climb out of the crib, but the older siblings continually found new ways to keep her confined. By one year she had pretty much given up trying to escape and was content to sit or rock in her crib hour after hour. The second year of life saw a general regression with increased hours of sleep and hours of rocking and head banging. By two and one half years of age, Sally was placed in a foster home and dramatic changes began to occur. This arrangement lasted only five months, however, and then Sally was placed in a children's home to await adoption. In these hectic surroundings she reverted back to her earlier behavior, and it was not until she was four years old that her current parents

---

[3] The motor theory of perception, which states in essence that we may perceive with our tongues what we hear with our ears, has many fascinating implications for speech and language clinicians. Compare the work of Berry (1969) with that of Lenneberg (1964) and formulate your own opinion on this issue.

adopted her. Sally's adjustment to their home was satisfactory but not dramatic, and speech development was very slow. Consistent with our diagnosis of environmental etiology, the therapy plan for Sally called for a total environmental language-enrichment plan and specific educational approaches to language development in the clinic. After only one and a half years of such therapy, Sally was ready for first grade and was showing near "average" performance in the first grade at last report.

Two techniques are essential in determining environmental etiological factors: the case history and the parental interview. The information gained from these two sources should provide the necessary clues. The strongest indicator would be a large discrepancy between language competence and language performance.

Some warning should be given regarding the frequent generalizations found in the literature about factors such as number of siblings, birth order, and bilingual homes. There is no conclusive evidence to date that these factors have an appreciable effect upon a child's basic language competence; it is possible that they do effect speech performance. Socioeconomic level encompasses far too many variables to be taken as a distinct factor.

Hearing acuity. Among the most obvious physical factors influencing language acquisition is hearing acuity. Deaf and severely hard-of-hearing children do not learn to perform in the language realm as well or as rapidly as do hearing children. Once again, however, we must be sobered by the fact that these children have to a large extent the basic symbolic resources of the hearing child and thus are quite capable of acquiring language if adequate stimulation can only be channeled into the central nervous system through some alternate route. Lenneberg (1967) makes a strong case for this. However, if we examine a five-year-old deaf child who has not had the opportunity to receive the language system due to his auditory deficit and the shortcomings of his environment, he does indeed suffer from language incompetence as well as diminished language performance. Whether you consider the problem to be due to the child's impairment or to the environment has little effect upon the final disposition of the case. Every child with language delay must undergo extensive hearing evaluations. For a complete discussion of audiological evaluations see Newby (1972) and others (O'Neill and Oyer, 1966; Davis and Silverman, 1970).

Differential diagnosis of children with language disorders requires careful analysis of historical information, intuitive observation of the child and his environment, skillful test administration and interpretation, and a thorough knowledge of normal and abnormal behavior. It is totally unreasonable to expect anyone to have all of the skills and knowledge necessary to make this diagnosis unilaterally. It is imperative that diagnosis be done by a team. The lack of interdisciplinary cooperation has resulted in far too many children being diagnosed by numerous "specialists," each viewing the child through his own professional biases, and each reaching different conclusions.

directing the remedial undertaking

As therapy approaches differ, so in fact do the uses clinicians make of the information provided from diagnosis. Some favor enhancing the strengths of the child; others prefer to direct their therapy efforts toward the weaknesses; many simply take the diagnostic information as an indication of where the child is at a given point in time and use that as a starting point for treatment.

In addition to searching for the strengths and weaknesses of the client, this last goal of diagnosis may also aid the clinician by: (1) determining the severity of the problem, (2) setting a baseline for remediation, (3) giving direction to grouping and scheduling consideration, (4) measuring progress, and (5) making a prognosis. Only by carefully interrelating data from the various diagnostic sources is it possible to obtain the information necessary for effective therapy.

In order to provide some organization to this area of diagnosis, the concepts of reception and expression have been coordinated to provide the schema outlined in Table 1.

TABLE 1   Schema for Diagnosis to Direct Remediation   *end of diagnostic part*

Reception	*Expression*
Auditory	Motor Maturation
sensation	gross motor
perception	speech motor
memory-symbolization	perceptual motor
conceptualization	Phonemic Acquisition
Visual	Syntax Acquisition
sensation	Vocabulary Acquisition
perception	
memory-symbolization	
Haptic	

reception—auditory modality

Sensation level.   The goal is to evaluate the auditory mechanism's ability to work as an efficient transducer in transmitting the stimulus energy to the central nervous system. Three test areas are included in this category:

AUDITORY ACUITY.   Tests of auditory acuity have been discussed elsewhere in this and other texts. The child who is unable to properly receive and transmit the acoustic signal to his central nervous system is a candidate for therapeutic procedures such as lip-reading, auditory training, speech therapy, and language development.

AUDITORY ATTENTION. Auditory attention has been variously defined but, in essence, refers to the ability to focus on a given message as a significant stimulus. Chalfant and Scheffelin state:

> Inattentiveness to auditory stimuli might be related to: (a) Low level or absence of hearing acuity; (b) distractibility involving competitive visual or auditory stimuli; (c) hyperactive behavior; (d) severe emotional disturbance; (e) severe mental retardation; or (f) inability to obtain meaning from auditory stimuli (1969: 11).

There are no well-developed techniques for evaluating a child's attention to auditory stimuli. The examiner must rely on observations of the child to determine if he shows awareness of sound by turning his head, changing his facial expression, or moving toward or away from the sound source. If a child is capable of receiving the sound signal but incapable of attending to that stimulus long enough for it to become meaningful, there will be severe impact on language development.

AUDITORY LOCALIZATION. Auditory localization is the ability to locate the direction of the significant sound in a perceptual field. In the more elementary form, localization refers simply to identifying the direction of any given sound; but its more complex form involves selecting a significant sound from a field of competing sounds. Informal tests of sound localization would be easy to develop and should add significant data to the diagnosis, since this ability no doubt helps the child to relate sounds to objects and persons and to develop the perceptual skills of discrimination.

Perception level. Berelson and Steiner (1964: 88) define perception as "the more complex process by which people select, organize, and interpret sensory stimulation into a meaningful and coherent picture of the world." Inherent in the concept of perception is the recognition of the constancies in a particular stimulus that allow the individual to distinguish that stimulus from all competing stimuli and to separate the significant sound from the background sounds. The following test areas are included under auditory perception:

FIGURE-GROUND DIFFERENTIATION. The ability to select and identify the relevant auditory stimuli from increasingly complex and competing background sounds is tested. It is quite possible to construct a test of figure-ground differentiation by using tape-recorded materials of varying amplitude, interest, and similarity with the stimulus signals. The Goldman-Fristoe-Woodcock Test of Auditory Discrimination (1970) is comprised of three portions: a training portion, a test of auditory discrimination in quiet conditions, and a test of auditory discrimination where a background noise 9 db less intense than the signal has been superimposed over the stimulus. The background noise consists of semi-intelligible noise recorded in a busy school cafeteria. The test includes a prerecorded test tape and a book of stimulus pictures. Norms are provided for individuals aged from three years, eight months, to over seventy years.

AUDITORY CLOSURE. Auditory closure is the ability to integrate the various separate units of a stimulus into a whole. In order for a listener to understand spoken language, he must be capable of making sense out of the sequentially presented sounds, syllables, words, phrases, and sentences. The skills of figure-ground differentiation, memory, and discrimination must in some way be coordinated to provide the listener with the meaning of the total message. Berry (1969) argues strongly that the perception of speech is syncratic in nature. That is, the child comprehends the whole of a given language stimulus before he can differentiate and analyze the parts. Whatever the order of development, however, it is important to identify this ability. Since our definition of closure stresses the ability to integrate separate units of a stimulus, we must test two somewhat different skills. These skills are sometimes labeled auditory blending (or synthesis) and auditory closure; however, we feel that they both belong under the heading of closure. Speech-sound synthesis is tested by having the child repeat words which have been spoken to him with each sound separated by slight time intervals. The sound blending subtest of the ITPA is an example of this type of measure. Van Riper (1972) presents a test of speech-sound synthesis as it pertains to articulation acquisition. The language diagnostician should follow up this type of testing with an analysis of the child's ability to synthesize larger samples of language such as sentences and paragraphs. Tests of closure which evaluate the child's ability to fill in missing parts in recreating the whole of the message evaluate a somewhat different but closely related skill. The auditory closure subtest of the ITPA measures this skill. In this test, words such as airplane are pronounced "air-pla-" and telephone is "tele-one." The child's task is to identify the word spoken, and the assumed skill involved is achieving closure from an incomplete stimulus. Sentence completion tasks which involve filling in blanks deal with closure at the contextual level. The Auditory-Vocal Association Test of the ITPA and the Intraverbal Test of the Parsons Language Sample use such techniques. Berry (1969) has devised an exploratory measure of linguistic closure for children from four to eight years of age.

AUDITORY DISCRIMINATION. Berry (1969) uses the term discrimination synonymously with perception. An individual's ability to identify differences in auditory signals has long been thought to be crucial to speech and language development. Speech clinicians have persistently relied on "ear training" in therapy because they strongly believe that the ear must discriminate before the mouth can articulate. Tests of auditory discrimination have been developed by Templin (1957); Wepman (1958); Mecham, Jex, and Jones (1969); Goldman, Fristoe, and Woodcock (1970); Berry (1969); and others.

> Following a rather thorough lecture on error identification as the most important aspect of auditory discrimination, we assigned a group of graduate students the task of applying this concept to language disorders. Compiling the best efforts of each class member, we devised a test which not only evaluated the child's auditory discrimination of his own articulation errors (when spoken by the examiner) but further analyzed errors of similar distinctive features. A second category tested the child's ability to discriminate errors of word order, semantic intent, and morphology. Clearly, the task involved more than discrimination since grammatical rules were involved.

The Lindamood Auditory Conceptualization Test (1971) deserves particular mention because it measures not only auditory discrimination but also the child's ability to determine the order of spoken sound patterns and the number of sounds in a stimulus. The test uses colored blocks, and the child manipulates these blocks according to the various auditory stimuli. We have found that the test is often difficult for children five years of age and younger, because it demands that the child understand the concept of same and different, numbers up to four, left to right ordering, and the concepts of first and last.

Memory-symbolization level. The ability to remember and recall the salient characteristics of auditory stimuli is vital to language functioning. Before a language sample can be reproduced, it must be received intact by the ear, stored and held for variable lengths of time, and recalled when needed. Language behavior involves the correct patterning of stimuli and the accurate reauditorization of that pattern. A word when recalled in improper or incomplete sequence may take any of a number of forms; and if that recall pattern is inconsistent from moment to moment, the learning of the symbol becomes an impossible task.

Obviously, most of the speech generated by the child is not a direct imitation of previously heard word sequences, but rather new and creative word combinations. The question then becomes, is the child producing properly ordered statements because he has an innate capacity for language functioning, or because he has ferreted out from the stimuli the common linguistic rules that guide language production? This controversial and stimulating question has not yet been answered. There is little controversy, however, over the need for recall for proper ordering of sounds within words. Questions do arise regarding the impact of the motoric system on auditory perception and recall, but we shall remain true to our course and pursue the study of auditory memory and recall without clouding the issue further. We shall briefly discuss seven different levels of auditory recall of varying complexity. Some of these measures no doubt tap skills other than simple recall since comprehension, attention span, and syntax are involved. This would imply that these tests flow up from the memory level as shown in Table 1, but we shall include them here for the purpose of clarity.

RECALL OF SPEECH SOUNDS. No standardized procedure with norms is available to test speech-sound recall. This ability is probably related more to articulation acquisition than to language alone. Winitz (1969) concluded from his investigation of relevant data that no definitive statement on the relationship of this skill to speech is possible. An important factor to keep in mind when testing this skill is the articulatory pattern of the child under examination. If the perception of sounds is related to their production, a child would be expected to have more difficulty recalling the sounds he does not articulate correctly. Metraux (1942) found that children with speech disorders have an easier time with vowels than consonants, which substantiates this premise.

RECALL OF SYLLABLES. It is curious that the syllable has not been used extensively in tests of recall since syllables are not "contaminated" by meaning. With no substantial data to rely on, the examiner is left to develop his own test of syllable recall. The same warnings regarding consonant errors apply in this case.

RECALL OF DIGITS. The Auditory Sequential Memory Test of the ITPA, the subtest of the Stanford Binet, and the Weschsler Intelligence Test use digits for measuring recall. Such tests suggest that the examiner space the stimuli from one half to one second apart. Generally children should be able to recall as many digits as they are years old up to six or so, which approximates the adult norm. Again, there are no definitive data to link this skill with any aspect of language functioning.

RECALL OF UNRELATED WORDS. Symbolic factors and comprehension complicate the task once words are involved, but it is assumed that this is more closely related to language functioning. Berry (1969) describes two tests of word recall suitable for children from seven to nine years of age, although norms suitable for universal interpretation are not available.

RECALL OF RHYTHM AND INFLECTION. Since much of the meaning of verbal utterance is carried by the prosodic elements of the passage, it is important to evaluate the child's ability to recall patterns of inflection and rhythm. Clapping, pencil-tapping, drums, and so on are used to measure a child's ability to follow rhythms, and inflection patterns can be produced either by using humming or words. Children as young as three years of age should begin to show rudimentary competence, although the exact norms are not available. We have informally tested children's abilities to understand melody patterns by "saying" common phrases using only the sound "ah" to control the prosodic elements. We often make this a multiple-choice task: "We are going to play a game, and I'm going to see how well you understand me when I talk a different language to you. This time I will either say 'How are you?' or 'My name is John.' . . . Ah . . . *ah* . . . ah . . . what did I say?"

RECALL OF SENTENCES. As the recall task begins to involve language units larger than the word, skills of syntax and verbal patterning become increasingly important. Although used for experimental purposes, the sentence-imitation tests devised by Slobin and Welsh (1967) as cited by McNeill (1970) present interesting information. These researchers investigated the child's ability to comprehend sentences through his ability to preserve meaning in repetition. Verbatim repetition of presented sentences was not expected. In this case, a correct response would be for the child to maintain the meaning of the sentence in his repetition. The skills involved imply syntactic development, comprehension, recall, and expression.

It is common to use directions as a method for measuring a child's ability to handle increasingly complex sentence forms. This measure of comprehension and recall demands no verbal response since the child is simply requested to perform a series of tasks: "point to the pencil, put the penny in the cup, and give me the crayon." Such tasks can be very simple or complicated, so the examiner is able to adapt the level of difficulty to the child.

RECALL OF STORIES. The recall of the content of stories is widely used to evaluate adult aphasics. Once again, linguistic comprehension is involved as well as longer-term retention and recall. Generally this testing takes the form of a narrative story followed by a question and answer period. It is also possible to ask the child to retell the story and establish some sort of criterion for judging those responses.

Berry (1969) suggests certain qualitative judgments which might be made of the child's responses, and it is obvious that certain techniques also lend themselves to quantitative measurement of the child's recall ability. It is possible to vary such attributes as the length of the story, content complexity, nature of the questions, and length of time between the story and the questions, in order to fit the measurement to the child.

> Chauncey was four when we first saw him for evaluation. The student clinician assigned to the diagnosis had written a short story about three ducks who didn't like to swim until late one spring day when their high and dry playground was flooded by heavy rains. Upon completion of the story, Chauncey was asked to recall the story. He stated: "Duckie not swim . . . play. Duckie all wet . . . swim fast." The student's accurate conclusion was that Chauncey had adequate recall for content although grammatical complexity was delayed.

Conceptualization. The abstraction process consists of leaving out details and attending to the similarities among perceptual experiences. As the child perceives differences and similarities in stimuli in his environment, he is increasingly capable of grouping these experiences into categories. This capability is the essence of concept development. Verbal concepts are formed when the child begins to respond to different words with the same or similar internal mediational behaviors (Kendler and Karasik, 1958). The exact relationship between concept formation and language has not been satisfactorily described; however, it is safe to assume that many language skills involve concept development—for instance, abstracting the qualities of certain words that make them nouns. The process is complicated as Staats indicates:

> The process of concept formation is seen as one which involves complicated principles of learning, communication, and mediated generalization. The relationship between the language process and the environmental process is complex. The language processes arise from a response to the environment but then in turn affect responses to other aspects of the environment (1968: 143).

As the child is exposed to a greater variety of experiences that isolate perceptual invariants, increasingly complex concepts become available. For this reason the testing of concept development becomes a theoretically limitless task. The relationship between language and concept formation is apparent in that language serves to store and transmit concepts; and the ability to manipulate symbolically experiential variables allows man to develop and refine concepts with ever-increasing complexity. Whorf (1956) points out, however, that language systems not only enhance concept formation but also define and limit them. To this extent, language both facilitates and restricts conceptualization.

Many of the diagnostic tests of language function are in effect measures of concept development—i.e., intelligence and achievement tests. The child's ability to solve problems, reason, recall, organize, plan, and deal in abstractions is all firmly based in language.

The author of the field research edition of the Basic Concept Inventory (Engelmann, 1967: 5) states: "The Basic Concept Inventory is a broad checklist of basic concepts that are involved in new learning situations in the first grade." Intended for culturally disadvantaged slow learners, the emotionally disturbed, and the mentally retarded, the test is based on the premise that learning involves concepts and knowledge of the child's ability to conceptualize is strategic to educational (and presumably remedial) undertakings.

The Boehm Test of Basic Concepts (1971) is a very useful measure to identify those children who have difficulty with concepts that are important for academic achievement. The fifty-item test measures the child's concepts of space, quantity, time, and miscellaneous items and can be given to groups of children. The test has value for children from five to eight years of age. As with many such measures, this test taps the child's vocabulary as well as his conceptualization and familiarity with the pictured items; it has met with wide acceptance and has a distinct value in directing the remedial effort.

Reception—visual modality

Sensation level. Visual acuity bears somewhat the same type of relationship to language development as does hearing acuity. That is, apparently the ability to develop symbolic concepts and the grammatical system of language is independent of the specific modality. Nonetheless, many of the adjunct language skills such as vocabulary development are related to the ability to see.

Perceptual level. Marianne Frostig's Developmental Test of Visual Perception (1964) is probably the best known and most widely used test of visual perception. This test measures five perceptual skills: eye-motor coordination, figure-ground, constancy of shape, position in space, and spatial relationships. The test manual describes the instrument as useful for either screening purposes for children in nursery school, kindergarten, and first grade or clinical evaluation of older children. Normative data are available for children between the ages of four and eight years. The test measures a child's perceptual competency and results in a perceptual quotient.

The Southern California Figure-Ground Visual Perception Test (Ayres, 1966a) provides a series of plates with superimposed pictures which the subject must identify. Developed for children aged from four to eleven years, this test provides normative data.

The Columbia Mental Maturity Scale (1959) may be used to measure visual perception, the child's ability to identify similarities and differences in stimuli that are categorized on the basis of color, size, and form. Although the test results in a mental age, Berry (1969: 288) points out that this "might more accurately be called a developmental quotient of visual perception."

Visual perceptual skills are often tested in relation to motor responses in what is termed visuomotor ability. The Hiskey-Nebraska Test of Learning Aptitude (1966) uses block patterns; Kohs (1923) described a test employing colored blocks which the child manipulates to match stimulus patterns. The Bender Visual-Motor Gestalt Test (1938) is a classic test of visuomotor behavior. This device requires the copying of designs from stimulus patterns. Interestingly, the test has also been widely used to diagnose brain damage, emotional disturbance, and other factors in its long and productive history. The Graham Kendall Memory-for-Designs Test (1960) requires the reproduction of fifteen geometric designs from memory and includes visuomotor integration and memory ability as well.

Memory symbolization level. Several measures of visual memory and symbolic functioning are available. The visual sequential memory subtest of the ITPA tests visual memory by demanding the recall of a sequence of stimulus patterns. Tests such as the Gates and MacGinitie Reading Tests (1965) measure visual comprehension and thus visual symbolic functioning.

Several tests reputed to measure cognitive ability involve some aspects of visual functioning at the perceptual, symbolic, and memory levels. The Columbia Mental Maturity Scale (1954), WISC (1949), WPPSI (1967), Goodenough Draw-A-Man Test (Harris, 1963), PPVT (1951), all include measures of visual functioning.

The rather obvious relationship between visual function and reading points up the importance of vision on one level, but the language-symbolic skills necessary for reading, for instance, do not depend entirely upon vision—witness the ability of the blind to read Braille. On the other hand, writers such as Luria (1966), Kephart (1960), and Barsch (1967) stress the importance of perception on motor ability and eventually on language functioning. Kephart (1960) emphasizes that perceptual motor skills are the foundations of higher cortical development in that higher forms of behavior develop out of motor learning. Barsch stresses the importance of movement patterns on learning.

reception—haptic modality

Haptic perception is essentially the result of central processing and the synthesis of tactile and kinesthetic information (Chalfant and Scheffelin, 1969). The impact of haptic perception on language function can be measured by the kind of information that the system provides. Chalfant and Scheffelin suggest that the haptic systems provide two major kinds of information.

The first category includes information about the environment such as: (a) geometric information concerning surface area—size, shapes, lines, and angles; (b) surface texture; (c) qualities of consistency such as hard, soft, resilient, or viscous; (d) pain; (e) temperature; and (f) pressure. In the second category, bodily movement provides information about the body itself such as: (a) dynamic movement patterns of the trunk, arms, legs, mandible, and tongue; (b) static limb positions or postures; and (c) sensitivity to the direction of linear and rotary movement of the skull, limbs, and entire body. Body movement also provides information about the location of objects in relation to the body itself.

The impact of this system on the perception of speech is not totally resolved. Liberman (1957) states that the perception of speech appears to be more closely related to the articulatory, or movement, patterns of the listener than to the acoustic stimulus, thus underlining the importance of the haptic system in speech perception. There is no final verdict, however, and auditory systems of perception will probably be found to have a very influential effect upon perception.

Examination of the haptic perceptual function ultimately involves the separation of touch and movement. Tactile perception is quite easily measured by having the subject identify the exact point of stimulation on the skin when all channels of input are interrupted except the tactile. Touching the tongue or palate with a tongue blade or similar object and then requesting that the subject indicate the exact point of contact gives some indication of the integrity of the touch system. Since the tongue must move to and from structures having various surfaces (teeth, hard palate, lips), it may be well to determine the ability of the oral structures to discriminate among various textures. Though resulting in no formalized and standardized test to date, the data from workers investigating oral discrimination of form (oral stereognosis) indicate that some relationship does indeed exist between oral discrimination ability and articulatory skill (Scott and Ringel, 1971). No doubt a test will be ultimately marketed that standardizes a technique where the subject identifies plastic shapes which are placed in the oral cavity. The Southern California Kinesthesia and Tactile Perception Tests (Ayres, 1966b) purports to measure these skills in children aged four to eight years. Even with the existence of this test, however, it is evident that there must be much more investigation into the nature of kinesthetic and tactile perception and their relationship with speech and language.

expression—motor maturation

The examining procedures for motor skills have been discussed in Chapter 3. Although a great deal is known about motor behavior and a similar wealth of knowledge is available on language function, there is little known beyond theory about the impact of motor function on language. At this point in the diagnostic process, the purpose in measuring the child's motor performance is to help establish the proper remedial program. If the examiner is willing to accept the theoretical postulate that motor skill is related to language function, then he should be willing to followup the testing with a program of motor and perceptual-motor therapy that will aid the child in gaining greater control over this function.

Although Table 1 identifies gross, speech, and perceptual motor subcategories, motoric control at any level requires coordinated control of movement through knowledge of the environment (sensory data from vision, hearing, and tactition), knowledge of the body's relationship with the environment (sensory data from proprioceptive, tactile, and kinesthetic receptors), knowledge of past experience and ability to relate that knowledge to the present circumstance (CNS functions of memory, organization, and integration), the ability to send specific and accurate innervating impulses to the muscles, and the ability of those muscle systems to respond appropriately. In order to speak, the child must not only perceive the acoustic signal of the word and recognize its unit, but he must also relate that word to the concept it represents and be able to control the musculature adequately for speech production. In this conceptual framework the separation of language performance from motor skills is not absolute.

Ayres (1964, 1968) has developed two tests which incorporate perceptual-motor tasks: The Southern California Motor Accuracy Test and The Southern California Perceptual-Motor Tests. The former test requires the subject to draw a line over a printed maze, and both speed and accuracy are incorporated into the scoring procedure. The latter tests involve imitation of postures, crossing the midline, bilateral motor coordination, right-left discrimination, and standing balance tests.

expression—phonemic acquisition

Articulation testing will be thoroughly discussed in Chapter 5. Articulation production is not separate from language functioning and language systems. The examination of articulation production must include a careful analysis of the linguistic systems that guide the sound productions of the child and of how well the child has learned or mislearned those systems. Just as there is a grammatical system that the child learns and incorporates in his production of syntactically accurate sentences, there is a plan that guides the learning of the sound system of speech. Articulation testing thus becomes more than a tabulatory process for identifying which sounds are in error; rather, it directs the remedial effort by identifying a broader breakdown in the idiosyncratic system that guides articulation performance. For too long speech clinicians have seen articulation testing as simply a procedure for identifying the existence of the problem, and now they must begin to organize and evaluate the data to help in other ways.

expression—syntax acquisition

The procedures available to measure the syntax performance of a child have been outlined earlier in this chapter. The most promising measures include Lee's Northwestern Syntax Screening Test (1969) and Lee and Canter's Developmental Sentence Scoring (1971) for the developmental sentence types.

Knowledge of the child's syntax structure has primarily two functions in directing the remedial effort. First, this knowledge will aid the clinician to enter the therapy process at the level most beneficial for the child; and second, through continuous reassessment procedures, this knowledge should help to inform the clinician of the impact of a given therapy procedure on the child's development.

expression—vocabulary acquisition

There is some question as to whether any formalized test is adequate to measure the expressive vocabulary of a child. Formal test data appear sterile when compared with everyday behavior. It is impossible to judge if the child's performance reflects a true paucity of vocabulary, unwillingness to interact in the test situation, or insecurity. Very often it is necessary to ask parents to keep a running diary of the child's verbal utterances.

For those who feel that a formal test may help to measure the verbal output of a child, the verbal expression subtest of the ITPA does an admirable job of evaluating not only the number of words a child speaks, but also the quality of verbal output.

Although simple quantitative data regarding a child's expressive vocabulary are of some value in planning a therapy strategy, there are other kinds of information available from this type of study which may be of additional value. The child's use of the various parts of speech, his morphological inflections, understanding of abstraction, and concepts such as color and size, all give the clinician data for planning.

Nation (1972) has devised a Vocabulary Usage Test for children between thirty-four and sixty-three months. The test is based upon the Peabody Picture Vocabulary Test and allows comparison between vocabulary comprehension and usage.

PROJECTS AND QUESTIONS

1. Compare the linguistic concepts of competence and performance with the traditional concepts of reception and expression.

2. How does the statement of the purposes of diagnosis presented in this chapter compare with those stated by Perkins (1971)?

3. Categorize as input, integrative, and output all of those behaviors which you feel are dependent upon language.

4. Another group of special educators, the learning disabilities (SLD, SLBP, LD) specialists, have shown an interest in language disorders. Formulate an argument which supports the proposition that speech clinicians are best qualified to work in this area.

5. Compare the chapters on normal language development presented in the 1954 and 1970 editions of Carmichael's *Manual of Child Psychology*. Do the differences reflect the changes in the types of information needed for understanding language functioning?

6. While many practicing speech clinicians have been struggling to update their knowledge of language disorders, the theoreticians have been moving beyond descriptive and developmental linguistics to the study of cognition and concept development. Look into the works of Piaget (1967) as they relate to these concerns.

7. Briefly list the psychological, physical, environmental, and intellectual requisites for language; contrast your list with the point of view presented by DeVito (1970).

8. What impact has behavior modification theory had on the use of the ITPA?

9. Outline a diagnostic evaluation for a language-deficient child, using no formalized tests.

10. What is the point of view presented by McGinnis (1963) regarding the early differential diagnosis of etiology in language-disturbed children?

11. A large number of clinicians are abandoning attempts to determine the etiology of language problems in favor of intensive study of current performance levels, useful reward systems, and task analysis. Formulate your own personal philosophy on the importance of etiology.

12. Summarize the cogent arguments presented by the psychologists in defense of the concept that language is a learned function.

13. Develop a twenty-stage task analysis of the skills necessary to generate a spoken sentence. Relate it to diagnosis.

14. Consult *ASHA Monograph* No. 14, and define what the authors mean by a "functional analysis" of speech and language.

15. What implication does the work of Shriner and Sherman (1967) have on your selection of appropriate language measures?

BIBLIOGRAPHY

AMMONS, R. and H. AMMONS (1958). *The Full-Range Picture Vocabulary Test.* Missoula, Mont.: Psychological Test Specialists.

ARTHUR, G. (1952). *The Arthur Adaptation of the Leiter International Performance Scale.* Washington, D.C.: Psychological Service Center Press.

AYRES, A. (1964). *Southern California Motor Accuracy Test.* Los Angeles: Western Psychological Services.

——— (1966a). *Southern California Figure-Ground Visual Perception Test.* Los Angeles: Western Psychological Services.

——— (1966b). *Southern California Kinesthesia and Tactile Perception Tests.* Los Angeles: Western Psychological Services.

——— (1968). *Southern California Perceptual-Motor Test.* Los Angeles: Western Psychological Services.

BANGS, T. (1961). "Evaluating Children with Language Delay." *Journal of Speech and Hearing Disorders,* 26: 6–18.

——— (1968). *Language and Learning Disorders of the Pre-Academic Child.* New York: Appleton-Century-Crofts.

BARATZ, J. (1968). "Language in the Economically Disadvantaged Child: A Perspective." *Journal of the American Speech and Hearing Association,* 10: 143–45.

——— (1969). "Language and Cognitive Assessment of Negro Children." *Journal of the American Speech and Hearing Association,* 11: 87–91.

BARRY, H. (1961). *The Young Aphasic Child: Evaluation and Training.* Washington, D.C.: Alexander Graham Bell Association for the Deaf, Inc.

BARSCH, R. (1967). *Achieving Perceptual-Motor Efficiency: A Space-Oriented Approach to Learning.* Seattle, Wash.: Special Child Publications.

BATEMAN, B. (1965). *The Illinois Test of Psycholinguistic Abilities in Current Research: Summaries of Studies.* Urbana: Institute for Research on Exceptional Children, University of Illinois.

BELLUGI, U. (1967). "The Acquisition of Negation." Unpublished Doctoral dissertation, Harvard University.

—— and R. BROWN, eds. (1964). "The Acquisition of Language." *Monographs of the Society for Research in Child Development,* 29: 5–191.

BENDER, L. (1938). "A Visual Motor Gestalt Test and Its Clinical Use." *Research Monograph No. 3, American Orthopsychiatric Association.*

—— and P. SCHILDER (1956). *Psychopathology of Children with Organic Brain Disorders.* Springfield, Ill.: Charles C Thomas.

BERELSON, B. and G. STEINER (1964). *Human Behavior: An Inventory of Scientific Findings.* New York: Harcourt, Brace, & World. Inc.

BERKO, J. (1958). "The Child's Learning of English Morphology." *Word,* 14: 150–77.

BERRY, M. (1969). *Language Disorders of Children.* New York: Appleton-Century-Crofts.

BEVERIDGE, W. (1957). *The Art of Scientific Investigation.* New York: W. W. Norton & Company Inc.

BLOOM, L. (1970). *Language Development: Form and Function in Emerging Grammars.* Cambridge, Mass.: M.I.T. Press.

BLOOMFIELD, L. (1933). *Language.* New York: Holt, Rinehart & Winston, Inc.

BODOR, D. (1940). "The Adjective-Verb Quotient: A Contribution to the Psychology of Language." *Psychological Record,* 3: 309–44.

BOEHM, A. (1971). *Boehm Test of Basic Concepts.* New York: Psychological Corporation.

BOSMA, J., ed. (1970). *Second Symposium on Oral Sensation and Perception.* Springfield, Ill.: Charles C Thomas.

BRAINE, M. (1963). "The Ontogeny of English Phrase Structure: The First Phase." *Language,* 39: 1–13.

BROWN, R. (1958). *Words and Things.* New York: The Free Press.

—— and U. BELLUGI (1964). "Three Processes in the Child's Acquisition of Syntax." *Harvard Education Review,* 34: 133–51.

BROWN, R. and J. BERKO (1960). "Word Association and the Acquisition of Grammar." *Child Development,* 31: 1–14.

BROWN, R. and C. FRAZER (1963). "The Acquisition of Syntax." In *Verbal Behavior and Learning: Problems and Process,* eds. C. Cofer and B. Musgrave. New York: McGraw-Hill Book Company, Pp. 158–201.

BZOCH, K. and R. LEAGUE (1971). *Assessing Language Skills in Infancy.* Gainesville, Fla.: Tree of Life Press.

CARROLL, J. (1964). "Words, Meanings, Concepts." *Harvard Educational Review,* 34: 178–202.

CARROW, M. (1968). "The Development of Auditory Comprehension of Language Structure in Children." *Journal of Speech and Hearing Disorders,* 33: 99–111.

CHALFANT, J. and M. SCHEFFELIN (1969). *Central Processing Dysfunctions in Children: A Review of Research.* Bethesda, Md.: U.S. Department of Health, Education, and Welfare.

CHOMSKY, C. (1969). *The Acquisition of Syntax in Children from 5 to 10.* Cambridge, Mass.: M.I.T. Press.

CHOMSKY, N. (1965). *Aspects of the Theory of Syntax.* Cambridge, Mass.: M.I.T. Press.

——— (1957). *Syntactic Structure.* The Hague: Mouton.

——— (1959). "Review of B. F. Skinner's *Verbal Behavior.*" *Language,* 35: 26–58.

Columbia Mental Maturity Scale (1959). New York: Harcourt, Brace & World, Inc.

CRABTREE, M. (1958). *The Houston Test for Language Development.* Houston: Houston Test Co.

DARLEY, F. (1964). *Diagnosis and Appraisal of Communication Disorders.* Englewood Cliffs, N.J.: Prentice-Hall, Inc.

——— and H. WINITZ (1961). "Age of First Word: Review of Research." *Journal of Speech and Hearing Disorders,* 26: 272–90.

DAVIS, E. (1937). "The Development of Linguistic Skills in Twins, Singletons with Siblings, and Only Children from Age Five to Ten Years," *Institute of Child Welfare, Monograph Series No. 14.* Minneapolis: University of Minnesota Press.

DAVIS, H. and R. SILVERMAN (1970). *Hearing and Deafness.* New York: Holt, Rinehart & Winston, Inc.

DAY, E. (1932). "The Development of Language in Twins." *Child Development,* 3: 179–99.

DEVITO, J. (1970). *The Psychology of Speech and Language.* New York: Random House, Inc.

DUNN, L. (1965). *Peabody Picture Vocabulary Test.* Minneapolis: American Guidance Service.

EISENSON, J. (1968). "Developmental Aphasia (Dyslogia): A Postulation of a Unitary Concept of the Disorder." *Cortex,* 4: 184–200.

———, J. AUER, and J. IRWIN (1963). *The Psychology of Communication.* New York: Appleton-Century-Crofts.

ENGELMANN, S. (1967). *The Basic Concept Inventory.* Chicago: Follett Educational Corporation.

FAIRBANKS, G. (1954). "Systematic Research in Experimental Phonetics: I. A Theory of the Speech Mechanism as a Servosystem." *Journal of Speech and Hearing Disorders,* 19: 133–40.

FISHER, H. and J. LOGEMANN (1971). *The Fisher-Logemann Test of Articulation Competence.* Boston: Houghton Mifflin Company.

FODOR, J. (1966). "How to Learn to Talk: Some Simple Ways." In *The Genesis of Language: A Psycholinguistic Approach,* eds. F. Smith and G. Miller. Cambridge, Mass.: M.I.T. Press. Pp. 105–23.

FOSTER, R., J. GIDDAN, and J. STARK (1969). *Assessment of Children's Language Comprehension* (Preliminary Manual). Palo Alto, Calif.: Consulting Psychologists Press, Inc.

FRANKENBURG, W., J. DODDS, and A. FANDAL (1970). *Denver Developmental Screening Test.* Denver, Colo.: University of Colorado Medical Center.

FRASER, C., U. BELLUGI, and R. BROWN (1963). "Control of Grammar in Imitation, Comprehension, and Production." *Journal of Verbal Learning and Verbal Behavior,* 2: 121–35.

FROSTIG, M., D. LEFEVER, P. MASLOW, and R. WHITTLESLEY (1964). *Marianne Frostig Developmental Test of Visual Perception.* Palo Alto, Calif.: Consulting Psychologists Press.

GATES, A. and W. MACGINITIE (1965). *Gates-MacGinitie Reading Tests.* New York: Teachers College Press.

GOLDMAN, R. and M. FRISTOE (1969). *Goldman-Fristoe Test of Articulation.* Circle Pines, Minn.: American Guidance Service, Inc.

———— and R. WOODCOCK (1970). *Goldman-Fristoe-Woodcock Test of Auditory Discrimination.* Circle Pines, Minn.: American Guidance Service, Inc.

GRAHAM, R. and B. KENDALL (1960). *Memory-for-Designs Test.* Missoula, Mont.: Psychological Test Specialists.

HARDY, W. (1962). "The Causes of Childhood Aphasia." In *Childhood Aphasia,* Proceedings of the Institute on Childhood Aphasia, ed. R. West. San Francisco: Society for Crippled Children and Adults.

———— (1970). *Communication and the Disadvantaged Child.* Baltimore: Williams and Wilkins.

———— (1965). "On Language Disorders in Young Children: A Reorganization of Thinking." *Journal of Speech and Hearing Disorders,* 30: 3–16.

HARRIS, D. (1963). *Children's Drawings as Measures of Intellectual Maturity.* New York: Harcourt, Brace & World, Inc.

HATTEN, J. and P. HATTEN (1971). "A Foster Home Approach to Speech Therapy." *Journal of Speech and Hearing Disorders,* 36: 257–63.

HAEUSSERMANN, E. (1958). *Developmental Potential of Preschool Children.* New York: Grune and Stratton.

HEAD, H. (1926). *Aphasia and Kindred Disorders of Speech.* New York: The Macmillan Company.

HISKEY, M. (1966). *Hiskey-Nebraska Test of Learning Aptitude.* Lincoln: University of Nebraska Press.

IRWIN, O. (1947). "Infant Speech: Variability and the Problem of Diagnosis." *Journal of Speech and Hearing Disorders,* 12: 287–89.

——— (1947). "Infant Speech: Consonantal Sounds According to Place of Articulation." *Journal of Speech and Hearing Disorders,* 12: 397–401.

——— (1947). "Infant Speech: Consonantal Sounds According to Manner of Articulation." *Journal of Speech and Hearing Disorders,* 12: 402–4.

——— (1960). "Infant Speech: Effect of Systematic Reading of Stories." *Journal of Speech and Hearing Research,* 3: 187–90.

JAKOBSON, R. and M. HALLE (1956). *Fundamentals of Language.* The Hague: Mouton.

JENKINS, J. and D. PALERMO (1964). "Mediation Processes and the Acquisition of Linguistic Structure." In *Monographs of the Society for Research in Child Development,* eds. U. Bellugi and R. Brown. 29: 141–69.

JOHNSON, W., F. DARLEY, and D. SPRIESTERSBACH (1963). *Diagnostic Methods in Speech Pathology.* New York: Harper & Row, Publishers.

JONES, L. and J. WEPMAN (1961)."Dimensions of Language Performance in Aphasia." *Journal of Speech and Hearing Research,* 4: 220–32.

KENDALL, D. (1966). "Language and Communication Problems in Children." In *Speech Pathology,* eds. R. Reiber and R. Brubaker. Amsterdam: North-Holland Publishing Company.

KENDLER, H. and A. KARASIK (1958). "Concept Formation as a Function of Competition Between Response Produced Cues." *Journal of Experimental Psychology,* 55: 278–83.

KEPHART, N. (1960). *The Slow Learner in the Classroom.* Columbus, Ohio: Charles E. Merrill, Inc.

KIRK, S. and J. McCARTHY (1961). "The Illinois Test of Psycholinguistic Abilities—An Approach to Differential Diagnosis." *American Journal of Mental Deficiency,* 66: 399–412.

——— and W. KIRK (1968). *Illinois Test of Psycholinguistic Abilities.* Urbana: University of Illinois Press.

KOHS, S. (1923). *Intelligence Measurement.* New York: The Macmillan Company.

LANDAU, W., R. GOLDSTEIN, and F. KLEFFNER (1960). "Congenital Aphasia. A Clinicopathologic Study." *Neurology,* 10: 915–21.

LEE, L. (1966). "Developmental Sentence Types: A Method for Comparing Normal and Deviant Syntactic Development." *Journal of Speech and Hearing Disorders,* 31: 327.

——— (1969). *The Northwestern Syntax Screening Test.* Evanston, Ill.: Northwestern University Press.

——— and S. CANTER (1971). "Developmental Sentence Scoring: A Clinical Procedure for Estimating Syntax Development in Children's Spontaneous Speech." *Journal of Speech and Hearing Disorders,* 36: 311–30.

LENNEBERG, E. (1967). *Biological Foundations of Language.* New York: John Wiley & Sons, Inc.

―――― ed. (1964). "Language Disorders in Childhood." *Harvard Education Review,* 34: 152–77.

LEREA, L. (1958). "Assessing Language Development." *Journal of Speech and Hearing Research,* 1: 75–85.

LIBERMAN, A. (1957). "Some Results of Research on Speech Perception." *Journal of the Acoustical Society of America,* 27: 117–23.

LINDAMOOD, C. and P. LINDAMOOD (1971). *Lindamood Auditory Conceptualization Test.* Boston: Teaching Resources.

LURIA, A. (1966). *Higher Cortical Functions in Man,* trans. B. Haigh. New York: Basic Books, Inc.

―――― (1958). "Brain Disorders and Language Analysis." *Language and Speech,* 1: 14–34.

McCARTHY, D. (1930). "The Language Development of the Preschool Child." *Child Welfare Monograph No. 4.* Minneapolis: University of Minnesota Press.

―――― (1954). "Language Development in Children." In *Manual of Child Psychology,* ed. L. Carmichael. New York: John Wiley & Sons, Inc. Pp. 492–630.

McGINNIS, M. (1963). *Aphasic Children: Identification and Education by the Association Method.* Washington, D.C.: Alexander Graham Bell Association for the Deaf.

McNEILL, D. (1970a). *The Acquisition of Language.* New York: Harper & Row, Publishers.

―――― (1970b). "The Development of Language." In *Carmichael's Manual of Child Psychology,* ed. P. Mussen. New York: John Wiley & Sons, Inc.

MECHAM, M. (1958). *Verbal Language Development Scale.* Beverly Hills, Calif.: Western Psychological Services.

MECHAM, M., J. JEX, and J. JONES (1969). *Test of Listening Accuracy in Children.* Provo, Utah: Brigham Young University Press.

―――― (1967). *Utah Test of Language Development.* Salt Lake City: Communication Research Associates.

MENYUK, P. (1964). "Comparison of Grammar of Children with Functionally Deviant and Normal Speech." *Journal of Speech and Hearing Research,* 7: 109–21.

―――― (1963a). "A Preliminary Evaluation of Grammatical Capacity in Children." *Journal of Verbal Learning and Verbal Behavior,* 2: 429–39.

―――― (1963b). "Syntactic Structures in the Language of Children." *Child Development,* 34: 407–22.

―――― (1968). "The Role of Distinctive Features in Children's Acquisition of Phonology." *Journal of Speech and Hearing Research,* 11: 138–46.

―――― (1966). Theories of Language Acquisition and Practices in Therapy." *Journal of the American Speech and Hearing Association,* 10: 200–201.

METRAUX, R. (1942). "Auditory Memory Span for Speech Sounds of Speech-Defective Children Compared with Normal Children." *Journal of Speech Disorders,* 7: 33–36.

MILLER, G. (1953). "What Is Information Measurement?" *American Psychologist,* 8: 3–11.

―――― (1965). "Some Preliminaries to Psycholinguistics." *American Psychologist,* 20: 15–20.

MOWRER, O. (1960). *Learning Theory and the Symbolic Processes.* New York: John Wiley & Sons, Inc.

―――― (1954). "The Psychologist Looks at Language." *American Psychologist,* 9: 660–92.

MUMA, J. (1971). "Language Intervention: Ten Techniques." *Language Speech and Hearing Services in Schools,* 5: 7–17.

MYKLEBUST, H. (1954). *Auditory Disorders in Children.* New York: Grune and Stratton.

MYSAK, E. (1959). "A Servo Model for Speech Therapy." *Journal of Speech and Hearing Disorders,* 24: 144–49.

NATION, J. (1972). "A Vocabulary Usage Test." *Journal of Psycholinguistic Research,* 1: 221–31.

NEWBY, H. (1972). *Audiology.* New York: Appleton-Century-Crofts.

O'NEILL, J. (1964). *The Hard of Hearing.* Englewood Cliffs, N.J.: Prentice-Hall, Inc.

O'NEILL, J. and H. OYER (1966). *Applied Audiometry.* New York: Dodd, Mead & Co.

OSGOOD, C. (1957a). "A Behavioristic Analysis of Perception and Language as Cognitive Phenomena." In *Contemporary Approaches to Cognition.* Cambridge, Mass.: Harvard University Press. Pp. 75–118.

―――― (1957b). "Motivational Dynamics of Language Behavior." In *Nebraska Symposium on Motivation,* ed. M. Jones, Lincoln, Nebraska: University of Nebraska Press. Pp. 348–424.

―――― and M. MIRON (1963). *Approaches to the Study of Aphasia.* Urbana: University of Illinois Press.

OSGOOD, C., G. SUCI, and P. TANNENBAUM (1957). *The Measurement of Meaning.* Urbana: University of Illinois Press.

OYER, H. (1966). *Auditory Communication for the Hard of Hearing.* Englewood Cliffs, N.J.: Prentice-Hall, Inc.

PERKINS, W. (1971). *Speech Pathology: An Applied Behavioral Science.* St. Louis, Mo.: C. V. Mosby Co.

PIAGET, J. (1952). *The Language and Thought of the Child.* London: Routledge and Kegan Paul.

———— (1952). *The Origins of Intelligence in Children.* New York: International University Press.

———— (1967). *Six Psychological Studies.* New York: Random House, Inc.

POOLE, I. (1934). "Genetic Development of Articulation of Consonant Sounds in Speech." *Elementary English Review,* 11: 159–61.

RINGEL, R. and S. EWANOSKI (1965). "Oral Perception: I. Two-Point Discrimination." *Journal of Speech and Hearing Research,* 8: 389–98.

RINGEL, R. and H. FLETCHER (1967). "Oral Perception: III. Texture Discrimination." *Journal of Speech and Hearing Research,* 10: 642–49.

ROUSEY, C. and A. MORIARTY (1965). *Diagnostic Implications of Speech Sounds: The Reflections of Development Conflict and Trauma.* Springfield, Ill.: Charles C Thomas.

SCHEIFELBUSCH, R., ed. (1972). *Language of the Mentally Retarded.* Baltimore: University Park Press.

————, R. COPELAND, and J. SMITH, eds. (1967). *Language and Mental Retardation.* New York: Holt, Rinehart & Winston, Inc.

SCHUELL, H., J. JENKINS, and E. JIMENEZ-PABON (1964). *Aphasia in Adults.* New York: Harper & Row, Publishers.

SCOTT, C. AND R. RINGEL (1971). "The Effects of Motor and Sensory Disruptions on Speech: A Description of Articulation." *Journal of Speech and Hearing Research,* 14: 819–28.

SHANNON, C. and W. WEAVER (1949). *The Mathematical Theory of Communication.* Urbana: University of Illinois Press.

SHELTON, R., W. ARNDT, and J. MILLER (1961). "Learning Principles and Teaching of Speech and Language." *Journal of Speech and Hearing Disorders,* 26: 368–76.

SHRINER, T. and D. SHERMAN (1967). "An Equation for Assessing Language Development." *Journal of Speech and Hearing Research,* 10: 41–48.

SIEGEL, G. and J. HARKINS (1963). "Verbal Behavior of Adults in Two Conditions with Institutionalized Retarded Children." *Journal of Speech and Hearing Disorders, Monograph Supplement,* 10: 39–46.

SKINNER, B. F. (1957). *Verbal Behavior.* New York: Appleton-Century-Crofts.

SLOANE, H. and B. MACAULAY (1968). *Operant Procedures in Remedial Speech and Language.* Boston: Houghton Mifflin Company.

SMITH, F. and G. MILLER (1966). *The Genesis of Language.* Cambridge, Mass.: M.I.T. Press.

SPRADLIN, J. (1963). "Assessment of Speech and Language of Retarded Children: The Parsons Language Sample." *Journal of Speech and Hearing Disorders, Monograph Supplement,* 10: 3–31.

———— (1967). "Procedures for Evaluating Processes Associated with Receptive and Expressive Language." In *Language and Mental Retardation,* R.

Schiefelbusch, R. Copeland, and J. Smith, eds. New York: Holt, Rinehart & Winston, Inc.

STAATS, A. (1968). *Learning, Language, and Cognition.* New York: Holt, Rinehart & Winston, Inc.

STARK, J. (1969). "Early Language Development and Use." *Journal of Communication Disorders,* 2: 48–56.

STRAUSS, A. and N. KEPHART (1955). *Psychopathology and Education of the Brain-Injured Child.* New York: Grune & Stratton.

STRAUSS, A. and L. LEHTINEN (1947). *Psychopathology and Education of the Brain-Injured Child.* New York: Grune & Stratton.

TEMPLIN, M. (1957). *Certain Language Skills in Children.* Minneapolis: University of Minnesota Press.

VAN RIPER, C. (1972). *Speech Correction: Principles and Methods.* Englewood Cliffs, N. J.: Prentice-Hall, Inc.

—— and J. IRWIN (1958). *Voice and Articulation.* Englewood Cliffs, N.J.: Prentice-Hall, Inc.

VETTER, H. (1969). *Language Behavior and Psycho-Pathology.* Chicago: Rand McNally and Co.

—— (1968). *Language Behavior in Schizophrenia.* Springfield, Ill.: Charles C Thomas.

WECHSLER, D. (1955). *Manual for the Wechsler Adult Intelligence Scale.* New York: Psychological Corporation.

WEINBERG, H. (1959). *Levels of Knowing and Existence: Studies in General Semantics.* New York: Harper & Row, Publishers.

WEPMAN, J. (1958). *Auditory Discrimination Test.* Chicago: Language Research Association.

—— and H. HASS (1969). "Surface Structure, Deep Structure, and Transformations: A Model for Syntactic Development." *Journal of Speech and Hearing Disorders,* 34: 303–12.

——, L. JONES, R. BOCK, and D. VAN PELT (1960). "Studies in Aphasia: Background and Theoretical Formulations." *Journal of Speech and Hearing Disorders,* 25: 323–32.

WEST, R., M. ANSBERRY, and A. CARR (1957). *The Rehabilitation of Speech.* New York: Harper & Row, Publishers.

WHORF, B. (1956). *Language, Thought, and Reality.* New York: John Wiley & Sons, Inc.

WINGATE, M. (1971). "The Fear of Stuttering." *Journal of the American Speech and Hearing Association,* 13: 3–5.

WINITZ, H. (1969). *Articulatory Acquisition and Behavior.* New York: Appleton-Century-Crofts.

WOLSKI, W. (1962). *The Michigan Picture Language Inventory.* Ann Arbor: University of Michigan Press.

WOOD, N. (1964). *Delayed Speech and Language Development.* Englewood Cliffs, N.J.: Prentice-Hall, Inc.

——— (1958). *Language Disorders in Children.* Chicago: National Society for Crippled Children and Adults, Inc.

ZIMMERMAN, I., V. STEINER, and R. EVATT (1969). *Preschool Language Scale.* Columbus, Ohio: Charles E. Merrill.

5

articulation disorders

Disturbances of speech-sound production—misarticulations—are probably the most common type of speech disorder. Most surveys show that the majority of children making up public-school caseloads present "functional" articulation disorders—i.e., there is no readily apparent organic basis for their sound errors (Powers, 1957a). In addition, individuals with neuromuscular impairment (such as paralysis of the facial muscles), orofacial deformity (such as cleft palate), or hearing loss also have difficulty producing speech sounds accurately.[1] The clinician, therefore, should have a thorough understanding of articulation and the disorders of articulation.

Articulation may be defined as an incredibly swift and complicated process whereby the lips, jaws, palate, and tongue modify or impede the breath stream to produce a repertoire of standard speech sounds. In other words, an individual performs a series of "valving" movements with his oral apparatus (physiological activity) producing audible events (acoustic signals) which have a shared significance (perception) for a community of speakers (Noll, 1970). Thus, an articulation error, or disorder, is a nonstandard production of one or more speech sounds.

[1] Might it be possible that the make-up of many public-school caseloads is an artifact of the type of screening tests employed? If the case-detection procedure consists solely of tasks which assess the adequacy of articulation, then only misarticulators will be identified. Further, under the pressure of state special education codes that specify a minimum caseload, there might be a tendency to select presumably less-involved clients for therapy.

There are three basic types of articulatory defects: *omissions* of sounds ("'kool" for "school"), *substitution of* one standard sound for another ("*th*oup" for "*s*oup"), and *distortions* (substitution of a nonstandard for a standard sound). Some writers list *additions* (the intrusion of an unwanted sound) as another type of articulatory disorder; in our experience, additions are generally results of emphasis ("*puh*lease close that door!") or idiosyncratic pronunciations ("I need some fil*um* to take photographs of the ath*uh*letes by the el*um* trees"). Persons generally misarticulate consonants more frequently than vowels.

Mispronunciations are also very common in people who speak English as a second language; but mispronunciations differ from articulation errors in that the former involve "inadequate" or "unusual" utterances of words or phrases, whereas misarticulation is characterized by deviant production of specific speech sounds (Egland, 1970). Mispronunciations can usually be corrected readily by ear, but articulation errors do not yield so swiftly to correction.

For a more extended treatment of articulation disorders, consult the work of Van Riper and Irwin (1958) and others (Milisen, 1954; Powers, 1957a; McDonald, 1964; Carrell, 1968; Winitz, 1969).

TESTING FOR ARTICULATION DISORDERS

The remainder of the chapter will deal with the various facets of assembling and utilizing information on clients presenting articulation errors. The discussion is divided into three segments: (a) case-detection screening (identifying the speech defectives in a large population); (b) predictive screening (determining which children will mature into good speech without therapeutic intervention); and (c) diagnostic articulation testing (determining the nature of the problem, planning and predicting the outcome of treatment).

case-detection screening

Commonly, public-school speech clinicians conduct surveys to identify those individuals with speech defects. The purpose of screening is to select children with significant communication problems by assessing a total population with a brief but discriminating testing procedure.[2] The objective, then, is *detection*, not *description* of persons with defective speech.

A screening test must be swift, yet discerning. The examiner must be able to detect individuals with impaired speech while rapidly passing over all

---

[2] Some speech clinicians rely on teacher- and self-referrals rather than a screening program. The reader will want to review our definition of a speech defect (Chapter 1, p. 2). In what sense could the screening process be iatrogenic? See Project 1 at the end of this chapter.

the normal speakers. Although brief, the detection process should provide a sufficient sample of each person's oral communication to permit critical judgment not just of his articulation but also his voice, rate, and language abilities. Since screening procedures and materials differ with various age groups, we shall describe methods for target populations: preschool and early elementary children (kindergarten through third grade), later elementary children (fourth through eighth grade), and older groups. See also the work of Black (1964), Irwin (1965), and Van Hattum (1969) for descriptions of screening programs used in school settings.

Preschool and early elementary children. There are essentially four ways to obtain a speech sample from a young child:

1. Observe him during free play, perhaps with other children. This procedure is very effective, but time-consuming.
2. Ask him questions. This involves too much talking on the part of the examiner, and some children are reluctant to answer questions (see Chapter 3).
3. Have him repeat words or phrases. This, too, requires unnecessary talking on the part of the clinician, and the examiner's model tends to influence the child's speech and thus does not provide a typical sample. Also, children rapidly tire of being parrots.
4. Have the child name colors, count, and identify pictures or objects. This is the most common method used; it is easy, takes very little time, and children seem to respond well to the tasks.

Most of the published diagnostic inventories cited later in this chapter include portions designed to serve as screening tests for children. For example, the first fifty items of the Templin-Darley Tests of Articulation (1970) are a useful screening device; the authors provide tables of norms which permit comparison of an individual child's score with others of the same age level.

Later elementary children. We generally use reading passages or sentences loaded with the most frequently defective speech sounds for screening children in grades four through eight. The vocabulary, of course, should be appropriate to the child's reading level. Here is a reading passage we devised for screening a group of sixth-, seventh-, and eighth-grade pupils:

> Marquette is the largest city in the Upper Peninsula of Michigan. Located on the south shore of Lake Superior, Marquette is a major shipping port. Long ore boats pass in the deep blue waters each day during the summer; the ships must go through the locks at the Soo to reach ports in the south. Pine trees march up from every shore. In winter the snow is deep and it is very cold. Fishing, though, is good all year long.

We find that children respond better to reading passages based upon their home area; it tends to personalize the routine nature of the screening procedure. The clinician may also choose from among several published reading passages for later elementary children (Avant and Hutton, 1962; Eisenson and Ogilvie, 1963: 185–86; Irwin, 1965: 391).

To obtain a sample of spontaneous speech, we again rely on questions: favorite hobbies, sports, and interests. Verbal puzzles and riddles are also effective but take more time. Actually, we find that later elementary children are often rather engaging conversationalists; they are sufficiently mature to enjoy relating to a new adult, but not old enough to resent being scrutinized. Indeed, they are often intrigued with the screening test and want to know how they have done. We usually try to provide a brief explanation, especially if we note articulation errors:

> Glen, a new fifth grader, distorted the /l/ and /r/ sounds. He put the copy of the reading passage down on the table, looked expectantly at the clinician, and asked how he had done. We told him that he seemed to say two sounds differently from most people and asked him if anyone else had ever mentioned it to him. He thought a moment and then revealed that some children in his last school had called him "Elmer Fudd." He added that his teachers sometimes admonished him to speak more clearly. We told Glen that we would see him later in the week and that together we would look at those troublesome sounds. The complete transaction took less than two minutes, but as we found out when therapy commenced, it had provided closure and reassurance for the child.

Older groups. Reading passages, sentences loaded with consonant sounds most frequently defective, and conversations are commonly used to obtain speech samples in screening programs for older individuals. The clinician can construct a reading passage of his own or use any of the several published versions which include "My Grandfather" (Van Riper, 1963: 484); "Arthur the Young Rat" (Johnson, Darley, and Spriestersbach, 1963: 233); "The Rainbow Passage" (Fairbanks, 1960: 127); and "Directions" (Anderson, 1953: 51).

Perhaps the best way to illustrate screening techniques for older groups is to present a portion of a memorandum which summarizes a program employed in a university:

> A. All students enrolling in teacher education—typically at the sophomore level—are seen individually for a brief screening interview in the speech clinic.
>
> 1. We urge referrals from our colleagues; a brief description of the major forms of speech impairment is sent to all instructors.
> 2. A notice is printed in the university bulletin to the effect that students may receive diagnostic and therapeutic services in the speech clinic without charge.
>
> B. The following reading passage and sentences are used; they are typed on plain white paper which is heat-sealed onto stiff tagboard and then laminated with clear plastic:

Reading Passage

I think I will hitch my wagon to a star, said Johnny Reed. I will show the world I can succeed. It takes more than luck to be a hero. I must try to make haste slowly. However, I will always be full of zip and vigor. Some days it is an effort to stay in the same place. I do not choose to run like that.

Sentences

Snow covered ski slopes.
The early bird gets the worm.
Duluth is the largest port city on Lake Superior.
The feather came off the hat.
She had a face that launched a thousand ships.
Each page of the soldier's journal is exciting.
Take the path to the left for Laughing Whitefish Falls.
We have chosen the road less traveled.

1. After introducing himself and explaining the nature of the screening task, the clinician requests the student to read the passage aloud. Generally, if the student's speech shows sufficient errors or differences, it will be noted during the oral reading. To clarify the issue, the student may be asked to read several of the sentences.

2. Finally, some questions are asked to elicit a sample of spontaneous speech. Queries such as, "What are you majoring in and how did you select that field?" or "If I were to come to your home area as a tourist, what are some things I might want to see?" are good starters.

C. A double filter system is used: senior and graduate level majors in speech pathology interview most of the students. When they hear something suspicious, they refer the student immediately to a faculty member, who then performs a rapid recheck.

D. Two forms are used: all students screened return a small green sheet containing their name, advisor, and a pass-fail designation to the education department. The examiners use another form (Figure 3) only for students who manifest a significant speech impairment.

E. Students judged to have speech problems are enrolled for group or individual treatment in the speech clinic.

The value of a screening program is contingent upon the follow-up. It is an infringement of a student's rights, not to mention a waste of the clinician's energy, to conduct elaborate screening programs unless we are prepared to work with those individuals identified as speech defective. Consult the publication by Peins and Pettas (1963) for an outline of a screening program and a follow-up speech improvement course on the college level.

Problems in screening. We have encountered several problems in conducting screening programs. Here are a few of the most salient challenges to the clinician:

1. THE ROUTINE NATURE OF THE TASK. Screening a large number of individuals makes it extremely difficult for the clinician to establish a genuine relation-

```
                    SPEECH SCREENING FORM

Name: _____  Local Address: _____

Date: _____  Academic Advisor: _____

        Voice Analysis:

        Pitch _____

        Loudness _____

        Quality _____

        Articulation Analysis:

            1.  r _____

            2.  l _____

            3. th _____

            4. th _____

            5.  s _____

            6.  z _____

            7. sh _____

            8. ch _____

            9.  j _____

            10.  Overall diction or pronunciation: _____

        Rate Analysis:

        Stuttering _____

        Comments _____

                                _____
                                Department of Speech Pathology
                                        and Audiology
```

FIGURE 3   Form Used in University Screening Program.

ship with each person being evaluated. However, it takes little time or energy to personalize the procedure; you never know whether the individual being screened might be your next client. Personal comments about a particular item of clothing or the individual's place of residence, a smile, or some small bit of humor can be helpful. When the testing is completed, many individuals want to know the results; it seems only common courtesy to tell them. In our experience, if the clinician is enjoying his job and shows it, if he treats each individual not as a subject but as an interesting and unique person, then he not only makes the child or adult feel better, he also makes the redundant task more palatable (Siegel, 1967).

Avoid stereotyped interactions with the individuals being screened; vary the wording of your questions to reduce monotony. Actually, brief screening encounters can be an excellent source of interviewing practice. Note the personal touch in this example:

> We recently watched for almost an hour while a graduate student screened several collegians. As each new student entered the room, she smiled graciously—and genuinely—and asked them to have a seat. She then introduced herself and outlined the screening procedure.
>
> *Clinician.* I'm Roberta Bolich. We are interested in getting a brief sample of your speech. First, I will ask you to read this passage and some sentences out loud; then I'll ask you some general kinds of questions.
> *Student.* Hey, like what's this for anyway? My grammar isn't too cool!
> *Clinician.* Well, we are not really interested in grammar as such. We're listening to all the education majors to see if anyone has a speech difference—sound errors, stuttering, hoarse voice, and so forth—which might interfere with their teaching. When we find someone who has problems, we set up a therapy program to help him.
> *Student.* Oh, I see. Then it's not really like a test, right? Okay, should I start reading this now?

2. THE TRAFFIC PROBLEM. Try to be considerate when you have scores of children milling around, irritated teachers casting baleful glances, and administrators impatient for therapy to commence. In order to screen large groups, it is necessary to make provisions for getting people in and out of the testing site as swiftly and quietly as possible. In public schools, we have used older children as guides and monitors; it is often helpful to have an extra room or space adjacent to the testing site as a waiting room. We feel that screening tests should be done individually and privately. However, some clinicians maintain that they get more authentic speech samples by bringing in several individuals at a time to provide an audience for each person being screened.

3. FEAR AND RESISTANCE. Young children are sometimes threatened by the prospect of speech screening. We find it helpful to go into kindergarten and first-grade classrooms before the screening and show the children exactly what

we plan to do. Even some college students are apprehensive about the "speech test," and it is necessary to reduce their uncertainty by appropriate explanations.

4. DEFINITION OF A SPEECH DEFECT.   In the past, many speech clinicians were overzealous in identifying speech disorders; even minor speech differences were characterized as problems, and the possessor was urged to enroll in treatment. Obviously, we cannot determine whether the individual has a speech defect on the basis of a brief screening interview; all we can specify is: *does he have a speech difference?* As we pointed out in Chapter 1, we must always scrutinize the individual to see if the difference constitutes a handicap. The proper focus of clinical speech pathology is people.[3]

predictive screening

A significant number of children entering kindergarten and first grade will not have acquired all the normal complement of consonant sounds (Pendergast, *et al.*, 1966). This places the therapist in a dilemma: at least half of these children will mature into normal articulation without therapeutic intervention—but which ones? Some of the children's speech differences are merely the results of late maturation and do not require treatment, but how do you separate the normal speakers from the potentially permanent lispers? Some clinicians simply delay treatment until the fourth or fifth grade (Roe and Milisen, 1942). However, if therapy is postponed for those who genuinely need assistance, it is possible that their speech errors will become habituated and more resistant to treatment; in addition, the child may be educationally and socially penalized if his speech pattern draws undue attention. A few therapists select certain children and not others, operating on an *ad hoc* basis. They then find it difficult to explain their selection process to teachers, parents, and administrators.

The opposite extreme is to work with all first-grade children who present articulation errors. The senior author wrote this memorandum to himself after visiting a public-school clinician in a remote area of Michigan's Upper Peninsula:

> R.'s caseload contains over 30 percent first graders, many of them with minor sound distortions. His annual case turnover is high but he is seeing no young stutterers or children with voice problems; R. said he was too busy to work with those "refractory" cases.

To work with every kindergartener or first grader with a frontal lisp is no solution at all; it is far too wasteful of therapeutic time and energy. A particularly effective local clinician has solved the problem. Here is her report:

[3] Although we have discussed speech screening in terms of articulatory defectiveness, the clinician also listens for disturbances in voice, rate, and gross language impairment.

When I first took the position as speech clinician in this school system, I discovered there were many early elementary children with mild-to-moderate speech differences which, if they persisted, could be potential problems. So, I started a three-pronged program: (1) First, I initiated a preschool screening and parent education project. I see all four-year-olds as part of a prekindergarten check and evaluate them for articulation, voice, rhythm, and language problems. Then, with a few selected children having difficulty, I perform demonstration therapy before the parents. I follow this up with parent education and counseling, gradually turning over the job to the mothers and fathers. (2) We also have a program of speech improvement for all children in kindergarten and first grade. There was some resistance from the teachers at the outset, but when they began to see the results, not only in speech and language development but also in reading readiness skills, speech improvement was made a part of the school curriculum. That has really helped. In 1959 when I first started, there were nineteen kindergarten children with articulation errors out of a total enrollment of sixty-two; last year we had only four. (3) The thing that helped us most, though, was using the Predictive Screening Test of Articulation (Van Riper and Erickson, 1968). I test all first graders during the first ten weeks of class. The test is easy and brief (ten minutes or less), and the results give me a basis for picking those children who need me most. Since we have a high incidence of speech defectiveness in this region, I use a cut-off score of 35. I feel less willy-nilly and more professional when I explain to teachers, parents, and administrators why I am working with Heino and not Susie!

Many clinicians now use the Predictive Screening Test of Articulation to identify children with potentially persistent problems. The purpose of the instrument is stated succinctly by Van Riper and Erickson (1968: 1):

We wish to emphasize that the basic purpose for which the Predictive Screening Test of Articulation has been devised is to differentiate children who will master their misarticulations without speech therapy from those who, without therapy, may persist in their errors. More specifically, the PSTA may be used to identify, among primary-school children who have functional misarticulations at the first-grade level, those children who will—and those who will not—have acquired normal mature articulation by the time they reach the third-grade level.

The Predictive Screening Test of Articulation consists of forty-seven items which were empirically shown to be predictive of articulatory maturation.[4] Most of the items assess the child's degree of stimulability: he is asked to repeat sounds, nonsense syllables, words, and a sentence after the examiner (see Figure 4). Item forty-five is meant to determine if he can move his tongue independent of his lower jaw, while number forty-six evaluates the child's ability to detect errors in the examiner's speech. The final task assesses whether the child can follow the examiner in a handclapping rhythm.

Van Riper and Erickson recommend a cut-off score of 34; they predict that children getting 34 or more items correct are likely to mature into good articulation:

---

[4] The Predictive Screening Test of Articulation is available at cost ($.50) from the Continuing Education Office, Western Michigan University, Kalamazoo, Michigan, 49001.

PREDICTIVE SCREENING TEST OF ARTICULATION (PSTA)

RESPONSE SHEET

Child's Name Lynn E. Birth date 1/19/64 Total Score 36

Grade 1 School Fisher Examiner Emerick

City Marquette State Michigan Date 9/15/70

Record the child's response to each item of the PSTA by
circling the 1 if his response is correct or by circling the
2 if his response is incorrect (or if no response is made).
Compute the child's total score by counting the number of
items where 1 has been circled. Enter this score in the
appropriate space at the top of the response sheet.

Item	Response Corr.	Incor.	Item	Response Corr.	Incor.
Part I			11. SHEEP	①	2
1. RABBIT	1	②	12. DISHES	①	2
2. SOAP	①	2	13. CHAIR	①	2
3. LEAF	①	2	14. MATCHES	①	2
4. ZIPPER	①	2	15. WATCH	①	2
			16. JAR	①	2
Part II			17. ENGINE	①	2
5. MUSIC	①	2			
6. VALENTINE	①	2	**Part III**		
7. TEETH	①	2	18. PRESENTS	1	②
8. SMOOTH	①	2	19. BREAD	1	②
9. ARROW	1	②	20. CRAYONS	1	②
10. BATHTUB	①	2			

FIGURE 4   PSTA Response Sheet Showing Test Results for a First-Grade Child.

140

	Item	Response Corr.	Incor.		Item	Response Corr.	Incor.
					Part IV		
21.	GRASS	1	②	39.	Sentence	①	2
22.	FROG	1	②				
23.	THREE	1	②		**Part V**		
24.	CLOWN	①	2	40.	(s)	①	2
25.	FLOWER	①	2	41.	(θ)	①	2
26.	SMOKE	①	2				
27.	SNAKE	①	2		**Part VI**		
28.	SPIDER	①	2	42.	SEESEESEE	①	2
29.	STAIRS	①	2	43.	ZOOZOOZOO	①	2
30.	SKY	①	2	44.	PUHTUHKUH	①	2
31.	SWEEPING	①	2				
32.	PLANT	①	2		**Part VII**		
33.	SHREDDED WHEAT	1	②	45.	LA-LA-LA	①	2
34.	TREE	1	②				
35.	DRESS	1	②		**Part VIII**		
36.	SLED	①	2	46.	Recognition	①	2
37.	SPLASH	①	2				
38.	STRING	1	②		**Part IX**		
				47.	Clapping Rhythm	①	2

FIGURE 4 Continued.

A cut-off score of 34 minimizes both types of error; those due to children predicted as being able to overcome their errors without therapy but who actually do not (false negative errors), and those due to children predicted as still having errors on third-grade entrance who instead will be error free (false positive errors) (1968: 4).

In practice, the final selection of a cut-off score may vary with the needs and orientation of the clinician as well as the nature of his program. A clinician who wished to exclude from therapy, for example, only those children virtually certain to demonstrate spontaneous acquisition of normal articulation by the third grade might well prefer to use a relatively high cut-off score. A clinician who is able to include only a limited number of first-grade children in his caseload, on the other hand, may wish to employ a cut-off score which is so low that there is virtually no chance that he will be devoting therapy time to a child who may not have required his attention. In any event, the clinician should regard the recommended cut-off score of 34 as a tentative one until he has demonstrated it to be an optimal cut-off score in his own situation (1968: 5).

The senior author tested his six-year-old daughter two weeks after she started first grade (Figure 4). She had eleven incorrect items—all involving the /r/ and /ɜ/ sounds—resulting in a total score of 36. By the end of the first grade she was using both phonemes inconsistently, and at the time of this writing she has completed second grade and possesses normal articulation.

The Predictive Screening Test of Articulation is very helpful; and in most instances, it is a sufficient basis for identifying those first-grade children who need our help. However, clinical decisions are not determined by test scores alone, and the worker is abrogating his responsibilities if he does not also use his professional judgment in selecting children for therapy.

There are some situations in which the clinician may decide to work with a child (and those in his environment) even though the best predictive indices suggest that the child does not need therapy. For example, the parents may be upset with the child's speech, or the child himself may be concerned about the way he talks, or he may present learning problems. The really important clinical decisions are not related to statistics or tests but are based on intelligent human judgment.

A significant amount of research has been directed toward the topic of prediction. The reader will want to consult the extensive review of the literature by Winitz (1969: 254–69) and Project 2 at the end of this chapter.

diagnostic articulation testing

In order to plan treatment, it is not enough to know if an individual has an articulation error. If we are to ascertain the individual's needs and plan for immediate treatment, we must do more than identify cases. Basically, we are concerned with four areas:

What sounds are in error? How many are produced in a defective manner? What type of errors does he have—omissions, substitutions, distortions? Where do the articulatory breakdowns occur in words—initially, medially, finally? Do the errors occur in all forms of utterance or only in rapid, connected speech?

How does the client misarticulate? That is, what are the specific muscle movement patterns that produce the errors? Are there any obvious dysfunctions?

How does his articulatory performance *vary*, and under what conditions does it vary? Does he improve when given a vivid visual and acoustic model to imitate? Does he have certain words or phonetic contexts in which he uttters his defective sound correctly, or closely approximating normalcy?

Why does he misarticulate? Are his deficiencies related to problems in discrimination, retention span, neuromuscular abilities, adequate speech models, stimulation, and motivation for good speech? If so, do these deficiencies perpetuate the articulation errors?

In other words, the diagnostician attempts to carefully describe the client's problem, identify if possible the precipitating and perpetuating factors, and synthesize all these data into a plan of therapy (Carrell, 1968). First let us consider how we go about obtaining a sample of the client's speech.

The initial task in diagnostic articulation evaluation is to evoke a sample of the client's speech. We must obtain a large enough sample—single-word utterance, oral reading, connected discourse—in order to accurately infer his typical articulatory performance.

We inspect a speaker's use of the forty or more phonemes of English speech. A phoneme is a sound family: there are lots of ways to say /s/—soup, blast, kiss—but they still all belong to the family of the /s/ phoneme. These variations are called phones. We don't usually notice any difference until a speaker varies his production too widely and substitutes, for example, a sharp, piercing whistle for the /s/.

The most common way of making a phonemic inventory is to have the client name objects or pictures, read sentences and prose passages loaded with particular sounds, and speak extemporaneously.[5]

Terry, a six-year-old child from a rural area, was seen recently for speech evaluation. Although somewhat uncertain and apprehensive when she entered the examining room, she rapidly warmed to the situation as the clinician sat calmly beside her commenting on the pictures in an appealing book for children. Then the clinician brought out a large hard-cover notebook and opened it at random, revealing colorful pictures in plastic sheets.

Clinician. This is my book; I made it myself, Terry. Aren't these pictures interesting? I bet you know all these things, don't you? Would you like to see all of them? Okay, let's go through the pictures one at a time, and I'll keep track on this piece of paper with Mr. Pencil here. Here's the first one. . . .

The clinician moved through the homemade articulation inventory, starting with items having sounds which children acquire early—/p/, /b/, /t/—and

---

[5] We prefer a method of testing articulation that permits spontaneous responses from the client. The research seems to suggest that clients are influenced by the examiner's articulation in a "say after me" model. See the study by Smith and Ainsworth (1967) and Project 3 at the end of this chapter.

then progressing to pictures evoking more difficult phonemes generally learned at age six or seven (Sander, 1972). On each page of the inventory were three pictures which contained the sound being tested in initial (beginning), medial (middle), and final (end) positions. Pictures had been chosen that were simple, common, colorful, current, real, and reasonably self-explanatory. On the back of each page the clinician had printed the sound being tested and brief comments or questions about the illustrations. The following transcript taken from a tape recording made during the diagnostic session reveals the flavor of the interaction between child and clinician.

Terry: Oh, I know, thatth a thanta tawth (Santa Claus); he tomth at twithmith time and bwingth wotth of toyth. . . .

Clinician: Right! Say, you are really good at naming these pictures. What's this one?

Terry: A bathkit, wooks wike an Eathto bathkit. Do you think there ith an Eathto bunny? My bwotho, Joey, he thatth there ithn't any Eathto bunny.

Clinician: Is that right? Well, I don't know. Look, we have one more picture on this page . . . you drink from a. . . .

Terry: Dwath, thatth a pwetty wed dwath.

Notice from this brief sample (the clinician was assessing the child's production of /s/) how the examiner guides Terry through the task. Praise and encouragement are offered. Sometimes the clinician may simply point to a picture and say, "What's this called?" or he may use an open-end sentence, "You drink from a ———" to evoke a response. It is more effective for the examiner to vary his prompters. Observe also that the child was doing more than uttering single words; in fact, we almost always get a sample of connected speech during the administration of the articulation inventory. With older clients, of course, our procedures differ:

Bill was a high-school senior when he came to us for help with what he called "my damn lisp." In our initial conversation with him, we noted that most of his sibilant sounds were distorted by lateral emission. Turning on a recorder, we had Bill perform the following tasks. First he read aloud these sentences, slowly and then swiftly:

Snow covered ski slopes.
His business was doing absolutely zero.
We each chomped on cheap chocolates.
She had a face that launched a thousand ships.
They took the soldiers before Judge Brown.

Indeed the /s/, /z/, /ch/, /sh/, and /dz/ were all distorted by lateral emission. We wanted a larger sample, however, so we had him read a passage from the school newspaper that he was carrying. Finally, we asked him to retell in his own words one of the "This Happened To Me" features taken from *Outdoor Life* magazine. This led to the discovery that hunting was a common interest and precipitated a rather lengthy discussion of the topic.

The student's first articulation inventory is generally a booming, buzzing confusion of stimuli. For that reason, we suggest that the beginning diagnostician listen for only one sound at a time. Tape-record, or better yet, video-tape

(Burkland, 1967) the session so that you can go back over the client's responses and check your reliability. With experience, you will be able to save time by testing more than one sound simultaneously (Irwin and Musselman, 1962; Fristoe and Goldman, 1968).

Many clinicians prefer to construct their own articulation inventory; we encourage the student to do so. Even if you decide never to use it, the experience of thinking in terms of phonemes tends to give focus to your clinical listening skills. Besides, there is often an intangible appeal to a homemade articulation test, an appeal that might make the difference in some diagnostic sessions.[6] There are several published articulation tests to choose from: Anderson, 1953; Cypreansen, Wiley, and Lasse, 1959; Bryngelson and Glaspey, 1962; Hejna, 1963; Fudala, 1970; Edmonson, 1960; Pendergast, *et al.*, 1966; Goldman and Fristoe, 1969; Templin and Darley, 1970; Ham, 1971; and Fisher and Logemann, 1971. Most of these inventories include stimulus pictures for testing children and structured sentences for older clients to read; filmstrips (Goldman and Fristoe, 1967) could also be employed. Several provide norms against which a child may be rated, and one (Fudala, 1970) features a method for scaling the degree of articulatory defectiveness.[7]

For detailed discussions of articulation testing see the work of Van Riper and Irwin (1958: 48–65) and others (Van Riper, 1963: 229–38; Powers, 1957b: 772–79; Johnson, Darley, and Spriestersbach, 1963: 80–99; Irwin, 1965: 82–3; Winitz, 1969: 237–73).

Making sense of the test results. It is not difficult to administer an articulation inventory. However, evaluating a client with an articulation disorder involves more than simply recording data into neat columns. In order to plan treatment, it is necessary to analyze the information: one must identify the types of errors, discover the location of the error in the communication context, discern if patterns exist, and scrutinize the variability of the client's performance. But before inspecting the parts so closely, we need to look at the whole.

Before making a detailed analysis of the client's articulation, we like to record our general impressions of his total communicative performance. Here is an example from the clinical notes of a graduate student:

> I don't know how Lloyd ever made it through high school. His speech is unintelligible unless you know the word he is saying. When he first came in and tried to tell me his name, I couldn't understand him; he had to take off his freshman beanie and show me the name tag. I made a recording of Lloyd reading "the Bamboo Passage," and here (in phonetics) is how he read the first sentence: "ʊkın æt ə ɔk ʌb æmbo ıt ız ad u ilib æt ıt ız ili ə mɛndʒ ʌb ə æs æmli." He omits almost all initial consonants, distorts the /l/ and /r/, and has several substitutions—he even substitutes /m/ for /p/.

---

[6] As Noll (1970) points out, an articulation inventory is not really a test but simply a set of stimulus pictures designed to evoke a particular word response from a child. The test, in a diagnostic sense, refers to the evaluation process of the listener, not to the picture items. In other words, the clinician is the diagnostic instrument.

[7] See Project 4 for a list of available articulation tests.

At first I thought he had a motor problem—he seemed to struggle a bit—but the more I watched and listened to him, it seemed like he was trying to put in those missing sounds but didn't know how. Maybe he is apraxic? I asked him to speed up, though, and his articulation got worse! He refused to try again. Anyway, I have never seen a case like this before, not an adult anyway. I have examined a couple of children, both around five years old, who had infantile articulation patterns. You know, Lloyd did sound a little bit like those kids.

I reviewed Lloyd's video tape and noticed several other things about his speech: (1) he keeps his jaws clenched tight when he talks—perhaps this is why he sounds nasal to me; (2) his whole posture is rigid and his face masklike—maybe he adopted this style of speaking as a coverup; (3) his rate is rather slow and his voice is flat and expressionless, but this, too, could be secondary to the severe articulation problem.

I think I'm beginning to get the feel for estimating severity. I read the article by Jordon (1960) and I found and made thermofax copies of the crude scales published by Powers (1957b: 778) and Milisen *et al.* (1954: 22). I don't completely understand the Wood Index (1949) or the Arizona Articulation Proficiency Scale (Fudala, 1970), but it seems like a numerical measure of severity would be handy sometimes.[8] Can we talk about it at our conference?

A PHONEMIC ANALYSIS. The first analytical task is to delineate which sounds the client is having difficulty with; this includes several facets and is termed a phonemic analysis (Van Riper, 1963: 221–23). A phonemic analysis identifies: (1) *which* sound is in error; (2) *what* type of defect it is—omission, substitution, or distortion; and (3) *where* the error occurs—the initial, medial, or final positions.[9]

Figure 5 presents an articulation inventory worksheet summarizing the results of an evaluation done with an eight-year-old second grader. The child's production of each phoneme was evaluated by having him name a series of pictures; each sound was tested in the initial, medial, and final positions (the column on the far left represents the ages at which the majority of children acquire the phoneme). Note the method of recording results:

√ = the sound was produced satisfactorily.
− = the sound was omitted.
s/sh = substitutions are recorded phonetically.
x = the sound was distorted; some clinicians recommend delineating the severity of a distortion as D_1 = mild, D_2 = moderate, D_3 = severe.

In the clinician's notes we discovered this cryptic message: *t/s* (I); *th/s* (M); −*s* (F). Can you put into words what the clinician wrote?[10] In order to show how the raw information is translated into workable messages, we now present a portion of the report we sent to the child's second-grade teacher:

[8] See Project 5.
[9] Is it possible to consider all articulation errors as substitutions? See Van Riper and Irwin (1958: 77–78). Is there a medial position? Consult Keenan (1961).
[10] /t/ substituted for /s/ in initial position; /θ/ substituted for /s/ in medial position; /s/ omitted in final position.

Name Ricky S.   Age 8 (6/1/56) Sex M Folder # 63-139
Clinician Helgeson   Date 4/7/63

DEV AGE		I	M	F	Stimulable
4 1/2	k	✓	✓	✓	
4 1/2	g	✓	✓	✓	
4 1/2	1	✓	✓	✓	
4 1/2	d	✓	✓	✓	
4 1/2	t	✓	✓	✓	
4 1/2	j	✓	✓	✓	
5 1/2	f	✓	✓	✓	
6 1/2	v	✓	✓	✓	
6 1/2	ʃ	S	S	S	Yes
6 1/2	ʒ	d	d	d	Yes
7 1/2	θ	t	t	t	Yes
7 1/2	+ʃ	✓	✓	✓	
7 1/2	dʒ	✓	✓	✓	
7 1/2	s	t	θ	-	Yes
7 1/2	z	d	ʒ	ʒ	Yes
7 1/2	r	w	w		Slight
7 1/2	ʒ	x	x	x	No

Key words:

Sounds most noticeably defective:

Sound discrimination:

Vocal phonics:

Oral examination:

Diadochokinetic rate:

Auditory memory:

Hearing:

Other observations:

FIGURE 5   Articulation Inventory Worksheet.

147

As you noted in your referral, Ricky has difficulty with several speech sounds. We asked him to name a set of pictures; the pictures were of common objects and contained each sound being tested at the beginning, middle, and end of the words. We found seven sound errors:

s/sh   He substitutes the /s/ for the /sh/—for example, "sip" for "ship."
d/th   He substitutes /d/ for the voiced /th/—for example, "dem" for "them."
t/th   He also substitutes the /t/ for the voiceless /th/, as "toot" for "tooth."
s   Ricky is inconsistent on the /s/. At the beginning of words such as "soup," he substitutes a /t/ and says "toup." In the middle of words he substitutes a /th/ ("bathkit" for "basket"). And he omits the sound when it is at the end of a word.
z   He is also inconsistent on the /z/. At the beginning of words, he substitutes a /d/ for /z/ ("debra" for "zebra") and substitutes the voiced /th/ for /z/ in the middle and at the ends of words ("buth" for "buzz").
w/r   Ricky substitutes the /w/ sound for /r/—for example, "wabbit" for "rabbit."
3   The vowel /r/ sound, as in "bird" and "word" is distorted. This is why, no doubt, you observed that he sounded "eastern."

Although at first inspection, substitution errors may seem random, further experience will reveal a definite regularity. Which phoneme is substituted depends, in part, on how alike the two sounds are—how much they *sound* alike and how much the *movements* that produce that phonemes are similar. Rarely will the /p/ sound be substituted for /r/; however, the /w/ sound is frequently used. You will want to study the work of Van Riper and Irwin (1958: 68–96) and Winitz (1969: 85) and review physiological and acoustic phonetics. Unusual substitutions do occur. We met one high-school teacher who substituted /f/ for /p/ and was outraged when his pupils laughed when he asked them after each test: "Flease, feofle, hand in your faters." He had a pronounced overbite with very large upper incisors, and it appeared as if he were making a fricative /p/. In the next unit we will discuss this area of kinetic analysis—how the client produces the error.[11]

A KINETIC ANALYSIS. In the last section we identified *what* sounds the client misarticulated. Now we must discuss *how* he is making the errors; what specifically is the individual doing to produce the phonemes in a defective manner? This is termed a kinetic analysis (Van Riper, 1963: 224–26). Let us provide an example:

We saw Robin, a university sophomore, for only a cursory appraisal before a weekend vacation. She distorted severely the /l/ and /r/ sounds, but there was something else about the way she produced the tongue-tip phonemes /ch/, /dz/, /t/, /d/, and even /n/ that had seemed strange. During the long drive, we remembered Powers' (1957a, p. 722) lucid description of the necessary motor requirements for accurate sound production and tried to relate it to Robin's misarticulation:

[11] Study the chart in Winitz (1969: 85). How many units of distinctive feature difference exist between the /p/ and /f/ phonemes? What other sounds might be substituted for /p/?

1. First, there must be *precision* of movement, precision in terms of *placement* of structures [that's part of Robin's problem, certainly]; movements must be in the right *direction* [she seems okay on that score]; there has to be the right *amount of contact surface* [now, there is a major factor in Robin's /l/ and /r/ distortion]; and the contacts between the articulators must be of the right shape [don't know about this, will have to see what she does when I get back].

2. Articulatory movements must also be made at the right speed. [Robin's rate is slow—yes, her specific articulatory movements are rather slow.]

3. The movements must be made with enough *energy* or *pressure*. [Maybe she has a health problem we don't know about, but her articulation certainly is not very crisp.]

4. [Lastly] there must be *synergy* of the sequential movements of speech, an optimum temporal-spatial integration of movements. [Does she put it all together? Have to scrutinize her more carefully but did notice rather flaccid gross motor behavior—and didn't she say something about having trouble in typing class and being generally clumsy?]

It finally dawned on us that Robin was trying to make the /l/ and /r/ sounds with her tongue tip down; and, since her tongue is so low in her mouth and the tip is forward, she dentalizes the other tongue-tip sounds.

We need always to start where the client is in order to help him change. We have to identify what he is doing so that we can alter it. How does one go about making a kinetic analysis? We use three methods: (1) We ask the client to tell us what he is doing. This is the least productive approach because most misarticulators—or for that matter normal speakers—simply cannot tell you what they are doing to produce certain sounds. However, as they progress in treatment, clients should become better informed about what is going on when they talk. (2) We watch what the client is doing. Does his mandible shift to one side when he utters sibilants? Does his tongue tip protrude between his incisors when he says the /s/ sound? What can we see? (3) With our trained ear and knowledge of motor phonetics, we try to duplicate with our own mouth what the client is doing. This is usually the best method of all. Often the client "teaches" us how to make his error, creating an objectivity and sharing that augers well for the outcome of treatment. An example of a clinician's search with a young child:

How do you do that? Let's see. I put my tongue tip out front, through the teeth "gate," right? Then what? Oh, I see, you squirt the air right through that tiny space around your tongue. Now, let me see if I can do it the way you do. How's that? Not quite the same, huh? Well, I have to learn how to do it the way you do so we can fix that sound up. Let's try again.

The kinetic analysis may also reveal obvious motor dysfunctions such as faccidity or spasticity of the oral musculature, and tremors. Indeed, we often perform a kinetic analysis during an oral peripheral examination (see Chapter 3).

The diagnostician must know all he can about motor phonetics, and it would be wise to review several books concerned with this topic. The publication by Carrell and Tiffany (1960) is an excellent point of departure. For additional information regarding the kinesiology of articulation, consult Van Riper (1963: 224–26) and others (Van Riper and Irwin, 1958: 72; Morley, 1965: 210–25; West, Ansberry, and Carr, 1957; 675–76; and Irwin and Duffy, 1955: 31).

IDENTIFYING SOURCES OF VARIABILITY. *Finding* a client's articulation errors and identifying *how* he produces them is only half the diagnostic task. We must also discover what circumstances improve his speech performance. Does he ever utter his defective sounds correctly? Inconsistency is an important clinical sign; if the client can make his error sound correctly on occasion —or significantly shift his production toward normalcy—the diagnostician considers this a favorable indicator for treatment. There are three reasons why clinicians are anxious to identify sources of variability in their clients' articulatory performances:

1. If the individual can make his error sound correctly under certain conditions, then we can assume he possesses normal capability to improve his articulation during treatment.

2. Inconsistency, especially if the client improves his performance when provided a good model, is a good prognostic sign. In our clinical experience, when we can identify sources of variability in a client's speech performance, we generally find that therapy progresses more rapidly.

3. If the client can modify his articulation performance under certain circumstances, we have a place to commence treatment. These correct productions provide a nucleus for therapeutic attention that may then be extended. The morale of both client and clinician is enhanced if some improvement can be made early in therapy.

We shall discuss four aspects of client variability: connected speech, response to stimulation, key words, and deep testing.

Connected speech. Most articulation inventories are designed to evoke naming responses, but not even the most taciturn of persons speaks only in single words. Speech flows—it is a dynamic, overlapping, incredibly swift activity; although careful listening may distinguish separate speech sounds, in spontaneous utterance each phoneme (phone) is influenced by the others that precede and follow it. This is called coarticulation and may extend across as many as four or five speech sounds (Noll, 1970: 289). Therefore, a complete picture of a client's articulation must include a sample of his spontaneous speech. A recent study supports this notion:

> The results of this study strongly suggest that analysis of connected speech describes a person's habitual articulation behavior more appropriately than does single-word testing. A connected-speech analysis enables one to determine the

physiological movement patterns which control both the syllabic and phonetic integrity of the individual's language system (Faircloth and Faircloth, 1970: 61).

We have already suggested several ways in which the clinician can obtain a sample of the client's connected speech; let us simply list some of the most common: (1) oral reading; (2) paraphrasing written material; (3) asking questions and holding a conversation; (4) extemporaneous, or impromptu, speaking; and (5) informal, off-guard spontaneous speech.[12]

Response to stimulation. What impact does the examiner's speech have upon the client's articulation errors? Given maximum attention from the client, can he then imitate the clinician's standard articulation product? Is there some modification in the direction of normalcy, or doesn't his articulation change at all? Consider again Figure 5, which depicts the results of an articulation inventory conducted with Ricky, an eight-year-old second grader. Note the column headed *Stimulable*. To illustrate this important diagnostic concept, we include a portion of the student examiner's protocol:

After I finished the articulation inventory and identified his sound errors, I went back and tested for stimulability. By that time Ricky was getting restless, so I made a game of it. I told him we were going to play follow-the-leader and began by having him model some of my gross motor movements. Then, I started to make some noises, an airplane, a siren, and so forth, and he continued to follow me. Finally, I moved to speech sounds—I started with sounds he could make, the /k/ and /g/—and told him to watch me closely and listen carefully. As you told me, I made the sounds in isolation three times and then nodded for him to imitate my production immediately. He seemed to like this. If he improved with the sounds in isolation, I moved to nonsense syllables and then to words. Anyway, here are the results:

Error Sound	Stimulable
sh	He produced a good /sh/ in isolation, in several syllables ("sha," "shi," "shu", "sho") but reverted to the /s/ when I moved to short words like "ship," "shoot," and "fish."
th	He copied my standard production of isolated syllables and even put them into words. I don't think this is a "defect" as such but rather a cultural thing.
th	Same thing.
s	He can make the /s/ easily, even in complex words like "first." I think we should start therapy with this sound.
z	Ditto. I believe we can correct both of these at the same time.
r	His error changed slightly, from a /w/ to a more lingual sound but only in isolation, not in syllables (I didn't try words).
ʒ	No response here at all, he didn't budge from his distortion. Guess we will need to search for key words and do a deep test.

[12] Is it possible for the clinician to obtain a really spontaneous speech sample free of examiner contamination or irrelevant stimuli? (See Laffel, 1965: 79.)

After we finished with the stimulability test, he still seemed interested in follow-ing-the-leader. So, I brought out the stethoscope and put it on him; he can make an almost acceptable /r/ with very intense and prolonged stimulation but the /ɜ/ didn't change at all. Guess I should have had him explore different tongue positions but we ran out of time.

⟶ Testing for stimulability (Milisen, 1954: 6–7) is an extremely useful diagnostic procedure. If a client can produce his error correctly by imitating a standard model—either in isolation, in nonsense syllables, or in words—then there are generally no serious organic obstacles that would prevent his eventual acquisition of the sound (Powers, 1957b: 779; Darley, 1964: 65).[13] Stimulability is also a useful prognostic sign; clients who can modify their articulation errors by imitating the examiner's standard production improve more swiftly in treatment than those who cannot. Finally, as illustrated in the case of Ricky, when the client has several defective sounds, the stimulability test provides the clinician with a place to begin treatment; it also suggests the *type* of therapy procedures to be used (Winitz, 1969).

⟶ Key words. The clinician should carefully note whether the client oc-casionally uses the correct sound in certain words. These "key words," as they are called, are valuable in therapy because

> . . . they provide for the person a model in his own mouth for the sound we seek to teach him. We can use these key words to help us perceive the character-istics of the standard sound, both acoustic cues and the postures and movements required for their production. They can be used in discriminating error words from normally spoken words (Van Riper, 1963: 231).

Key words give us a starting point:

> Steve produced a defective /r/ on all the items in the phonemic inventory—single words, blends, and sentences. Near the end of the session, however, he be-gan to talk about space travel (a Gemini space shot had gone off that morning) and out popped "rocket" uttered with a normal /r/ sound. We talked further and noted several other /r/ words, all related to space travel, that Steve said normally. Apparently, the experience of hearing these terms repeated again and again in the context of an exciting vicarious adventure, prompted him to utter them correctly. We started therapy with a unit about space travel; we uttered, and had Steve utter, the key words over and over as we pretended to be astro-nauts. We used an auditory training unit to heighten his self-hearing; we had him prolong the /r/ sound as he monitored himself with earphones. Gradually, we shifted to more prosaic modes of travel, railroads, cars, and trucks. We strengthened the /r/ and expanded the list of key words. By then Steve had an internal model with which he could scan his speech. His recovery was incredibly swift.

[13] A similar proposition has been made about stuttering: stutterers are fluent in some circumstances, and therefore they must not have organic impairment. Is this truer of stuttering than of articulation disorders?

Deep testing. We pointed out previously that in spontaneous, on-going speech, each sound is influenced and altered by the phonetic context in which it occurs. Phonemes are uttered differently in the company of other phonemes, even as people behave differently depending upon their circumstances and companions. Most articulation tests permit only a superficial assessment of a client's articulation of a given sound; they provide a small sampling of the many possible phonetic environments in which the case's misarticulated sound can occur. The evidence is clear that misarticulators are inconsistent (Spriestersbach and Curtis, 1951; Curtis and Hardy, 1959) and that these inconsistencies are of great importance for treatment. As speech clinicians we are not just interested in identifying what the client *cannot* do, we must also search diligently for what he *can* do. It is often necessary, then, to delve beneath the surface with a more comprehensive deep-testing device.

Several writers (Powers, 1957b: 778; Curtis and Hardy, 1959; Van Riper, 1963: 232–34) have stressed the importance of more thorough articulation testing. McDonald (1964) devised a sensitive testing instrument, the Deep Test of Articulation, which allows the examiner to evaluate a client's misarticulation of any defective sound in a systematic way and in all possible phonetic contexts. McDonald describes the Deep Test in these words:

> In a "Deep Test of Articulation" the phonetic environment of a sound is manipulated to cause the sound to be articulated as it is preceded by each of the consonants and vowels and followed by a vowel, and as it is preceded by a vowel and followed by each of the consonants and vowels (1964: 129).

Here is a portion of a transcribed session in which the examiner is administering the /s/ portion of the McDonald instrument to a second-grade boy with a lateral lisp:

> *Clinician.* Okay, Tony, we are ready to start with the numbered pages. You understand now that you are to make a funny big word from the names of the objects on the two pictures, like we did in the example "tub-vase," without stopping between the word? Fine! Here is the first one:

1. housepipe	no change
2. housebell	no change
3. housetie	improvement—moderate
4. housedog	improvement—moderate
5. housecow	no change
6. housegun	no change

Note that the word *house*, with a final /s/, is tested as it precedes all other phonemes; the examiner listens carefully to identify any changes in the client's misarticulation. Then, the examiner reverses the procedure so that /s/ follows all other phonemes, thus:

1. cupsun

2. tubsun

3. kitesun

For older clients, McDonald has prepared a series of sentences to be read aloud. The diagnostician will want to be familiar with this test.

We do not routinely administer the Deep Test of Articulation during a diagnostic evaluation of a child. Rather, we prefer to use the test during the initial stages of treatment, exploring with the client for loci of improved, or at least altered, sound production.

A LINGUISTIC ANALYSIS.   In the past few years, linguists and speech pathologists interested in language have provided us with a new way of looking at articulation disorders. For some time, clinicians had observed that children with functional sound errors seemed to be deficient in language skills. Research (Vandemark and Mann, 1965; Ferrier, 1966; Shriner *et al.*, 1969) tended to support this notion. But now, experts in linguistics point out that individuals with articulation defects do not have a "broken-down" sound production facility; they do not, in other words, simply possess an incomplete, happenstance system of speech sounds (Compton, 1970). On the contrary, careful phonological analysis reveals that many articulatory defectives do indeed have logical and coherent principles underlying their idiosyncratic use of speech sounds (Fisher and Logemann, 1971). According to McReynolds and Huston:

> When articulation errors occur, they may consist of a phoneme system organized differently from the adult phoneme system. The more the systems differ, the more severe the child's articulation problem. The child's system may be complete for the child and as lawful as the adult's, but it is his own system, and his rules are at variance with the adult or the standard system (1971: 155–56).

In terms of diagnosis, then, we shift our focus from the child's sound error per se to the underlying patterns his errors follow (Compton, 1970: 319). What are the elements comprising his sound system? What are the rules he employs in using the speech sounds in his particular repertoire?

> A phonologic pattern is defined as occurring when one or more relationships are discovered between phonemes that have at least one major articulation feature in common (Weber, 1970: 137).

We recently examined a child who substituted plosives for all the fricative consonants. The misarticulation of the fricative sounds was viewed as a surface reflection of an underlying phonological principle—the child's system did not include friction as a "manner of articulation." Instead of teaching one sound at a time, we sought to include the principle of friction within his system of phonology. Weber (1970) provides many additional examples in his excellent article on patterns of deviant articulation.

What are the advantages of a linguistic analysis? Generally speaking, there are two: (1) it provides a model for understanding articulation disorders in many children; and (2) it provides a basis for more efficient therapy. We have discussed the first advantage but the latter needs amplification.

Therapy directed toward one sound often improves others that are phonetically similar (Elbert, Shelton, and Arndt, 1967). Considered within the framework of underlying phonological principles, it makes sense that training in features common to many sounds would result in greater improvement in misarticulation than specific training for each sound error.

Let us illustrate our discussion with a case recently seen for evaluation:

Audrey, age four years, seven months, was referred to us by a local school clinician. Her speech was unintelligible. Her developmental and medical history was unremarkable. Her oral peripheral organs were judged to be structurally and functionally normal. Her hearing was within the normal limits for pure tone and speech reception. Her verbal intelligence (Peabody Picture Vocabulary Test) was low normal. Her receptive language seemed normal—she was able to follow rather complex directions. There was some history of familial discord and perhaps reduced environmental stimulation; her parents were estranged and the father left the home for several months, necessitating the mother's employment outside the home.

We administered parts of the Templin-Darley Tests of Articulation (1970) and the McDonald Deep Test of Articulation (1964). We found that the child possessed only six phonemes, /m/, /p/, /b/, /t/, /d/, and /h/. Here is a delineation of her errors:

Standard Sound	Substitution
k	t, h
g	d, h
θ	t
ð	d
n	d

All the rest were substituted by a voiceless, glottal fricative, /h/.

Following the suggestion of Weber (1970) and Beresford and Grady (1968), we examined the child's phoneme system by employing three major articulation features—*place* of articulation, *manner* of articulation, and *voicing* (Fairbanks, 1960: 58) as shown in the following diagram:

	Labial	Labio-dental	Dental	Alveolar	Palatal	Velar	Glottal
Glide							
Semivowel							
Nasal	m						
Stop	p,b			t,d			
Fricative							h

Audrey had not acquired several aspects of the features that distinguish sounds such as place and manner of articulation. She recognized voicing-unvoicing in the plosives /pb/ and /td/, but yet she substituted the voiceless fricative /h/ for all the glides and other fricatives. Her particular phonological system did not include friction, glides, semivowels, and so on. Rather than working on sounds in therapy with her, we concentrated on those features her system omits, following Compton (1970), McReynolds and Huston (1971), and Weber (1970). Finally, we gave her some perceptual categories whereby she can contrast language units: a "hip" versus "ʃip" kind of thing."

Audrey's articulation was viewed in terms of underlying patterns rather than individual errors. Although she was unintelligible, according to our standard, she did have an organized system for using her limited supply of sounds. All sounds can be contrasted with one another by the use of "distinctive features." A /p/ differs from an /r/ sound in at least three ways—*voicing, place* of articulation (bilabial versus palatal), and *manner* of articulation. /p/ is a stop-plosive, /r/ is a semivowel. We decided that if Audrey had several sound errors, all with the underlying problem of confusion in the feature of manner or place of articulation, then we needed to work with her so that she could come to recognize that feature. She would then be able to make all the error sounds that are related to that feature confusion. There are other distinctive features; the best discussion of them can be found in Winitz (1969: 79–96) in the list below.

We made the following suggestions for therapy to the referring clinician:

1. Instead of teaching her sounds, teach some of the features that classify sounds —specifically, teach her the concept of friction as it relates to changes at the place of articulation.

2. Use real words, like "hip" and "ship" to show her how meaning is changed by altering place of articulation, from glottal to lingual-palatal. Teach her to discriminate auditorily in this way in order to enlarge her categories for distinguishing among phonemes.

3. Stress vocal phonics.

4. Use tongue exercises to help her explore the geography of her mouth.

5. Remember how young she is, and once you thoroughly understand what you want to do, simplify everything for her.

The following list of readings will be very helpful:

ALBRIGHT, R. and J. ALBRIGHT. "Application of Descriptive Linguistics to Child Language." *Journal of Speech and Hearing Research,* 1 (1958): 257–61.

BERESFORD, R. and P. GRADY. "Some Aspects of Assessment." *British Journal of Disorders of Communication,* 3 (1968): 28–35.

COMPTON, A. "Generative Studies of Children's Phonological Disorders." *Journal of Speech and Hearing Disorders,* 35 (1970): 315–39.

CORDER, S. "Linguistics and Speech Therapy." *British Journal of Disorders of Communication,* 2 (1966): 119–30.

CROCKER, J. "A Phonological Model of Children's Articulation Competence." *Journal of Speech and Hearing Disorders,* 34 (1969): 203–13.

FLEMING, K. "Guidelines for Choosing Appropriate Phonetic Contexts for Speech-Sound Recognition and Production Practice." *Journal of Speech and Hearing Disorders,* 36 (1971): 356–67.

FRY, P. B. "The Phonemic System in Children's Speech." *British Journal of Disorders of Communication,* 3 (1968): 13–19.

HAAS, W. "Functional Phonetics and Speech Therapy." *British Journal of Disorders of Communication*, 3 (1968): 20–27.

―――. "Phonological Analysis of a Case of Dyslalia." *Journal of Speech and Hearing Disorders*, 28 (1963): 239–46.

McREYNOLDS, L. and K. HUSTON. "A Distinctive Feature Analysis of Children's Misarticulations." *Journal of Speech and Hearing Disorders*, 36 (1971): 155–66.

MENYUK, P. and S. ANDERSON. "Children's Identification and Reproduction of /w/, /r/, and /l/." *Journal of Speech and Hearing Research*, 12 (1969): 39–52.

WEBER, J. "Patterning of Deviant Articulation Behavior." *Journal of Speech and Hearing Disorders*, 35 (1970): 135–41.

WINITZ, H. *Articulatory Acquisition and Behavior*. New York: Appleton-Century-Crofts, 1969.

DYSLALIA, DYSARTHRIA, AND DYSPRAXIA.   Some children who have been diagnosed as having functional articulation disorders—no readily discernible organic basis for their sound errors—may, on close examination, possess subtle neurological impairments. Not long ago, a local school clinician sent the senior author this note:

> I am concerned about some children in my caseload who don't improve in therapy. It makes the youngsters feel like failures to be seen year after year with little or no improvement. Have you studied this problem? How can we recognize those clients with mild or minor physical abnormalities that underlie their articulation disorders?

Prompted by the clinician's concern, we searched the literature for information on the persistence of articulatory disorders. Although we found the cupboard relatively bare (Dickson, 1962; Wilbeck, 1963; Eberline, 1963; Foster, 1963; Palmer, Wurth, and Kinchloe, 1964) we were now sufficiently intrigued to explore the issue as a clinical research project. The following abstract describes the nature of the investigation:

> The proposed investigation explores the variables involved in success and failure of articulation therapy with school-age children. More specifically, the purpose of this research is to specify the reasons why some children presenting functional disorders of articulation do, and others do not, achieve normal speech following an extended period of remediation in school. By exploring a wide range of variables—physiological, psychological, educational, and so on—the ultimate purposes of this study are to: (1) specify subtypes within the "failure" population; (2) determine which variables are the most powerful in the persistence of articulation errors; and (3) create a schema, or profile, for charting the various factors involved in the success and failure of articulation therapy.

Our research is incomplete, but the preliminary results do identify clusters of variables. Although each child had been diagnosed as having a "functional" disorder of articulation, the cases comprising the "persistent" group (those students who did not alter their defective sound production in one school year of treatment) showed more signs of possible organic impairment—including mild or marginal motoric disability.[14] Here is a list of cues, or indicators, frequently found among the children who did not make progress in therapy:[15]

1. Motor behavior on the slow and incoordinated end of the normal range
2. Dysrythmia of tongue movements
3. Drooling
4. Abnormal chewing and swallowing
5. Protruding and retracting of the tongue not accomplished swiftly
6. Reading problems
7. Difficulty attending (frequently says, "huh?" but no measured hearing loss); listening in noise is often even more difficult
8. Reverses sounds, leaves out phonemes in longer words
9. Tends to reverse letters when writing
10. Cannot sound out words (vocal phonics)

We are also impressed with the great overlap between groups on many of the dimensions studied. Differential diagnosis is not an easy task. To assist you in distinguishing between the three major categories of articulatory disorders—dysarthria, dyspraxia, and dyslalia—we include Table 2 prepared on the basis of our experience and a survey of the literature. We urge you to carefully study the monumental work of Darley, Aronson, and Brown (1969a; 1969b) as well as other sources (Morley, 1965: 178–260; Milisen, 1966: 137–49; Carrell, 1968: 74–84; Luchsinger and Arnold, 1965: 715–35; West and Ansberry, 1968: 180–207; Peacher, 1962: 638–69).

ADDITIONAL EVALUATIONAL ACTIVITIES

Diagnosticians often give additional tests to a client who presents an articulation disorder. We shall consider briefly only five aspects which clinicians frequently assess: sound discrimination, auditory memory span, vocal phonics, oral sensory discrimination, and parental attitudes and adjustments. The reader will want to review Chapter 3 regarding examination procedures commonly undertaken with clients.

sound discrimination testing

Some children with articulatory disorders have difficulty distinguishing sounds from one another. Although the research is far from unequivocal (see reviews by Van Riper and Irwin, 1958: 23–36; and Winitz, 1969: 180–98) on

---

[14] Three groups were studied: a group with persistent articulation disorders as defined above; a second group of children who did improve during a year of treatment; and a third group of normal-speaking children.

[15] Items 1, 2, and 5 appear to be the most persistent.

this, there is sufficient evidence to require sound discrimination testing for each case, especially children with multiple sound errors (Sherman and Geith, 1967).

We recently evaluated a second-grade boy who, in addition to having several defective sounds (/s/, /z/, /ch/, /dʒ/, and /ʒ/) was a poor reader. The child had repeated first grade and the teacher told us, "Bernie doesn't know 'Dick' from 'down'." After scrutinizing Bernie's audiogram—his hearing for pure tone was within normal limits—we decided to administer a rather comprehensive battery of sound-discrimination tests.

We wanted to see how the child would do on an *interpersonal* measure of discrimination, and we selected the Templin Short Test (1943) and the Wepman Auditory Discrimination Test (Wepman, 1958). The Templin instrument features paired nonsense syllables that the examiner utters and the child indicates if the pair are "same" or "different." Bernie seemed bored with this task but he made only seven errors—which is well below the norm for his grade level. The Wepman test consists of word pairs (for example, pat/pack, coast/toast, badge/badge) which are read to the client who judges whether they are the same or different (see the research of Vellutino, DeSetto, and Steger, 1972). Again, Bernie performed well, missing only two items (thimble/symbol and clothe/clove).

Recalling the conclusion which Aungst and Frick (1964: 83) reached in their research in sound discrimination, "The ability to discriminate between paired auditory stimuli presented by another speaker is unrelated to the ability to judge one's own speech production as correct or incorrect," and the advice that the clinician should tailor his discrimination assessment procedures to his particular client (Spriestersbach and Curtis, 1951), we moved to more sensitive tasks.

We devised an *interpersonal* test of discrimination: we uttered short words (for example, "sail," "ship," "earth," "chop") twice, once using Bernie's errors and once correctly. His job was to "catch" the mistakes. We mixed the order of errors and correct sounds and used five word pairs for each defective phoneme. At first he didn't understand the task, so we gave him several examples. He liked "catching" us and did very well except for the /ʒ/ list, where he missed three of the five items.

Finally, we concluded the examination with three *intrapersonal* tests of auditory discrimination (Aungst and Frick, 1964): Bernie and the examiner made a short tape recording wherein they both named a set of stimulus pictures. The clinician simulated the child's error on some items and uttered others correctly. When the tape was played back, the child was asked to compare his production to that of the clinician. He missed seven of fifteen items and requested several playbacks of the recording.

We then had the child name another set of pictures (some containing his error sounds, others without any error sounds) and asked him to tell us immediately if he had said it "right" or "wrong." He was unable to do this task, shrugged, and played with the electrical cord on the machine after naming each picture.

After a short break, we listened to the tape made during the test of instantaneous judgement just described. We asked Bernie to tell us which words were said correctly and incorrectly. Even on this test of delayed judgment, he experienced considerable difficulty, missing thirteen of twenty items.

Our projected treatment plan for Bernie included this note:

We must turn on his self-hearing, using a stethoscope and auditory trainer. Adapt some of the procedures suggested for using delayed, simultaneous, and

TABLE 2 Differential Diagnosis of Dysarthria, Dyspraxia and Dyslalia*

	Dysarthria	Dyspraxia	Dyslalia
Definition	Distinct patterns of speech disturbance due to weakness and slowness. Incoordination of speech muscles. Oral movements are disrupted and reflect different types of neuropathology. Articulation, phonation, resonation, and prosody may be impaired.	Articulation errors, in the absence of muscle slowness, weakness, incoordination, due to disruption of cortical programming for the *voluntary* production of speech sounds.	Articulation errors without apparent organic disability.
Medical history	Often diagnosed as neuropathology.	May be apparent or diagnosed neuropathology.	Generally unremarkable.
Development of speech	Generally delayed.	May be delayed.	May be slower than normal.
Oral peripheral examination	Obvious defectiveness: slow, weak, and incoordinated. *Vegetative* functions (sucking, chewing) disturbed, as well as speech movements.	No obvious dysfunction except when requested to execute *voluntary* movement. Vegetative functions performed adequately.	Generally unremarkable. May be slower than normal.

Articulation	Simplification:
	  a. distortions
	  b. substitutions.
	Errors consistent.
	More complex units (clusters of consonants) are more difficult.
	Errors consistent with neurological record.
		Complication:
		  a. transpositions, reversals
		  b. perseverative and anticipatory errors
		  c. fewer distortions, more substitutions.
		Errors erratic.
		Fewer errors in spontaneous performance.
		Inconsistency is key sign.	

TABLE 2 (Continued)

	Dysarthria	Dyspraxia	Dyslalia
Repeated utterance	Same performance.	Makes repeated attempt and may achieve correct performance.	May improve depending on amount of auditory-visual stimulation.
Rate	Deterioration of performance with increased rate. Slow rate of speech.	Performance improves at faster rate. Disturbances of prosody: stuttering-like struggle reactions.	Generally does poorer at increased rate. Normal rate of speech.
Response to Stimulation	May alter performance slightly to match auditory-visual model. Best responses to demonstration of specific articulatory gestures.	Best performance if client sees and hears model.	Variable, may demonstrate normal capacity.
Associated disabilities	Reading, spelling, and writing problems.	Reading, spelling, and writing problems.	More frequent difficulties with language arts than in normals; may be secondary to speech disorder.
Treatment	Assistance in making compensatory adjustments.	Direct training in listening and repeating.	

* Adapted from Morley (1965: 258–59) and the research of Johns and Darley (1970).

anticipatory feedback (Van Riper and Irwin, 1958: 124–31). He has got to learn to scan his own sound production so that he can compare and match it to our standard model (Woolf and Pilberg, 1971).

In some cases, the diagnostician will want to administer additional tests to evaluate auditory perceptual skills. The instruments devised by Goldman, Fristoe, and Woodcock (1969) and Kimmel and Wahl (1970) are useful in this regard.

auditory memory span

A few of our clients with articulation disorders have considerable difficulty retaining information in "immediate memory." In some instances, a child simply cannot seem to attend to a series of items presented auditorily— an ability necessary for the acquisition of speech—and repeat them back. As with sound discrimination, the research on the relationship between articulatory defectiveness and auditory memory span is not conclusive (Winitz, 1969: 178–80; see also the work of Locke, 1969). However, we commonly include an assessment of retention span in an evaluation of clients presenting error sounds.

To test for auditory memory span, the examiner may use digits, speech sounds, nonsense syllables, and sentences of progressively longer length. Items such as digits are presented one per second; the client either repeats the items or writes them down. Norms may be found in various source books (Berry and Eisenson, 1956: 503; Van Riper, 1963: 477–78; Irwin, 1965: 396–97). Baker and Leland (1959) have published a test of auditory memory span that employs words and syllables. The clinician should be aware that anxiety tends to reduce retention span.

Clients with limited auditory memory span experience considerable difficulty in therapy. Happily, however, in our experience specific training in the retention of longer and longer units often meliorates the condition.

vocal phonics

Van Riper (1963: 479–80) has devised a simple test for determining a client's ability to *analyze* (break a word down into its sound elements) and *synthesize* (assemble a word from its component sounds) language units. We find vocal phonics to be an extremely useful concept not only for diagnostic purposes, but also for therapy. Children who do poorly in vocal phonics, especially synthesis tasks, need considerable training in this aspect, along with conventional articulation therapy.[16]

---

[16] We have kept careful records over the past eleven years on our university students, generally sophomores, who have difficulty with an introductory course in phonetics. At the outset of the course, we administer a test of vocal phonics; those who do poorly, missing more than three of ten items, tend to have trouble learning phonetics, particularly transcription skills.

Most children are delighted with games involving mystery or guessing and find tests of phonetic analysis and synthesis particularly intriguing. Here is how one clinician introduced a test of vocal phonics (synthesis) to a young child:

Do you know that I can stretch words out like rubber bands? Watch me say the name for this thing (points to nose) and s-t-r-e-t-c-h it way out: n . . . o . . . z. What did I say? That's right, nose . . . n . . . o . . . z. Now, you did very well and let's see if you can put back together some words that I am going to stretch way apart. P . . . aɪ, ʃ . . . u.

 oral sensory discrimination

Recently, the relationships between oral-tactile kinesthesia and speech proficiency have received considerable research attention (see Project 2, Chapter 3, pp. 77–78). Unfortunately, most of the work is still experimental, and as yet clinicians have no diagnostic tools and procedures for evaluating speech defective clients. However, it is possible to improvise:

We encountered Julie while certifying caseloads in a rural area of Upper Michigan. The public-school clinician had been working with the child for three years —Julie was now in the fourth grade—but with only minimal results. Although she exhibited no gross abnormality of the oral area, her lalling persisted; the clinician reported that Julie seemed uncertain of movements and positioning of her tongue when asked to assume various articulatory postures. Remembering the work of McCall (1969), we decided to do some gross clinical testing of the child's lingual-tactile sensation and perception.

First, we assessed tactile *sensitivity*—could she detect the presence of a stimulus? Using a cotton wisp, we lightly brushed Julie's tongue at various locations; interestingly, she made more errors on the right than on the left side, and her responses became progressively more certain and swift as we moved away from the tip toward the dorsum. Next, we tested for tactile *localization*—could Julie identify the precise spot we touched with a surgical stick? Using a schematic drawing of the tongue, the child attempted to locate the exact point of stimulation. Again, we noted that Julie was more accurate away from the tongue tip and on the left side.

We also wanted to evaluate *tactile acuity*—could she detect minimal changes in stimuli? The only materials we could find to assess this dimension of lingual sensitivity were an old set of stainless steel weights borrowed from the chemistry teacher. Sterilizing them carefully in alcohol, we placed them gently on Julie's tongue (at the midline) and asked her to judge their relative weight. She had no difficulty with this admittedly gross task, nor did she experience any difficulty identifying various *textures* (emery board, eraser, cotton, polished block of marble). Recalling some research (Ringel, Burke, and Scott, 1968) which showed that speakers with articulation defects experience more difficulty identifying shapes orally (*oral form recognition*), we searched about the school for suitable stimulus objects to use with Julie. The only items we could find were some small plastic letters and a number of small bracelet charms. Julie may simply have been fatigued at this point, but she did miss over half the items presented. We had borrowed a pair of calipers from the metal shop to test for *two-point discrimination,* but Julie was tired and we abandoned the evaluation.

Julie was referred to a neurologist, who confirmed our impression of lingual-sensory deficit. The speech clinician altered his therapy with the child to include tongue exercises, point-to-point matching in the oral area, oral object identification, and compensatory articulatory positioning. The child is still in therapy, but at our last visit showed significant improvement.

parental attitudes and adjustments

We must have some information about the parents of our clients. What role, if any, have they played in the child's articulation disorder? Although we quite agree with McDonald (1962) that disturbed families often tend to develop handicapped children, we are not particularly impressed by research efforts comparing parents of articulatory-defective children with parents of normal-speaking children (Bloch and Goodstein, 1971). Only a few parents of cases with whom we have worked actually neglected or psychologically abused their children. There were some evil parents who seemed not to care about their offspring, a few who tormented their children with their own private demons, and some who propelled and pushed them like pawns in the status game. But most parents are simply people with their own distinct needs and interests. We must come to realize that parents are not just vehicles to further our therapeutic goals. When we find those who do have problems that impinge upon our client's treatment program, it is our responsibility to see that they get the help they need; we should not just criticize them and thus explain away our own failure.

The best way to find out about our client's parents is to talk with them (Emerick, 1969). On occasion, we have administered one of the published attitude and adjustment inventories (Schaefer and Bell, n.d.; Wiley, 1955; Roth, 1961; Wyatt, 1964), but we have never felt comfortable using them. We prefer interviewing. The specific areas of exploration will depend, of course, upon the particular case being evaluated. There are, however, several general areas of inquiry: the amount and type of stimulation the parents provided during the child's speech development; the parent's expectations regarding the child's development, particularly his acquisition of speech; the child's communication patterns at home; the child's need for speech; how the family deals with the child's speech difference at home; how the parents have tried to help the child's defective articulation. In addition, the clinician is interested in evaluating the speech models the parents provide for their child.

PROGNOSIS

In Chapter 3 we discussed prognosis in a general way, defining the concept as professional premonitions regarding a client's potential for treatment.

Now we will consider two aspects of clinical forecasting in articulation disorders: (1) determining the most effective place to begin therapy; and (2) delineating factors involved in predicting the outcome of therapy.

Where should we begin therapy? If a client has several sound errors, which one (or more than one) should we treat first? In a real sense, we have already answered this query; the data we obtain by performing the various diagnostic procedures outlined above will no doubt lead the clinician to an auspicious starting point. Let us review the factors we consider in deciding where to begin. On the basis of our experience, we have ranked the factors listed below according to their clinical importance; however, each client must be examined carefully to determine the relative impact each of these aspects will have on his particular problem:

1. We prefer to select the most stimulable sound error.

2. We consider the client's preference: Which sound error does he most wish to eliminate?

3. We determine which sound error, if improved, would make the client's speech pattern less conspicuous. Three major considerations are: the relative *frequency* in the spoken language of the various sounds in error (the /s/ sound occurs more frequently than /ch/); the *nature* of the error (lateral distortions are more conspicuous than t/th substitutions); and the *type* of error (omissions are the most conspicuous, then substitutions and distortions).

4. We like to select a sound that is phonetically easier. The /th/ is easier to produce than the /r/ because it involves fewer oral adjustments.

5. We prefer to start with the most visible sound. If a client has errors on both /f/ and /r/, for example, we would usually begin with the /f/ sound.

6. We consider the norms for consonant sound maturation when working with children. If a six-year-old misarticulates /k/, /g/, and /s/, therapy would generally begin with the plosives since a child of that age should have acquired /k/ and /g/ but not necessarily /s/.

It is easy to present such a list, but it is quite another thing to weigh the various factors and reach a decision for a real client. Turn back to the case of Ricky (pp. 146–48 and Figure 5). Considering the aspects we have listed, determine if you agree with the student clinician's selection of the sound error with which to begin therapy. Many clinicians prefer to conduct trial therapy and select a particular sound—or underlying pattern of sound errors—only after extensive clinical scrutiny of the case.

Prognosis also means predicting the outcome of therapy. What are the prospects for success? We do not have any final answers, but treatment does seem more effective if the following factors obtain:

1. If the client can correctly produce his error sounds when provided a standard model (stimulability)

2. If the client has few errors—the more sounds misarticulated, the poorer the prognosis

3. If the client is inconsistent in his sound error
4. If the client can synthesize sounds into words (vocal phonics)
5. If the client is motivated to improve his speech
6. If the client's mental age is within normal limits
7. If the client's auditory memory span is within normal limits
8. If the client can locate his own errors
9. If the client does not have other speech or language abnormalities
10. If the client's parents, teacher, and peers are willing to cooperate
11. If the client is relatively free of negative personality traits
12. If the client is not receiving powerful reinforcement for abnormal speech
13. If the client can come frequently to therapy
14. If the client shows swift improvement during trial therapy
15. If the client has personal assets from which he derives satisfaction
16. If the client is relatively free from health problems

Again, it is rather easy to prepare lists; it is a far more difficult task to *apply* these variables, weigh them carefully, and then make a prediction for a given client. We have long hungered for a better way to identify patterns in the hundreds of variables involved in clinical success and failure with our clients.

A graduate student attempted to devise such a prognostic paradigm: he prepared a chart whereby the diagnostician could array, under a small number of categories, the various factors listed above. By assigning weights to each factor, and dividing the data into three categories, *motivation, opportunity,* and *capacity,* he felt that patterns would emerge more clearly. See if you can extend and improve upon this admittedly crude but heuristic model:

Motivation	*Opportunity*	*Capacity*
Utility of the speech change	Family cooperation	Stimulability
Cost to the client	Frequency of therapy	Motor ability
Self-estimate regarding probability of success	Distance to be traveled for therapy	Intelligence
History of achievement	Others	Severity of the problem
Current level of aspiration		Auditory abilities
Importance of oral communication		General health and vitality
Secondary gains derived from defective speech		Others
Others		

PROJECTS AND QUESTIONS

1. Can persons not trained in speech pathology identify speech defects as accurately as experienced clinicians? If they cannot, how does that influence our definition of a speech defect? Does group pressure affect listeners' judgment? Review the following studies before responding to the questions:

DIEHL, C. and C. STINNETT. "Efficiency of Teacher Referrals in a School Speech Testing Program." *Journal of Speech and Hearing Disorders,* 24 (1959): 34–36.

MILLER, G. and W. TIFFANY. "The Effects of Group Pressure on Judgments of Speech Sounds." *Journal of Speech and Hearing Research,* 6 (1963): 149–56.

OYER, H. "Speech Error Recognition Ability." *Journal of Speech and Hearing Disorders,* 24 (1959): 391–94.

SIEGEL, G. "Experienced and Inexperienced Articulation Examiners." *Journal of Speech and Hearing Disorders,* 27 (1962): 28–35.

2. Examine how other tests predict spontaneous improvement in young children: The Templin-Darley Tests of Articulation (1970); A Screening Deep Test of Articulation (McDonald, 1968); Carter and Buck (1958). Could you employ the word-repetition task devised by Elbert, Shelton, and Arndt (1967) as a test of prediction? What does Renfrew (1966) mean by the persistence of an open syllable? and of what relevance is this to predicting articulatory maturation?

3. Does the examiner's articulatory model influence the response of a child being tested? Consult the review of research on this by Winitz (1969: 241–44). Can you identify any circumstances in which it might be preferable to administer an "imitative" articulation inventory?

4. Below is a list of published articulation inventories. Inspect at least five of them. Read the study by Shanks, Sharpe, and Jackson (1970) before critically examining the various tests of articulation.

The Arizona Articulation Proficiency Scale. Revised edition. J. Fudala. Beverly Hills, Calif.: Western Psychological Services, 1970.

Bryngelson-Glaspey Speech Improvement Cards. B. Bryngelson and E. Glaspey. Chicago: Scott-Foresman Company, 1962.

Developmental Articulation Test. R. Hejna. Ann Arbor, Mich.: Speech Materials, 1963.

The Evaluation of Sounds: An Articulation Index for the Young Public School Child. D. Ham. Springfield, Ill.: Charles C Thomas, 1971.

The Fisher-Logemann Test of Articulation Competence. H. Fisher and J. Logemann. Boston: Houghton Mifflin Company, 1971.

Goldman-Fristoe Test of Articulation. R. Goldman and M. Fristoe. Circle Pines, Minn.: American Guidance Service, 1969.

The Laradon Articulation Scale. W. Edmonston. Denver, Colo.: Laradon Hall, 1960.

Photo Articulation Test. K. Pendergast, S. Dickey, J. Selmar, and A. Soder. Danville, Ill.: Interstate Printers and Publishers, 1969.

Templin-Darley Tests of Articulation. Second edition. M. Templin and F. Darley. Iowa City: Bureau of Educational Research and Service, University of Iowa, 1970.

5. There are several ways to judge severity. We can use an index (Wood, 1949; Fudala, 1970), a crude rating scale (distortion = 1, substitution = 2, omission = 3), or simply count the number of error sounds. There is even an ordinal scale for rating the severity of a given error sound (Milisen, 1954:

22). But what are some crucial qualitative aspects of severity? For example, a lateral lisp is usually more conspicuous than a *w/r* substitution. See if you can devise a scale that considers several qualitative dimensions.

6. We tend to spend so much time scanning for speech defects that we lose our perspective on normalcy. Study the following two articles:

MARGE, M. "A Factor Analysis of Oral Communication Skills in Older Children." *Journal of Speech and Hearing Research,* 7 (1964): 31–46.

SNOW, K. "A Detailed Analysis of Articulation Responses of Normal First-grade Children." *Journal of Speech and Hearing Research,* 6 (1963): 277–90.

7. Develop arguments both for and against the following statement: "Articulation tests have not yet been developed to the point where specific and detailed teaching instructions may be programmed on the basis of the test protocols" (Winitz, 1969: 252).

8. What criteria should be employed in selecting speech-screening devices? See Nichols, A., "Utility Factors in Articulation Screening: Efficiency of Selection and Cost," *Journal of Communication Disorders,* 1 (1968): 16–25.

9. Design a test of auditory discrimination that fulfills the following three criteria: (a) demands an immediate response from the child; (b) includes self-listening tasks; and (c) interrupts the child's oral motor responses (rehearsal of faulty articulatory patterns) with which he listens.

10. Trace the concept of "functional articulation disorder" in the literature. Start with Powers (1957a: 707–9) and Roberts (1967). Do speech clinicians use the term "functional" in the same sense that the medical profession uses "idiopathic"?

11. Make an abstract of Locke, J., "Questionable Assumptions Underlying Articulation Research," *Journal of Speech and Hearing Disorders,* 33 (1968): 112–16.

12. All clients with articulation disorders are not alike. Are there subtypes within the total population of clients with sound errors? See Prins, T. D., "Analysis of Correlations Among Various Articulatory Deviations," *Journal of Speech and Hearing Research,* 5 (1962): 152–60.

13. Apraxic, dysarthric, and dyslalic individuals are all presented with a lighted match close to their lips and requested to blow it out. Describe their performance. Then, an unlit match is again presented to each client and the request is made to "pretend that the match is burning and blow it out." How would their performance differ?[17]

14. Behavior modification is currently a popular method of treatment in the helping professions. How, for example, would an operant-conditioning clinician evaluate a child presenting an articulation defect? Would he limit himself to the actual articulatory behavior and establish baseline, or level of performance, data?

BIBLIOGRAPHY

ALBRIGHT, R. and J. ALBRIGHT (1958). "Application of Descriptive Linguistics to Child Language." *Journal of Speech and Hearing Research,* 1: 257–61.

---

[17] Dr. Daniel Boone first brought this test to our attention.

ANDERSON, V. (1953). *Improving the Child's Speech*. New York: Oxford University Press.

AUNGST, L. and J. FRICK (1964). "Auditory Discrimination Ability and Consistency of Articulation of /r/." *Journal of Speech and Hearing Disorders*, 29: 76–85.

AVANT, V. and C. HUTTON (1962). "Passage for Speech Screening in Upper Elementary Grades." *Journal of Speech and Hearing Disorders*, 27: 40–46.

BAKER, H. J. and B. LELAND (1959). *Detroit Tests of Learning Aptitude*. Indianapolis: The Bobbs-Merrill Company, Inc.

BERESFORD, R. and P. GRADY (1968). "Some Aspects of Assessment." *British Journal of Disorders of Communication*, 3: 28–35.

BERRY, M. and J. EISENSON (1956). *Speech Disorders*. New York: Appleton-Century-Crofts.

BLACK, M. (1964). *Speech Correction in the Schools*. Englewood Cliffs, N.J.: Prentice-Hall, Inc.

BLOCH, E. and L. GOODSTEIN (1971). "Functional Speech Disorders and Personality: A Decade of Research." *Journal of Speech and Hearing Disorders*, 36: 295–314.

BRYNGELSON, B. and E. GLASPEY (1962). *Speech in the Classroom* (with speech improvement cards), 3rd ed. Chicago: Scott, Foresman & Company.

BURKLAND, M. (1967). "Use of Television to Study Articulation Problems." *Journal of Speech and Hearing Disorders*, 32: 80–81.

CARRELL, J. (1968). *Disorders of Articulation*. Englewood Cliffs, N.J.: Prentice-Hall, Inc.

CARRELL, J. and W. TIFFANY (1960). *Phonetics: Theory and Application to Speech Improvement*. New York: McGraw-Hill Book Company.

CARTER, E. and M. BUCK (1958). "Prognostic Testing for Functional Articulation Disorders Among Children in the First Grade." *Journal of Speech and Hearing Disorders*, 23: 124–33.

COMPTON, A. (1970). "Generative Studies of Children's Phonological Disorders." *Journal of Speech and Hearing Disorders*, 35: 315–39.

CORDER, S. (1966). "Linguistics and Speech Therapy." *British Journal of Disorders of Communication*, 2: 119–30.

CROCKER, J. (1969). "A Phonological Model of Children's Articulation Competencies." *Journal of Speech and Hearing Disorders*, 34: 203–13.

CURTIS, J. and J. HARDY (1959). "A Phonetic Study of Misarticulation of /r/." *Journal of Speech and Hearing Research*, 2: 244–57.

CYPREANSEN, L., J. WILEY, and L. LASSE (1959). *Speech Development, Improvement, and Correction*. New York: Ronald Press.

DARLEY, F. (1964). *Diagnosis and Appraisal of Communication Disorders*. Englewood Cliffs, N.J.: Prentice-Hall, Inc.

———— A. Aronson, and J. Brown (1969a). "Differential Diagnostic Patterns of Dysarthria." *Journal of Speech and Hearing Research,* 12: 246–69.

———— (1969b). "Clusters of Deviant Speech Dimensions in the Dysarthrias." *Journal of Speech and Hearing Research,* 12: 462–96.

Dickson, S. (1962). "Differences Between Children Who Spontaneously Outgrow and Children Who Retain Functional Articulation Errors." *Journal of Speech and Hearing Research,* 5: 263–71.

Eberline, L. (1963). "Persistence of Articulatory Disorders." Unpublished Master's thesis, Texas Women's University.

Edmonson, W. (1960). *The Laradon Articulation Scale.* Denver, Colo.: Laradon Hall.

Egland, G. (1970). *Speech and Language Problems.* Englewood Cliffs, N.J.: Prentice-Hall, Inc.

Eisenson, J. and M. Ogilvie (1963). *Speech Correction in the Schools,* 2nd ed. New York: The Macmillan Company.

Elbert, M., R. Shelton, and W. Arndt (1967). "A Task for Evaluation of Articulation Change: 1. Development of Methodology." *Journal of Speech and Hearing Research,* 10: 281–88.

Emerick, L. (1969). *The Parent Interview.* Danville, Ill.: Interstate Printers and Publishers.

Fairbanks, G. (1960). *Voice and Articulation Drillbook,* 2nd ed. New York: Harper & Row, Publishers.

Faircloth, M. and S. Faircloth (1970). "An Analysis of the Articulatory Behavior of a Speech-defective Child in Connected Speech and Isolated-word Responses." *Journal of Speech and Hearing Disorders,* 35: 51–61.

Ferrier, E. (1966). "An Investigation of the ITPA Performance of Children with Functional Defects of Articulation." *Exceptional Children,* 32: 625–29.

Fisher, H. and J. Logemann (1971). *The Fisher-Logemann Test of Articulation Competence.* Boston: Houghton Mifflin Company.

Fleming, K. (1971). "Guidelines for Choosing Appropriate Phonetic Contexts for Speech Sound Recognition and Production Practice." *Journal of Speech and Hearing Disorders,* 36: 356–67.

Foster, S. (1963). "Language Skills for Children with Persistent Articulatory Disorders." Unpublished Master's thesis, Texas Women's University.

Fristoe, M. and R. Goldman (1968). "Comparisons of Traditional and Condensed Articulation Tests Examining the Same Number of Sounds." *Journal of Speech and Hearing Research,* 11: 583–89.

Fry, P. (1968). "The Phonemic System in Children's Speech." *British Journal of Disorders of Communication,* 3: 13–19.

Fudala, J. (1970). *The Arizona Articulation Proficiency Scale,* rev. ed. Beverly Hills, Calif.: Western Psychological Services.

GOLDMAN, R. and M. FRISTOE (1967). "The Development of a Film-strip Articulation Test." *Journal of Speech and Hearing Disorders,* 32: 256–62.

—— (1969). *Goldman-Fristoe Test of Articulation.* Circle Pines, Minn.: American Guidance Service.

—— and R. WOODCOCK (1969). *Goldman-Fristoe-Woodcock Test of Auditory Discrimination.* Circle Pines, Minn.: American Guidance Service.

HAAS, W. (1968). "Functional Phonetics and Speech Therapy." *British Journal of Disorders of Communication,* 3: 20–27.

—— (1963). "Phonological Analysis of a Case of Dyslalia." *Journal of Speech and Hearing Disorders,* 28: 239–46.

HAM, D. (1971). *The Evaluation of Sounds: An Articulation Index for the Young Public School Child.* Springfield, Ill.: Charles C Thomas.

HEJNA, R. F. (1963). *Developmental Articulation Test.* Ann Arbor, Mich.: Speech Materials.

IRWIN, J. and J. DUFFY (1955). *Speech and Hearing Hurdles.* Columbus, Ohio: School and College Service.

IRWIN, R. (1965). *Speech and Hearing Therapy.* Pittsburgh: Stanwix House.

—— and B. MUSSELMAN (1962). "A Compact Picture Articulation Test." *Journal of Speech and Hearing Disorders,* 27: 36–39.

JOHNS, D. and F. DARLEY (1970). "Phonemic Variability in Apraxia of Speech." *Journal of Speech and Hearing Research,* 13: 556–83.

JOHNSON, W., F. DARLEY, and D. SPRIESTERSBACH (1963). *Diagnostic Methods in Speech Pathology.* New York: Harper & Row, Publishers.

JORDON, E. (1960). "Articulation Test Measures and Listener Ratings of Articulation Defectiveness." *Journal of Speech and Hearing Research,* 3: 304–19.

KEENAN, J. (1961). "What Is Medial Position?" *Journal of Speech and Hearing Disorders,* 26: 171–74.

KIMMEL, G. and J. WAHL (1970). *Screening Test for Auditory Perception.* Johnstown, Pa.: Mafex Associates.

LAFFEL, J. (1965). *Pathological and Normal Language.* New York: Atherton Press.

LOCKE, J. (1969). "Short-term Auditory Memory, Oral Perception and Experimental Sound Learning." *Journal of Speech and Hearing Research,* 12: 185–92.

LUCHSINGER, R. and G. ARNOLD (1965). *Voice-Speech-Language.* Belmont, Calif.: Wadsworth.

MCCALL, G. (1969). "The Assessment of Lingual Tactile Sensation and Perception." *Journal of Speech and Hearing Disorders,* 34: 151–56.

MCDONALD, E. (1964). *Articulation Testing and Treatment.* Pittsburgh: Stanwix House.

———— (1968). *A Screening Deep Test of Articulation.* Pittsburgh: Stanwix House.

———— (1962). *Understand Those Feelings.* Pittsburgh: Stanwix House.

McReynolds, L. and K. Huston (1971). "A Distinctive Feature Analysis of Children's Misarticulations." *Journal of Speech and Hearing Disorders,* 36: 155–66.

Menyuk, P. and S. Anderson (1969). "Children's Identification and Reproduction of /w/ and /r/." *Journal of Speech and Hearing Research,* 12: 39–52.

Milisen, R. (1966). "Articulatory Problems." In *Speech Pathology,* eds. R. Rieber and R. Brubaker. Philadelphia: J.B. Lippincott, Co.

———— *et al.* (1954). "The Disorder of Articulation: A Systematic Clinical and Experimental Approach." *Journal of Speech and Hearing Disorders,* Monograph Supplement 4.

Morley, M. (1965). *The Development and Disorders of Speech in Childhood,* 2nd ed. Baltimore: William and Wilkins.

Noll, J. D. (1970). "Articulatory Assessment." In *Speech and the Dentofacial Complex: The State of the Art.* American Speech and Hearing Association, Report No. 5. Pp. 283–98.

Palmer, M., C. Wurth, and J. Kinchloe (1964). "The Influence of Lingual Apraxia and Agnosia in 'Functional' Disorders of Articulation." *Cerebral Palsy Review,* 25: 7–9.

Peacher, W. (1962). "Dysarthria-Lesions of the Nervous System Causing Articulatory Disorders." In *Voice and Speech Disorders: Medical Aspects,* ed. N. Levin. Springfield, Ill.: Charles C Thomas.

Peins, M. and M. Pettas (1963). "A College Speech Improvement Course." *Speech Teacher,* 12: 37–40.

Pendergast, K. *et al.* (1969). "An Articulation Study of 15,255 Seattle 1st Grade Children with and without Kindergarten." *Exceptional Child,* 33: 541–47.

Powers, M. (1957a). "Functional Disorders of Articulation—Symptomatology and Etiology." In *Handbook of Speech Pathology,* ed. L. Travis. New York: Appleton-Century-Crofts.

———— (1957b). "Clinical and Educational Procedures in Functional Disorders of Articulation." In *Handbook of Speech Pathology,* ed. L. Travis. New York: Appleton-Century-Crofts.

Renfrew, C. (1966). "Persistence of the Open Syllable in Defective Articulation." *Journal of Speech and Hearing Disorders,* 31: 370–73.

Ringel, R., K. Burke, and C. Scott (1958). "Tactile Perception: Form Discrimination in the Mouth." *British Journal of Disorders of Communication,* 3: 150–55.

ROBERTS, D. (1967). "The Term Dyslalia: Its Uses and Value." *Journal of the Australian College of Speech Therapists,* 17: 44–52.

ROE, V. and R. MILISEN (1942). "The Effect of Maturation upon Defective Articulation in Elementary Grades." *Journal of Speech and Hearing Disorders,* 7: 37–50.

ROTH, R. (1961). *The Mother-Child Relationship Evaluation.* Beverly Hills, Calif.: Western Psychological Services.

SANDER, E. (1972). "When Are Speech Sounds Learned?" *Journal of Speech and Hearing Disorders,* 37: 55–63.

SCHAEFER, E. and R. Q. BELL (n.d.). *Parental Attitude Research Instruments and Normative Data.* Bethesda, Md.: National Institute of Mental Health.

SHANKS, S., M. SHARPE, and B. JACKSON (1970). "Spontaneous Responses of First-grade Children to Diagnostic Picture Articulation Tests." *Journal of Communication Disorders,* 3: 106–17.

SHERMAN, D. and A. GEITH (1967). "Speech Sound Discrimination and Articulation Skill." *Journal of Speech and Hearing Research,* 10: 277–80.

SHRINER, T. *et al.* (1969). "The Relationship Between Articulation Defects and Syntax in Speech Defective Children." *Journal of Speech and Hearing Research,* 12: 319–25.

SIEGEL, G. (1967). "Interpersonal Approach to the Study of Communication Disorders." *Journal of Speech and Hearing Disorders,* 32: 112–20.

SMITH, M. and S. AINSWORTH (1967). "The Effect of Three Types of Stimulation of Articulatory Responses of Speech Defective Children." *Journal of Speech and Hearing Research,* 10: 333–38.

SPRIESTERSBACH, D. and J. CURTIS (1951). "Misarticulation and Discrimination of Speech Sounds." *Quarterly Journal of Speech,* 37: 483–91.

TEMPLIN, M. (1943). "A Study of Sound Discrimination Ability of Elementary School Pupils." *Journal of Speech and Hearing Disorders,* 8: 132.

TEMPLIN, M. and F. DARLEY (1970). *The Templin-Darley Tests of Articulation* 2nd ed. Iowa City: University of Iowa Bureau of Educational Research and Service.

VANDEMARK, A. and M. MANN (1965). "Oral Language Skills of Children with Defective Articulation." *Journal of Speech and Hearing Research,* 8: 409–14.

VAN HATTUM, R., ed. (1969). *Clinical Speech in the Schools: Organization and Management.* Springfield, Ill.: Charles C Thomas.

VAN RIPER, C. (1963). *Speech Correction: Principles and Methods,* 4th ed. Englewood Cliffs, N.J.: Prentice-Hall, Inc.

———— and R. ERICKSON (1968). *Predictive Screening Test of Articulation.* Kalamazoo, Mich.: Western Michigan University Press.

VAN RIPER, C. and J. IRWIN (1958). *Voice and Articulation.* Englewood Cliffs, N.J.: Prentice-Hall, Inc.

VELLUTINO, E., L. DeSETTO, and J. STEGER (1972). "Categorical Judgment and the Wepman Test of Auditory Discrimination." *Journal of Speech and Hearing Disorders,* 37: 252–57.

WEBER, J. (1970). "Patterning of Deviant Articulation Behavior." *Journal of Speech and Hearing Disorders,* 35: 135–41.

WEPMAN, J. (1958). *Auditory Discrimination Test.* Chicago: Language Research Associates.

WEST, R. and M. ANSBERRY (1968). *The Rehabilitation of Speech,* 4th ed. New York: Harper & Row, Publishers.

———— and A. CARR (1957). *The Rehabilitation of Speech,* 3rd ed. New York: Harper & Row, Publishers.

WILBECK, M. (1963). "An Investigation of Certain Factors in Children with Persistent Functional Articulation Disorders." Unpublished Master's thesis, University of Houston.

WILEY, J. H. (1955). "A Scale to Measure Parental Attitudes." *Journal of Speech and Hearing Disorders,* 20: 284–90.

WINITZ, H. (1969). *Articulatory Acquisition and Behavior.* New York: Appleton-Century-Crofts.

WOOLF, G. and R. PILBERG (1971). "A Comparison of Three Tests of Auditory Discrimination and Their Relationship to Performance on a Deep Test of Articulation." *Journal of Communication Disorders,* 3: 239–49.

WOOD, K. (1949). "Measurement of Progress in the Correction of Articulatory Speech Defects." *Journal of Speech and Hearing Disorders,* 14: 171–74.

WYATT, G. (1964). *Language Learning and Communication Disorders in Children.* New York: The Free Press.

6

stuttering

Stuttering is a baffling disorder for both client and clinician. It is amazing that such an ancient, universal, and obvious human problem should defy precise description; despite countless scientific investigations, the basic nature and cause of stuttering still remain a mystery.

It has been our experience that most clinicians diligently seek information about stuttering by attending conferences, searching for descriptions of ongoing therapy, and requesting to observe master clinicians treating clients. Perhaps this is a good place to review the fund of reliable truth we do possess on stuttering.

Sifting through the huge mounds of written material to find facts about stuttering is like sluicing poor placer dirt: the reader has to do an incredible amount of winnowing before even small specks of truth emerge (Hoffer, 1969). Perhaps revealing more temerity than good sense, we present below a list of "facts" about stuttering gleaned from the literature and an extensive clinical practice. For purposes of exposition we have eschewed lengthy lists of references. Each item can be documented, however, even though some might disagree with our particular selection or interpretation:

Characteristics - "Facts" about stuttering

1. Stuttering as a disorder has existed throughout recorded history (and probably before).
2. Stuttering is found among all peoples of the world; its relative incidence

and its forms vary across cultures (the most commonly reported incidence in the United States is slightly less than 1 percent).

3. Stuttering is a disorder of childhood, generally having its onset before the age of six; rarely does it begin in older persons, and when it does it may be a distinct subtype of the disorder (for example, neurotic stuttering).

4. Stuttering is found more frequently among males.

5. The overt characteristics of stuttering tend to be more severe among males.

→ 6. Stuttering exhibits a familial incidence pattern.

7. Stuttering may be precipitated (and perpetuated) by certain environmental events, particularly the impact of significant others—usually the parents.

8. Stuttering tends to appear more frequently in children described as "sensitive," who may be more vulnerable or susceptible to stress.

9. Stuttering tends to appear more frequently in children who were slower in acquiring speech or who manifested speech inadequacies (articulation errors) other than fluency breakdowns.

10. Stuttering, in its developed state, has both overt and covert dimensions.

11. Stuttering is intermittent in occurrence. Many stutterers exhibit a decrease in blocking with repeated oral readings of the same material; moments of stuttering tend also to occur consistently on particular words.

12. The basic speech characteristics of stuttering consist of part-word repetitions (phonemic, syllabic) and prolongations. These oscillations and fixations may be audible or silent and tend to occur more frequently at the beginning of an utterance and on longer words.

13. Stuttering tends to change in form and severity as the individual matures.

14. Stuttering tends to exhibit cycles of frequency and severity in a given individual.

15. Stuttering is apparently "outgrown" by a significant number of individuals.

16. Stuttering, in its developed form, consists largely of escape and avoidance behavior; that is, much of the overt abnormality results from the individual's attempt to cope with the emission of the basic speech characteristics described in Number 12.

17. Stuttering is also characterized by speech and voice abnormalities other than dysfluency—narrow pitch range, vocal tension, lack of vocal expression —which can be detected in nonstuttered speech.

18. Stuttering, in its developed form, is often associated with an expectancy or anticipation of its occurrence.

19. Stuttering is a personal problem; individuals who stutter report fear, frustration, social penalties, dissatisfaction with themselves, lower level of aspiration, felt loss of social esteem. There is a tendency for problems common to all human beings to become associated with the speech disturbance.

20. Stuttering is a social-psychological event. The acoustic and visual phenomena that occur during the motor act of stuttering are noxious stimuli in a communicative context, and listeners tend to react in various explicit or implicit ways. The stutterer tends in turn to react to these listener responses.

For more detailed discussions of stuttering, the reader should consult the work of Van Riper (1971) and others (Beech and Fransella, 1968; Bloodstein, 1969; Sheehan, 1970; Emerick and Hamre, 1972.) We now turn to a controversial but important consideration: is it possible to identify types of fluency disorders? Does the diagnostic label *stuttering* impart a linguistic unity to a disorder that may encompass several disparate types of fluency disturbances?

Stuttering wears a variety of sad and confining disguises. Although the research is negligible in this area, clinically we have seen several distinct subtypes—for example, interiorized and exteriorized stutterers (Douglass and Quarrington, 1952), predominantly clonic and predominantly tonic stutterers, clients who feature escape techniques, and those who are addicted to avoidance. We find these distinctions useful in planning therapy. Several observers have noted and attempted to classify subgroups of stutterers but, as yet, no one system has been accorded widespread acceptance (see Project 1).

For differential diagnosis, we are concerned not only with types of stutterers but also with varieties of fluency disturbance. There are several kinds of fluency breakdowns that can be confused with stuttering. In our clinical experience we have seen individuals with five rather distinct forms of abnormal disfluency:

5 Forms of Abnormal Disfluency

1. *Episodic stress reaction.*   It is well known that most speakers exhibit some degree of disfluency—revisions, interjections, word and phrase repetitions, and the like. Furthermore, everyone occasionally stutters (part-word repetitions and prolongations) at some point. Stress, particularly communicative stress, tends to increase a speaker's disfluency; Van Riper (1963) speculates that there is a positive relationship between communicative stress and progressive deterioration of speech:

> With minor stress, repetitions of sentences or phrases occur; with more stress, words are repeated; with even more pressure, the oscillating occurs on syllables. When complete disruption occurs but the urge to speak still remains, first prolongations of an audible sound ("mmmmmmother") are shown and finally even this breaks down to a silent posture (Van Riper, 1963: 320).

Other forms of stress, such as battle conditions (Gavis, 1964; Grinker and Spiegal, 1945) or intense excitement, can also precipitate a fluency breakdown.

Fluency breakdowns due to episodic stress show a number of consistent identifying features: an acknowledged source of intense or prolonged stimulation; tension overflow throughout the body (including the oral area), which may also produce a tremulous voice; an exacerbation of "normal" disfluency —broken words, incomplete phrases, interjections, repetitions of whole words; some part-word repetitions, usually syllabic but always with the correct vowel, never with the /ə/ vowel replacement; no avoidance, fear, rarely any penalty —perhaps some embarrassment after the incident is over. Finally, the most crucial characteristic is that the disfluency decreases markedly or stops when (or shortly after) the stress terminates. It is likely that all but the most stoic of persons have experienced an episodic fluency breakdown.

—> 2. *Neurotic or hysterical stuttering.*   Most stutterers, particularly confirmed adult cases, acquire a negative feeling tone about their problem.[1] One of our clients summarized it succinctly when he said, "Stutterers are bugged because they are plugged." A few stutterers, however, show symptoms of a primary neurosis—they are "plugged because they are bugged." For these individuals, stuttering is a maladaptive solution to an acute psychological problem:

> Colleen, an eighth-grade parochial-school pupil, began to stutter suddenly following the death of her parents in an automobile accident. She collapsed upon hearing the tragic news and remained mute, almost transfixed and catatonic, for several hours. During the planning for the funeral and the extended period of the wake, she started to stutter—a monotonous repetition of the initial syllable of words. She showed no struggle, no avoidance behavior. She looked directly at the auditor when she spoke and smiled bravely. We followed this case closely until the remission of stuttering two months later, and her disfluency was always the same—it never varied in form or severity from situation to situation. When she read a passage several times, she did not show the typical reduction (adaptation) in stuttering. School documents, as well as interviews with several relatives, indicated that Colleen had had no prior speech difficulty. One maternal aunt whom we interviewed did recall, however, that the girl had several "spells" of uncontrolled weeping and laughing during her first menses a year before. The child had received an incredible amount of attention and solace after her parents' death—perhaps even more so because of her "stuttering—from sympathetic adults.

Neurotic stuttering is characterized by a sudden onset (often in an older child), a monosymptomatic speech pattern, little situational variation, and seeming unconcern or indifference; the individual may be experiencing chronic stress or a sudden acute emotional upheaval; there may be a history of neurotic symptoms (Van Riper and Gruber, 1957: 16; Freund, 1966: 139–40).

—> 3. *Fluency breakdowns following brain injury.*   We have observed disfluency in clients suffering from Parkinson's disease, some types of cerebral palsy, and other neurological impairments. Several aphasics with whom we have worked, particularly those clients who show good progress in word-finding but have residual syntactic difficulty, exhibited fluency breakdowns superficially similar to stuttering:

> Miss Horn had suffered an aneurysm in the Circle of Willis leaving her hemiplegic, apraxic, and with mild expressive aphasia. When we examined her, almost a year after the cerebral vascular episode, her speech pattern resembled clonic stuttering. She would begin a word, repeat a phoneme or syllable several

[1] Wingate (1971) dismisses the fear component in stuttering with a gratuitous admission that it may be a factor in some cases. It is easy to disregard fear as an essential feature of stuttering since quite a few clients deny it themselves. "It doesn't bother me" is a common remark. However, the verbal denials are often contradicted by a client's behavior once a trusting clinical relationship is developed.

times, back up and try again; if blocked once more, a repetition might rever-
berate almost endlessly. She frequently pounded on the table as if to time her
utterances. We could discern no evidence of fear or avoidance, just severe frustration. Interestingly, when she spoke or read swiftly her fluency increased
dramatically; she also talked quite freely when distracted from closely monitoring the act of speaking. Here is a sample of her speech taken from a tape recording during a group therapy session: "I can't—I can't (sigh) . . . I-I-I-I have tr-
trouble with my, ah, with my speech . . . and, ah, my leg is, is, you know,
stiff. . . ."

The disfluencies noted are rather typical—whole-word repetitions, revisions,
interjections, broken words, gaps in the flow of speech. This client had difficulty formulating messages and then programming the proper motor sequences to utter the thought; unlike stutterers who have difficulty getting
started, Miss Horn's fluency breakdowns occurred at any point in a sentence
(see Luchsinger and Arnold, 1965: 711).

→ 4. *Stuttering among the retarded.* Some observers have reported a
rather high prevalence of stuttering among mentally retarded, especially mongoloid, children (Van Riper, 1971: 42–45). We are frankly puzzled by these
reports since our experience agrees quite closely with the findings of Sheehan, Martyn, and Kilburn (1968) and Martyn, Sheehan, and Slutz (1969). We
found only one stutterer in a population of 217 severely retarded children
(ages four to twelve) in a residential hospital. It was our impression that the
group of children evaluated, which included a large number with Down's
syndrome, simply did not have a sufficient flow of speech on which to stutter;
the majority were limited to one- or two-word utterances or an assortment
of unintelligible grunts. Interestingly, we did observe stuttering emerge in
two mongoloid children during a language-building program.

We have seen several stutterers among public-school special education
("educable") pupils; it is our impression that the relative incidence of stuttering in this group is similar to that in most published surveys for normal
school-age populations. Their stuttering behavior exhibited the following
characteristics: (1) an uncomplicated, typically clonic or repetitive, pattern;
(2) little word or sound fear; (3) no anticipation of difficulty—most of these
clients showed little awareness of their disfluency; and (4) almost no avoidance behavior (except sullen withdrawal). Frustration and struggle were the
predominant features. These children responded best to a treatment program
that stressed a direct attack on the motor act of stuttering, employing mirror
work and imitation of the clinician.

→ 5. *Cluttering.* Cluttering is sometimes confused with stuttering:

Ralph was referred to us as a stutterer by his critic teacher during his semester
of student teaching. When we examined him, he revealed no fears or avoid-
ances, exhibited only a few part-word repetitions, and had no fixations; he said

that he enjoyed talking, did a lot of it, and that he was asked frequently to repeat, "especially when I talk fast." His speech was swift and jumbled, it emerged
in rapid torrents until he jammed up, and then he surged pell mell on again in
another staccato outburst. In spontaneous talking, his message was characterized
by disorganized sentences; he would start to tell us something, lose the train of
thought, and then change the content in midsentence. He slurred sounds and
omitted and transposed words and phrases; he said "plobably," "posed," and
"pacific" for "probably," "supposed," and "specific." He gave the overall impression of being in haste. When we asked him to slow down and speak carefully, there was a dramatic improvement, but he soon forgot our admonishment
and reverted to his hurried, disorganized style. Ralph was an impatient, impul-
sive young man, always on the go. His course work was characteristically done
in a great, almost compulsive, rush.

The distinguishing features of cluttering and stuttering have been succinctly summarized by Weiss (1964, see particularly p. 69) and Freund (1966:
140–44). The diagnostician should be aware, however, that some stutterers
may also exhibit features associated with cluttering; and it may be necessary
to determine which fluency problem is primary (generally cluttering) or the
most problematical.

Each of the fluency disorders described above requires distinctly different clinical management, even though the objective distortion of the speech
signal may be somewhat similar. The diagnostician must keep in mind that a
speech disorder involves more than a disturbance in the acoustic characteristics of an individual's oral output (see Project 2).

In order to better reveal the diagnostician in action, the remainder of
the present chapter will be devoted to case presentations. We shall describe
the assessment of a young child reportedly beginning to stutter, the evaluation
of the school-age child, and conclude with a lengthy case study of an adult
client.

EVALUATION AT THE ONSET OF STUTTERING

Experienced clinicians agree that the problem of stuttering is much easier
to prevent in children than to treat in chronic adult clients. Indeed, the
early detection and management of children beginning to stutter is one of the
most significant contributions a speech clinician can make. The diagnostician
must seek answers for a great many questions: Is the child stuttering? If he is
stuttering, how far has the disorder progressed? When did it begin? What
factors were associated with the onset of the problem? How aware is the child
that his speech is blocked? How do listeners attempt to help him, and how
does he respond to their efforts? How can we alter the child's environment to
prevent the problem from getting worse?

Throughout this volume we have repeatedly suggested that diagnosis
and therapy are not separate undertakings. The careful assessment of a

client's problem is often therapeutic; only by working with an individual for a period of time do we truly come to know the dimensions of his problem. This is particularly true in the management of children beginning to stutter. In order to illustrate the activities of the diagnostician-therapist, we present below a case study of a four-year-old child brought to the clinic as an "incipient" stutterer. Our account is chronological and reports what was done from the initial contact to the termination of treatment.

the case of Craig Ryan

Late one day in midsummer we received a call from an anxious parent. Mrs. Ryan had that afternoon consulted a local pediatrician about her son, Craig, who, she said, was beginning to stutter. The physician conducted a physical examination and then suggested that the mother call the speech clinic.[2] Mrs. Ryan told us that her four-year-old son had begun to stutter six weeks before, during the time that several guests were staying at the house. She continued:

> It seems to come and go—one day he will be talking fine and the next day he may have a lot of trouble. At first we just ignored it, but when he kept on stuttering we—me, mainly—asked him to "slow down" and "take it easy." He seems to get very upset when I do that, and the other day he told me that he couldn't talk. What can we do?

We agree with Wyatt (1969) that the onset of stuttering is a crisis situation in which swift intervention is absolutely essential. Accordingly, we hastily revised our appointments and promised to see Mrs. Ryan and Craig at 9:00 the next morning. We praised her for calling and suggested that Craig did not need to know the real purpose of the visit to the speech clinic; we advised her to simply tell him that she had to see some people at the university and he could come along and play a few of the interesting games they had for children.

In planning for the assessment, we assigned an undergraduate student to observe Craig and Mrs. Ryan in the clinic waiting room. He was to unobtrusively watch the parent-child interaction and submit a descriptive report to us before we interviewed the mother. Here is what he wrote:

> Mrs. Ryan gave Craig several things to play with—a puzzle, a little box with toy animals in it, and a number of picture books—that she had apparently brought

---

[2] In many cases the physician is the first professional to be consulted (Emerick and Teigland, 1965). We had contacted each pediatrician in the community personally, discussed briefly the onset of stuttering, and outlined the role of the speech pathologist in dealing with the problem. We enlisted their support in the early identification of children beginning to stutter and gave them a pamphlet that covered the subject.

with her. I didn't hear any speech breaks. But, then, he didn't talk very much; it didn't seem like he had to in that situation. He did make some car noises. Once he wandered down the hall toward the speech science lab and she called him back. He obeyed quickly.

Before examining a child individually, we like to chat informally with both the youngster and the parent. We do this primarily to observe if the parents are reacting in an overt way to the child's speech. When the child is asked a question, do the parents attempt to answer for him? Do they point out instances of stuttering to the examiner? Do they signal their presence by non-verbal behavior—gestures, postures, and the like? How does the child respond to this? We made a brief tour of the speech clinic, ignoring Craig and chatting with Mrs. Ryan. Ushering them into a playroom, we invited the child to sample the toys while we talked with his mother. Gradually, we edged closer to the boy and casually began to join his play, commenting on what his cars were doing and asking him some questions. Soon he was chattering to the clinician. No disfluency was observed until Craig, wishing to direct the examiner's steam shovel, uttered the word "I" with five easy rhythmical repetitions. Mrs. Ryan leaned forward in her chair and nodded toward us. Craig did not appear to notice either his disfluency or his mother's nonverbal cue. Would his speech change if his mother left? How would he respond to stress?

On a prearranged signal, a graduate student came in and asked Mrs. Ryan if she would like to see the rest of the "school." Craig glanced up briefly as his mother left but continued playing and talking with the examiner. No increase in disfluency was noted. Diagnosticians observe two clinical rules when examining young children thought to be starting to stutter: they use indirect means of obtaining a speech sample, and they never do anything that might bring the child's disfluency to his attention (Silverman, 1972). Employing play as a vehicle, it was very easy to engage Craig in conversation. With some more reluctant children we have used puppets or extended periods of self-talk (see Chapter 3). But we also must have some idea of the impact of stress upon the child's fluency. Slowly and subtly at first, we began to hurry the play and to interrupt Craig in midsentence with our own message. We asked him a question and before he could finish his answer, we asked another. Then, when he tried to respond or direct the examiner's attention to some facet of our joint play, we looked away from him and purposely dropped toys on the floor and noisily scurried to pick them up. We gauged the communicative stress carefully, watching for changes in the child's speech. Following this, we once again resumed an easy, relaxed style of interaction with the youngster. We abandoned the play for a moment, feasted on a piece of candy, and went to get a drink of water. Returning to the room with Craig, the examiner pointed to a log building set and said, "We really should build a garage for the cars and fire truck . . . but, golly, I have to do some school things first. Say, if you helped me, maybe we could get done faster, okay?" Craig eagerly volunteered to "help" administer a hearing screening test, a vocabulary intelligence measure, and several tasks to assess motor skills. We thanked the child for coming in to see us and started him on the garage-building project with a student clinician while we prepared for the interview with Mrs. Ryan. But first, while our impressions of Craig were clear and fresh, we recorded these observations:

> Craig is doing some "stuttering" but he is not yet a stutterer. In addition to normal disfluency (mostly word and phrase repetition, interjection), he did have some syllable repetitions: as many as five repetitions per word, usually not more than three. The repetitions occurred on the initial word of an utterance, most often when he was attempting to direct my play activity. During spontaneous speech, he repeated on five or six words per hundred. The repetitions were easy and rhythmical—same tempo and speed as the rest of his utterances. No evidence of tension, fear, or avoidance. He speaks with no forcing or airflow stoppage. When communicative stress was introduced, the disfluencies increased markedly—as many as ten to fifteen repetitions, mainly on small words, pronouns like "I," "me," and "you." They were faster, but there was still no tension or struggle. But his face did flush and his eyeblink rate increased; his motor activity also seemed to become somewhat rigid or depressed. My impression is that "listener loss" produced the most stress, then "interruption," "hurrying," and finally "questioning." His hearing is normal, and he scored in the 98th percentile on a vocabulary intelligence measure. Motor behavior seems adequate: gait, stance, throwing, block-building, and skipping—all appeared normal.

We checked our observations with those of a graduate student who had monitored the entire diagnostic session behind a one-way mirror. Her findings are summarized on a clinical worksheet (Figure 6) designed to facilitate identification of children beginning to stutter. (See Van Riper, 1971: 28, for a clinical schema to differentiate stuttering and normal disfluency; consult also the checklist devised by Cooper, 1972.)

Initial interview with Mrs. Ryan. The initial interview with a parent of a child beginning to stutter is of critical importance. We must establish our professional competence, demonstrate our genuine interest, and convince the parent that we can be trusted. In short, our primary task in this initial contact is to build a relationship for subsequent counseling sessions. We also listen carefully to the parent's presenting story (see Chapter 2, pp. 31–32): How do they see the child and his problem? In their view, what might have caused it? What do they identify as their role in the onset of the child's stuttering? What expectations and apprehensions do they have regarding the nature and outcome of treatment? Let us emphasize here that this is *their* story. Hear them out. It is not the proper time to take a lengthy case history; there will be plenty of time for a careful review of the background of the problem in subsequent interviews when the parent can then profit from an objective review of the situation. Guilt, which is almost always present in these sessions, must not be engendered by the interviewer's questions or commentary.

We prefer to record these initial interviews; this frees us from the onus

Name: <u>Craig Ryan</u> Birthdate: <u>5/27/65</u> Date: <u>7/9/69</u> File: <u>#69-320</u>
Observer: <u>P. Van Hollenbeck</u> Situation: <u>"joint play"</u>

1. <u>Repetitions</u>: whole word <u>x</u> syllabic <u>x</u> phonemic <u> </u>

   a. Frequency of repetitions: No. per word <u>   3   </u>
                                 No. per hundred words <u>   6 </u>
   b. Speed of repetitions: <u> same tempo as rest of speech </u>
   c. Coarticulation
       (is appropriate vowel used in repetition?): <u> okay   </u>
   d. Evidence of tension: <u> none </u>
   e. Other: <u> </u>

2. <u>Prolongations</u>: syllabic <u> </u> vocalic <u> </u> consonant <u> </u>
                articulatory posture <u> </u>
   a. Frequency of prolongation: <u> none noted </u>
   b. Evidence of tension: <u> </u>
   c. Change in pitch: <u> </u>
   d. Stoppage in phonation (silent prolongations): <u> </u>
   e. Repetitions end in prolongations or silent postures: <u> </u>
   f. Other: <u> </u>

3. Response to Communicative Stress:

   a. Type of stress: b. Response:
      <u>loss of listener   </u>   <u>long string of repetitions</u>
      <u>hurrying him   </u>   <u>fewer repetitions on "I"</u>
      <u>interruptions   </u>   <u> </u>
      <u>overlapping questions</u>   <u> </u>

4. Awareness:

   a. Eye contact: <u> ? couldn't see </u>
   b. Facial flushing: <u> yes </u>
   c. Motor behavior: <u> sort of "froze" </u>
   d. Eyeblink rate: <u>   23   </u>   <u> 37 (during stress)</u>
                 base rate   disfluency
   e. Verbalizes about speech problem: <u> not observed </u>
   f. Behavior following disfluency: <u> keeps on talking </u>

5. Advanced features:

   a. Evidence of frustration: <u> none </u>
   b. Evidence of avoidance: <u> none </u>
   c. Breathing disturbance: <u> none </u>
   d. Facial contortion, extraneous body movements: <u> none </u>
   e. Tremors: <u> none </u>

6. Other observations: <u>He really seems to like to talk! When you</u>
<u>stepped out of the room for a minute, he admonished the toy</u>
<u>soldiers and chattered away to himself. It almost seems as if</u>
<u>he feels his listener is going to flee.</u>

FIGURE 6   Clinical Worksheet: Onset of Stuttering.

of note-taking, and we can devote our entire attention to the respondent. It also permits repeated review of the session. Here is a resume of our initial interview with Mrs. Ryan:

> Margaret Ryan is an attractive, meticulously groomed woman in her early thirties. She began by explaining that her husband—the only dental surgeon practicing in the city—could not make the conference due to prior commitments. It was slightly embarrassing, she revealed in a faintly jocular but condescending manner, for a member of the medical community to consult with paramedical (her word) services. Craig, the fourth of her five children, began to stutter quite suddenly; before that time he was considered a normal speaker. She attributed the repetitive speech initially to excitement stemming from a hectic weekend when several guests stayed in the house:
>
> "I'm active in Eastern Star and during our regional meeting in late May, I invited eleven women to stay at our house. Although we have a very large home— it's on Ridge Street—things were pretty busy to say the least. Sunday morning when I was helping to get breakfast (I have a college girl who lives in and does housework and baby-sitting), Craig wanted to tell me something. I was so busy I only half-listened to him, and he followed me around the kitchen trying to get my attention. That was when it started. He began to repeat words and parts of words over and over again. We told him to slow down and take it easy and he seemed to be okay. But then it came back."
>
> Mrs. Ryan described Craig as a "good child, always willing to please." According to her report, he is an "active" youngster who plays well with other children in the neighborhood. She added that Craig is "sensitive," and when we asked what she meant, she said:
>
> "He seems very aware—much more so than the other children—of people's feelings, especially their reactions to him. Sometimes, even before the stuttering, he would burst into tears if someone laughed at him or teased him."
>
> Mrs. Ryan revealed that she is "quite worried" about Craig. None of her children has ever had any kind of speech problem. She confided, somewhat hesitantly, that her brother had stuttered "until he finished high school," and she had always felt sorry for him and embarrassed that a Crowe would have a speech impediment. She added:
>
> "You probably aren't familiar with our family name, Crowe, since you are new to the area. My grandparents settled in Granite Harbor in 1883, and my parents still live in the family mansion overlooking Lake Superior."
>
> Rapport was readily established but seemed superficial throughout the interview. Mrs. Ryan appeared to want to impress, rather than inform. Her manner was patronizing. She dropped the names of several prominent persons in town and wanted to make sure the interviewer knew that she was a member of an old Granite Harbor family and lived on Ridge Street, an exclusive section of town. Near the end of the session, however, she did admit to some feelings of guilt: she wondered aloud if her being "very involved" in civic affairs might have something to do with Craig's stuttering. She said that she is "extremely busy" and does not spend much time with the children. Mrs. Ryan then solicited the interviewer's approval by suggesting that "*quality* of interaction with one's children is more important than *quantity*." Several times during the interview, the respondent asked the examiner's impression of Craig's speech problem. As we pointed out in Chapter 2, it is more effective to obtain information before providing it, so each time we demurred and delayed our response until the close of the session. A parent must have closure, however, and here is what we said:

"Craig does indeed have some breaks in his speech, more than normal for a child his age. He is doing some stuttering but it is still the 'good kind': he is not struggling or avoiding and, most important, he doesn't seem to be very aware that talking is tough. We want to prevent that and I cannot do anything without your help. We need to find out why he is repeating words and syllables; we need to know when he does it, under what circumstances. In many cases like this, if we identify and alter certain environmental situations, the child stops stuttering. Craig's speech will only get worse if we ask him to stop or change the way he is talking. Talking is automatic, and the more he tries to think and plan how he is speaking, the more tangled up he will get. You were very wise to bring him in now before the fear and frustration had a chance to develop. Why don't we meet tomorrow, and together we can begin to review Craig's background and then decide how to gather information on what is happening now. I would like to meet soon with Dr. Ryan, too."

Plan of treatment. The therapeutic management of children beginning to stutter is largely indirect: we work for changes in the environment through parental counseling and education.[3] In the case of Craig Ryan, our treatment plan included four basic goals:

1. to deal with parental emotions and resistance;
2. to obtain a careful case history;
3. to review the nature and onset of stuttering; and
4. to provide general and specific suggestions for altering the home situation and parent-child interaction.

For purposes of discussion, we will consider each goal separately, although it is rarely possible to do this in clinical practice. Note the interplay of diagnosis and therapy as we review our activities relative to the four goals.

HANDLING EMOTION AND RESISTANCE.   There was a distinct change in Mrs. Ryan's demeanor when she returned for the second session. No longer quite so supercilious and condescending, she reported that she had done a lot of thinking about her part in the onset of Craig's stuttering:

Maybe I'm too involved. In addition to Eastern Star, I'm an officer in the League of Women Voters, I belong to the County Historical Society, and I'm active in a local ecology group. It has crossed my mind before—maybe I was not spending enough time with the children, but I always felt community service was expected of me. Noblesse oblige, you know. Last night my father took me

[3] Most parents with whom we have worked responded well to the program of counseling and education (*Phase One*) illustrated by the case of Craig Ryan (Schuell, 1949). In a few instances, however, it has been necessary to become more directive (*Phase Two*), spelling out exactly how the household must be reorganized (Johnson, 1961; see also Van Riper, 1961: 110–11). In only a small number of cases have we had to move to *Phase Three*: some adamant parents became amenable to counseling and recommendations only after stormy sessions with several adult stutterers. Although we do not like to, it is also possible (and occasionally necessary) to work directly with the child (Van Riper, 1963: 371–73).

aside and suggested, in his own understated, patrician manner, that I see a psychiatrist, because I was obviously doing something wrong with Craig.

We let Mrs. Ryan talk it out, nodding occasionally and expressing our interest and understanding. When she had finished, we searched for the right words:

> Most parents feel a bit guilty when their children begin to stutter. They sense that they may have caused the problem—a notion which unfortunately is reinforced by many laymen. Parents, especially mothers, are blamed for everything negative about their youngsters. And stuttering is such a highly visible problem; the neighbor kid might wet the bed every night, but no one else need know. No doubt you were also a bit surprised when I indicated that I would be seeing you and not Craig. I'm very glad that you told me how you feel and that you are open and honest, because it's difficult to deal objectively with a problem when feelings get in the way. An undercurrent of guilt or resentment makes the problem very difficult to clear up. As I pointed out yesterday, you were most wise to bring Craig in now when we, you and I as a team, can sort out and eliminate those things that produce the speech breaks. We can't change what happened, but that's not nearly so important as what's going on right now. We can alter the present. Why don't we get started by reviewing all the aspects that we can think of?

THE CASE HISTORY. We seek more than information when we compile a case history. A parent's careful review of the many factors involved in his child's problem tends to foster objectivity. It also shifts the focus away from a general impression of "trouble" to observation of specific behavior. We include a portion of our case history of Craig Ryan:

> *History of speech problem.* Craig began to "stutter" about six weeks ago. His mother attributes the initial speech disfluency to the excitement of several weekend guests. No prior history of speech, hearing, or language difficulty. In fact, he was judged to be a good speaker. Both parents offered advice to "slow down," which seemed to help at first but which now the child rejects. Disfluency consists of syllabic repetitions that seem to appear for a time and then subside. No negative reactions from playmates and adult visitors. Craig is reported to have said that he could not talk, following a recent siege of disfluency.
> *Developmental history.* Normal (fourth) pregnancy. No untoward conditions associated with delivery. Described as "good" baby, slept and fed well. Sat up at three months, walked at ten months, and spoke first word at eleven months. Usual childhood colds and flu, but no high fevers. Mother characterizes the child as "sensitive" to the opinions and reactions of others, especially adults. Vulnerable to teasing and criticism, "thin-skinned." Gets along well with siblings but prefers to play with neighbor children his own age.
> *Family.* Margaret Ryan, age thirty-three. Married twelve years. Housewife. Graduated from well-known Eastern liberal arts college. Parents well respected, prominent in the community. Active in civic and social affairs: member of local ecology group, officer in League of Women Voters, on board of trustees of county historical society, and past matron of local chapter of Eastern Star. Articulate in speech, patrician in manner. Describes advantages provided *for* children but

mentioned only church attendance as something done *with* the five children.

Dr. Len Ryan, age thirty-eight. Dental surgeon. Describes himself as a "hard scrambler." Born and raised on a small farm in rural area of Upper Michigan. Father deceased; mother, senile, resides in a nursing home. Worked his way through college. Proud of the fact that he learned to discipline himself and do without to become a professional. Confided that he drives himself for perfection; tries not to expect it of others, but is frequently disappointed when people don't "measure up." Very busy professionally, but manages to work with the Wilderness Society for preservation of natural areas. Enjoys the out-of-doors, avid back-packer and canoeist. Feels that his wife's parents look down on him because of his "lack of social polish." He volunteered that he has a "good" marriage. Proud of his wife's background and civic involvement. Little sharing with children. Craig has four siblings: twin girls age eleven, another girl age nine years, baby brother, two years old. The three girls are all active, bright, and involved with their own sets of friends. None has a speech problem. One other person resides in the Ryan home, a university sophomore woman who baby-sits and helps with the housework in return for board and room. We talked to this girl one day between classes. She speaks very swiftly and in long, complicated sentences. She is very fond of the two-year-old brother.

THE NATURE AND ONSET OF STUTTERING.   The second interview with Mrs. Ryan was devoted mostly to obtaining a case history (we met with Dr. Ryan late that afternoon). By this time, she was insistently curious: What is stuttering? What causes it? What did we mean when we said that Craig still had the "good kind" of stuttering? We gave her a copy of a short pamphlet (Emerick, 1970) written for parents whose children are beginning to stutter and asked that she read it carefully and discuss the material with her husband.[4] Perhaps, we warned, portions of the booklet might make them feel a bit guilty; we reminded Mrs. Ryan that our purpose was to convey information, not to point an accusing finger. Finally, we asked both parents to record their observations regarding Craig's speech breaks:

> It is often helpful if we put down on paper some of the things we see and hear about the way our child is talking. It will help obtain a clearer picture of the child's situation. Try to be as objective and honest as you can in making your observations. Use the chart (Figure 7) at the end of the pamphlet. In the four squares you record what you observed (and the date) with respect to the questions listed along the border. For example: Mrs. E. made an effort on January 19, to study Mary's nonfluency. She found that the child was mainly repeating first sounds of words (muh-muh-Mommy). Mrs. E. put this information, with the date, in one of the four blocks opposite the first question. She then followed down the page and put her other observations about Mary's reactions in the rest of the blocks opposite the questions.
>
> It will be helpful to you to see under what circumstances the child is experiencing the most speech interruptions. To whom was he talking? What was he talking about? What happened immediately before he began to talk? What hap-

---

[4] There are several excellent publications concerning the onset of stuttering (Lassers, 1945; Pennington, 1955; Johnson, 1959; Robinson, 1960; Murphy, 1962; Mulder, 1960; Sander, 1959).

SPEECH CHART		
What type of speech inter-ruptions did the child have (repeating sounds or words; hesitations, changing his sentences)?	date: .... date:	date: .... date:
Did he appear to be tense or struggle with the speech interruptions?	date: .... date:	date: .... date:
Did he seem to be aware that he was having the interrup-tions; did he react to them? If so, how did he react?	date: .... date:	date: .... date:
To whom was he talking when the speech interruptions were noted?	date: .... date:	date: .... date:
What was he talking about?	date: .... date:	date: .... date:
What had happened immediately prior to his speaking (was he interrupted, ignored, ex-cited, frustrated, tired)?	date: .... date:	date: .... date:
What was happening--what was the listener doing--when the child was talking? (Did they offer advice, look away, become tense, etc.?)	date: .... date:	date: .... date:

Record number of times:						
1. Demand for speech						
2. Child told "no" or "don't"						
3. Child was interrupted while talking						
4. Parental conflict or tension						
5. Gave child speech advice, such as "stop and start over," "take a deep breath," "slow down."						

FIGURE 7   Form for Recording Parental Observations of Speech Interruptions.

pened when he was trying to talk? If, for example, you note that the child's speech interruptions occur most frequently when he is competing with his brothers and sisters for speaking time, then you will readily see what needs to be corrected in order to help him. Using this chart, we will be able to find the reasons for an increase in the child's speech interruptions. Once we know *how* and *why* the child is hesitating, we are less apt to label his behavior as stuttering; we concentrate less on the speech and more on the circumstances. Also, we can then take steps to smooth out the circumstances that seem to increase the child's speech interruptions.

Some parents find it difficult to do things with their children, to share on the children's level (Kinstler, 1961). Mrs. Ryan's conception of parenthood was doing *for* her children—providing educational opportunities, music and dance lessons, bicycles, just about anything they desired. She did little *with* Craig or his siblings. Somewhat reluctantly at first, Mrs. Ryan began to implement our suggestions. She arranged a daily "special time" with Craig when they could share some simple activity: playing cars, building forts, or grooming the family dog. She even arranged for Craig to help her bake a special pastry, lick stamps for the ecology group's membership renewal mailing, and sort out a collection of antique bottles. To her surprise, Mrs. Ryan soon began to enjoy her son's company, and it was obvious that Craig relished these moments. "And he stutters so little now," Mrs. Ryan reported happily during our fifth conference.

Since he was unable to attend all the interviews, we invited Dr. Ryan on a hike near town, and suggested that Craig might enjoy coming with us. We suspected that a mutual interest could be developed here. Incredibly, Dr. Ryan had never considered his son as a potential companion in his outdoor adventures. "The girls didn't want to come along and so I got used to going by myself," he commented. We climbed to a huge slab of stone which provided a magnificent view of Lake Superior. Craig and the clinician sat silently contemplating the lake while Dr. Ryan talked about pollution.

Craig shifted closer to his father and asked what could be done to save the beautiful lake and they talked quietly for a long time. Dr. Ryan called to thank us the next morning and added that he was taking Craig on an overnight canoe trip on a local river.

The primary focus of this book does not permit a complete account of this phase of counseling with the Ryan family. We have therefore included only fragments to illustrate the clinician's role in modifying the home and parent-child relationship (see Project 3).

ALTERING HOME AND PARENT-CHILD INTERACTION.   We held six additional counseling interviews with the Ryans during the remainder of the summer school session. These meetings were devoted to analyzing the parents' observations of Craig's speech behavior; we also made a number of suggestions designed to improve parent-children communication and reduce fluency disruptors. The best suggestions came from the parents themselves. Mrs. Ryan, for example, made this report at the fourth interview and then devised a method of self-checking:

> You know, I found out what a token listener I am with Craig . . . maybe with others, too! The other day I came home from a meeting, and he followed me into the den trying to tell me something. I was still thinking about the meeting, opening my mail, and trying to catch fragments of the news on the radio. Craig started stuttering very badly, and then I realized I had been nodding and saying "ummmm" to him when he was trying to ask a question. I have to learn to be a better listener. So my husband and I talked it over: we decided to institute a policy where the listener has to paraphrase what the speaker has said before he can reply.

We suggested that Mrs. Ryan find someone else to take over some of her civic and social obligations temporarily and arrange to spend even more time with Craig:

> Do something simple like shopping, or even better a quiet visit to the Presque Isle Zoo. Don't take the other children, just Craig. Be there completely, listen to him. Do some self-talk, using short, simple sentences about what he is seeing and experiencing. Refrain from asking him questions. Top off the experience with an ice cream cone or some other treat.

Outcome of treatment. By the end of summer school, Craig was exhibiting no signs of stuttering except occasionally at the family dinner table. We loaned Mrs. Ryan a portable recorder and asked her to tape the flow of conversation at the evening meal. When we played back the tape, it was obvious that the communicative competition was severe even with the clinical monitor present. Everyone, including the two-year-old, clamored to tell the events of his day. We helped Mrs. Ryan devise some family ground rules that would give all parties a fair and equal chance to talk.

When we called early in the fall semester to check on how Craig was doing, Mrs. Ryan reported that he had not stuttered for several weeks and that they had decided to send him to a nursery school. We learned later that Craig stuttered briefly when he started nursery school, but it lasted for only two days and was of mild proportions. For the past three years we have checked Craig's progress through a public-school clinician, and no recurrence of stuttering has been noted. His present teacher, in fact, considers him an exemplary speaker.

Prognosis. We are very impressed with the efficacy of treatment for young children beginning to stutter. When the clinician can intervene before the child develops fear and avoidance reactions, and if the parents are amenable to counseling, the prognosis for recovery is excellent. Our own records on 143 cases, admittedly limited and incomplete, reveal an astounding success ratio of 87 percent. There are several factors that the clinician must consider when estimating a client's prospects for recovery:

1. How long has the child been stuttering? The older the child is and the longer his exposure to adverse environmental reactions, the poorer his prognosis.
2. What type and intensity of environmental reactions has the child been exposed to? Our cases who experienced slapping or other forms of physical abuse had the worst prognoses.
3. Is the child aware that he has difficulty speaking? (See Figure 6.) The more heedful the child is of his speech interruptions, the less positive the prognosis.
4. What type of speech disfluency characteristics are present? The more features present (see Figure 6)—in particular, cessation of phonation, stoppage of air-flow, and disturbance in coarticulation—the poorer the prognosis.
5. How amenable are the parents to counseling? The presence of parental psychopathology is an extremely poor sign for prognosis.
6. What is the child's level of intelligence? We have had more limited success with "slow" children.
7. Are there organic or neurotic factors that figure in the onset of stuttering? Chances for recovery are more limited if either is present.

Our clinical success or failure with children beginning to stutter is also related to the characteristic pattern of factors present at the onset of stuttering. Apparently, there are several ways of becoming a stutterer, and a careful scrutiny of 143 cases seen over the past fifteen years revealed four basic patterns (see Van Riper, 1971: 104–117):

PATTERN ONE. The most typical form (77 cases) of onset in our clinical experience is that of the bright, alert, and sensitive child (Robinson, 1964: 59) who may have low frustration tolerance. This child began to talk early and was considered normal in all respects. The parents are not unusually demanding or rejecting but often are very busy and involved people; most often they are simply not properly informed about speech development in young children. The child cannot seem to keep up with the pace of the house or may be overwhelmed trying to match the fluency of others; there are many fluency disruptors present. Our records show complete recovery in all cases we treated.

PATTERN TWO. This pattern was the next most frequent (34 cases) in our clinical sample. The child is average or above in intelligence but may have an articulation problem. The parents are typically ambivalent and inconsistent in their child-rearing; they may have implicit or explicit standards that are unusually high. The mother tends to be malcontent. Some critical episode such as changing schools or the birth of a sibling may precipitate the stuttering:

> Bobby, age three, was an only child. His mother was seven months pregnant when he suddenly began to stutter following an altercation with his father over finishing all the food on his plate. The father, a navy veteran, was an exceptionally perfectionistic and demanding individual. He insisted that the home be vacuumed and scrubbed daily and flew into a rage if items were not in their proper place. He actually conducted a daily inspection of Bobby's room and

chalked up demerits (no dessert) if his shoes and toys were not lined up in a military manner. Mrs. Baker was completely overwhelmed and dominated by her husband; she even talked about him to Bobby in hushed and reverent tones as "our father." We must confess that we failed miserably to alter the home situation, and our latest check revealed that Bobby is now stuttering quite severely.

Despite our failure in the case described briefly above, the prognosis in Pattern Two is quite good. The significant variable is parental cooperation. In some cases, the parents have been seen jointly by a family service agency.

PATTERN THREE. A significant number (23 cases) of children exhibited a third type of onset. The child is almost always "slow" or below average not only in intelligence but in many other respects. He is usually delayed in speech and language development. Often there is a history of disease or injury; the child may show signs of neurological impairment such as motor clumsiness, mixed cerebral dominance, and slow diadochokinetic rate. The general impression is that of inadequacy—a lack of capacity to think and talk—not only in the child but also in the parents (Andrews and Harris, 1964). The parents—almost one-third of our Pattern Three cases were being raised by only the mother—seem to be marginal persons who have produced marginal children. They have low socioeconomic status. Almost in every case, the child was said to have stuttered since he began to speak. Prognosis is only fair or guarded in these cases. Therapy is generally more prolonged than in Patterns One and Two, and our success ratio is less than 50 percent.

PATTERN FOUR. This final mode of onset is relatively rare (9 cases). The child is usually normal or above in intelligence. The onset of stuttering is sudden and severe and always seems to follow some traumatic episode.

Theophilis, age six, began to stutter severely when the tip of his right index finger was nipped off in an automatic barn cleaner. His father, a successful dairy farmer and part-time Pentecostal preacher, had warned the boy not to play in the barn. Indeed, he had filled the boy with fears of sin and hellfire; he prayed over and protected the child from evil in a thousand intricate ways. Easily excited and disorganized by emotional stimuli, the boy feared the dark, wet his bed almost nightly, and altogether was a miserable, cowed little boy.

Prognosis in these Pattern Four cases is poor. We can only report one unequivocal success among the nine cases we have seen. These children and their families needed so much more than we could offer; we now refer them to a skilled child psychologist.

We have often wondered how much we actually did for some of these cases. Would they have gotten better without our help, due simply to the passage of time and some internal recovery potential in the child? Did we do any good? In most instances, however, the recovery from stuttering occurred too swiftly after the initiation of therapeutic practices (two weeks to several months) to be attributed to spontaneous recovery (Wingate, 1964; Shearer and

Williams, 1965; Sheehan and Martyn, 1970). Consult the work of Wyatt (1969: 310–12) for a list of variables contributing to and inhibiting progress.

EVALUATION OF THE SCHOOL AGE CHILD

Appraising and treating elementary-school stutterers is particularly challenging. This group of children, approximately seven to twelve years old, is no longer beginning to stutter; they are not simply repeating and hesitating. They struggle noticeably when speaking and attempt to avoid or disguise their difficulty; they are frustrated and bewildered by their behavior. The self-perpetuating cycle has started, and it is now necessary to deal directly with the stuttering.

The clinician is faced with several thorny problems when planning an examination of a young stutterer (Van Riper, 1964): (1) Young children frequently lack the insight and cooperation necessary to analyze their problem objectively and rationally. (2) Children are reluctant to freely verbalize their internal feelings. (3) Children can face unpleasant and feared experiences only with great difficulty; the desire to escape is very strong. (4) The speech therapist is associated in the child's mind with the teaching personnel, who may in some cases be penalizing or disturbing listeners. In addition, the clinician may find himself identified with authority figures; this tends to undermine a trusting relationship. (5) Lastly, and perhaps most significantly, the child usually has no choice about entering therapy; most likely he is brought for evaluation by his parents, referred by a teacher, or identified by a speech clinician.

Some therapists continue to deal with young stutterers as if their problem were incipient or primary. They talk in hushed voices about rhythm problems and report that they are "watching" a child who stutters. Parents and teachers are advised to refrain from using the word "stuttering." Literature concerning the onset of stuttering is sent home which, in the absence of counseling and follow-up, merely increases the parents' guilt. This leads to an elaborate conspiracy of silence that only makes matters worse:

> To pretend that there is no speech defect when it is obvious to the child and everyone else is folly, since this pretense will only make him feel he is doing something unclean, as well as unspeakable (Van Riper, 1961: 114).

In their uncertainty lest they do something harmful and create "stuttering," such clinicians do nothing at all. The emperor has no stuttering problem. Perhaps this is one reason why the children, taking their cue from their elders, so frequently *act* as if they were not greatly concerned about their speech (Silverman, 1970).

These youngsters respond to an honest, straightforward clinical approach. Note the frank, direct style employed in this example:

This is the way one public-school speech therapist began the first session with a stutterer whose first utterance in asking if this was the speech room revealed that he was in the advanced stages of the disorder. Note how the therapist takes the attention off the child and reveals himself. Note how he shows that his intention is not to punish but to understand what it is like to stutter. Note how he shows that he is willing to put the stuttering in his own mouth without fear or distress. Observe also how he indicates some measure of professional competence. There are many other ways of doing these things, and you will have to find those which fit you and fit the child in front of you.

"Hello. I suppose you're wondering what's going to happen today. You know that I am a speech-correction teacher and that my job is to help you get rid of your stuttering. But you don't know what kind of person I am except that I'm a stranger and you often have more trouble talking to a stranger. And you don't know how much I'll make you talk or how much stuttering you'll have. So you're probably a bit scared. You don't have to be, because today I'm going to do most of the talking.

"You noticed that I didn't ask your name. That's because I know that saying your name is often one of the hardest things there is to do. How did I know that? It's because I have worked with other kids who've stuttered—a lot of them. And it's because I had to do a lot of stuttering myself when I was learning to be a speech-correction teacher. I had to go into stores and stutter like this [Demonstrates] and like this . . . and like this . . . and many other ways, too. I had to know how it looked and how it felt. And at first, I was sure scared and embarrassed—especially when I had to do it on the phone or to one of my classmates. Once, it almost seemed to run away with me and I couldn't stop. So I think you'll find that I can understand how you feel when you stutter. I also learned how to help the stutterer and I want to help you. So let's get started.

"The first thing I've got to do is to know *how* you stutter. Let me give you some samples and ask you if you've ever had that kind of stuttering. How about this kind? [Therapist illustrates a very severe and unusual form of stuttering.] You don't have that kind? Good! One of the kids I worked with had that kind when we first started. How about this kind? . . . Or this? . . . [Therapist gradually shows models of decreasing abnormality and unfamiliarity.] But I bet you've often had some like this, haven't you? [Illustrates.]

"Well, I've got a vague idea about how you stutter, but I don't know how it feels, and I've got to know that. So look at this picture and tell me—after you put it down—what's happening in the picture. And if you stutter, fine! I can see what we've got to work with. Go ahead.

"You probably noticed that when you stuttered on those two words that I was stuttering right along with you, but silently. I was trying to understand just what you were doing and to know how it felt. I don't think I quite got it, but it was something like this. . . . On that word "boy" you pressed your lips together and off to one side . . . like this . . . and then they began to quiver as you forced . . . like this . . . and then you popped your mouth open like this . . . and the word came out. Let me have another to study. Say "banana-banana-banana" very swiftly. . . . O.K. Same kind of stuff, eh? I bet you felt as though your lips were glued together. Let me try it again. . . .

That's enough stuttering for today. Now let me outline for you exactly how we're going to work on this problem together (Van Riper, 1964: 30–31).

The diagnostician must then prepare a description of the child's stuttering pattern: How frequently does he block? How severe are the disfluencies?

How complex is the moment of stuttering? We also note any avoidance behavior, fear reactions, or signs of penalty and frustration. Word or sound fears are occasionally present, and we have often noted apprehension about certain speaking situations (for example, classroom recitation). Any observed or reported variations in the frequency and severity of stuttering are recorded. Here is a portion of a diagnostic report regarding an eight-year-old child:

> His blocks are mainly tonic or fixative, but he came jerking and bouncing out of them with a series of rapid Moro reflexes of his chest, neck, and shoulders. During the worst of them he covered his mouth with his hand and lowered his head. He stuttered on about 15 percent of the words in a reading passage; he seemed to stutter less during spontaneous speech. His blocks last as long as eight seconds with an average duration of two to three seconds. He did not have the well-developed avoidances, sound fears, word fears, or the elaborate covert aspects that characterize confirmed adult stutterers. But he was frustrated by his speech barriers. Although he still had some periods of comparative fluency, especially during school vacations, these were becoming more and more infrequent.

A comprehensive case history is also useful. We are particularly interested in the history of the speech problem, the role of the parents in the onset and persistence of the stuttering, and some notion of how the child fits into the family situation. We quote again from the report on the same child:

> According to his mother, Mark began to stutter when he was about three years old. She traced the cause for the problem back to the child's first year of life. When he was eight months old, Mark had an extremely high fever of unknown etiology which precipitated a series of severe convulsions. The parents were told that the child probably had sustained "minimal brain damage" and that they should watch his development closely for signs of abnormality. Apparently they did watch closely; they heard the disfluency known to characterize the speech of children. Mark was taken to a pediatrician, and the parents were told that Mark would "grow out of it"; they decided they should help him grow out of it faster by suggesting that he stop and start over again, think what he was going to say, take a deep breath—all the old home remedies for stuttering. Mark's problem had grown steadily more severe, especially since he had started kindergarten. Although he was a bright boy—an IQ of 121 was obtained on a comprehensive intelligence measure—he was doing poorly at school; he refused to participate in oral activities and was teased by several of his classmates.
>
> Mrs. Swenson, Mark's mother, is a physically large and psychologically dominating woman in her late thirties. A teacher by profession—she holds a permanent certificate in secondary education with a major in English and a minor in speech—she tends to be direct and didactic in her relationships with others. Before her marriage, she taught in the local high school and still substitutes on occasion. Each spring she promotes, directs, and judges an oral interpretation contest in the community. Mrs. Swenson enjoys a reputation in the community as an excellent public speaker; she served as president of the P.T.A. for four consecutive years. I found her to be an accomplished speaker although quite rapid in rate and very complex in style; she actually seemed to derive oral pleasure when she could use a word like "germane," "anachronistic," or "recalci-

trant." Mark's stuttering is, for her, both a personal and a professional failure, and she is convinced that the neighbors and teachers in the small town blame her for the child's problem.

Mark's father is a very busy manager of a drive-in restaurant, one of a national chain that features an inexpensive hamburger. After several abortive phone calls, two broken appointments, and one fleeting conversation beside a sputtering grill, he finally consented to an interview in the clinic. He came primed. The first thing he said when he arrived—ten minutes late—was, "I have a very loving relationship with my son." Yet after discussing his relationship with Mark it soon became apparent that Mr. Swenson preferred his oldest son who is a skilled Little League athlete at ten. Although he told of pitching practice and other athletic activities carried out with the oldest son, he could not think of one thing he had done with Mark. He airily dismissed this by indicating that Mark likes fishing and nature study and, "Who has time for driving to the lake or chasing bugs?" Mr. Swenson refused to sit down during the interview and paced back and forth, smoking incessantly. To all my attempts to explain Mark's problem, he countered, "You're the expert" and rejected any notion that he might have a role in the child's speech therapy. When asked how he reacted when Mark stuttered, he said that he pretended it didn't exist and hoped that if he persisted in this behavior it might go away.

Mark is a middle child. In addition to the older brother who excels at whatever he tries (he is a star baseball pitcher, top student, and successful newspaper carrier), there is a four-year-old sister, a precocious imp with puckish dimples and huge brown eyes. According to Mrs. Swenson, the sun rises and sets on little Gigi.

We do not routinely refer young stutterers for psychological testing; it almost always is not indicated (Bloch and Goodstein, 1971) and such evaluation can be assaultive.[5] We are interested, however, in how the child sees himself in relation to his speech problem. To determine this we use informal procedures —three wishes (Silverman, 1970), play therapy and puppetry, skits and role playing (Chapman, 1959), and drawings (Sheehan, Cortese, and Hadley, 1962).

Finally, we like to administer screening tests of motor ability, verbal intelligence, and auditory functioning. School performance reports and results of achievement tests are also examined.[6] Be sure to work closely with the young stutterer's teacher. She can be very helpful since she sees so much more of the child's behavior—how he learns, his assets and liabilities, his relationship with his peers, how he reacts when he stutters, and how he responds to others' reactions to his stuttering. Communication is a two-way street, so also make certain that you share information with the teacher. Here is an informal

---

[5] It is best to inform a client, particularly the older stutterer, that you may need to look at his problem from several perspectives and referral to other professionals may be necessary. Do not wait until therapy is stymied by lack of motivation or resistance to refer the person for psychological evaluation. The client can only interpret your action as assaultive and punitive.

[6] Dr. Hal Luper has been looking at stuttering in young children as a language problem. Administering various tests of language abilities, in particular the Northwestern Syntax Screening Test (Lee, 1969), he found that some young stutterers revealed significant linguistic deficiencies, particularly in encoding skills. He reports good therapeutic results by using language training.

report a school speech clinician sent to a third-grade teacher regarding a young stutterer in her classroom:

> Thank you for sending Becky down to me. I'm glad you mentioned that she seemed quiet in class, that she never volunteered and said "I don't know" a lot when asked direct questions. She has learned to hide her stuttering, has interiorized the problem, and is very adept at avoiding for one so young. You might have a frank talk with her some day soon; tell her you know she has some trouble talking and that you are willing to take all the time she needs to say what she wants to say. You will probably notice this semester that she will seem to get worse, she will be stuttering more. We expect this. We have to bring the stuttering out in the open before we can change it, before she can learn to do it easier and smoother. Stutterers often get worse before they get better, and this can be alarming to those around them. Why don't I stop after school tomorrow and we can chat about what I plan to do in therapy? I think she can make good progress, and I sure will appreciate all the help you can give me.

Since 1962 when we set out to devise a therapy program for young stutterers (Emerick, 1970), we have seen a total of seventy-three children and have consulted with public-school clinicians about many others. According to our records, and they are frankly incomplete in follow-up, fifty-one children made a total recovery and are no longer considered stutterers by parents, peers, or teachers; an additional twelve children made considerable improvement or are still undergoing treatment; the ten remaining youngsters made little or no improvement. What factors are crucial for improvement? What variables should the diagnostician consider when making a prognosis?

According to our records, the most significant improvement in therapy was noted in those cases where the following factors obtained:

1. No prior record of unsuccessful treatment (children identified and treated unsuccessfully as "primary" stutterers did poorly in our program; an absence of treatment seems more conducive to success than a history of therapeutic failure)
2. *Cooperative parents, willing to participate meaningfully in a program of counseling*
3. More severe stuttering pattern; mild stutterers showed little improvement
4. *A predominantly clonic stuttering pattern featuring struggle and escape* (children who had become adept at avoidance generally had more difficulty)
5. Cooperative teachers and other school personnel
6. *No other significant problems* (reading difficulty, a scholastic problem independent of stuttering, etc.)
7. When *the child has other resources* (expertise in scouting, athletics, music)
8. When group therapy can be utilized
9. *When it is possible to schedule intensive therapy* (at least three, preferably four, contacts a week)
10. When the child can tolerate imitating various stuttering patterns (not necessarily his own) demonstrated by the examiner

All of the factors listed are significant prognostically; however, Items Two, Four, Six, Seven, and Nine loom as the most critical to recovery.

For an account of therapy for young stutterers, including case studies of clinical successes and failures, see the publication by Emerick (1970). You will find much that is helpful also in the excellent contributions of Chapman (1959) and others (Van Riper, 1964; Goven and Vette, 1966; Simpson, 1966; Stennett, 1967; Fox and Connelly, 1970; Williams, 1971).

ASSESSMENT OF THE ADULT STUTTERER

The following case report was compiled in preparation for a unique summer institute in stuttering therapy sponsored by the Speech Foundation of America (Starkweather, 1972). It is presented to illustrate common assessment procedures employed with adult stutterers. Although he was an unusually difficult and severe case, the client did possess characteristics common to all stutterers.

We heard about Joe Dupreas through a local vocational counselor who had been attempting to prepare him for employment. He sent us this note:

> Joe Dupreas, a nineteen-year-old high-school graduate, is the most severe stutterer I have ever talked with—I can barely understand him. He had speech therapy while attending junior and senior high school in Hubbell but with little improvement. He's been involved in some minor scrapes—reckless driving, possession of alcoholic beverages—but basically he seems like a nice kid. He wants to get away from home; his father reportedly derides Joe because of his speech defect and his chronic unemployment. Joe doesn't have a chance—he has no skills and his stuttering problem is very severe. He doesn't say much, but I think he is just about ready to give up.

We sent a letter to Joe that outlined the summer institute and asked if he could come down to Marquette for a preliminary interview.

the initial interview

A few days later we received a scrawled note from Joe telling us he could not come to Marquette. His driver's license had been revoked, and he would not ask his father to make the trip. So we decided to meet him in Hubbell.

We had arranged to meet in the Intermediate School District office building. The only available space was the office supply room, and all during our brief chat we were constantly interrupted by secretaries. Although it was far from an ideal setting, something significant passed between Joe and the clinician during that first brief encounter.

A handsome, dark-haired young man, Joe shook hands limply and perched on the edge of the only chair in the room. We told him at great length about the institute, painting vivid pictures of the fishbowl nature of the situation, the intensity of the daily schedule, and the agony of prolonged self-confrontation. It was going to be a difficult experience, and we needed someone who could stand the pace, a man who above all else wanted to change his speech and would drive single-mindedly toward the goal. Could he do it? Joe didn't blink. He just said rather softly, stuttering severely, that he felt he could handle it. He claimed that his speech difficulty did not bother him so much now, at least not to the degree it had in school. His major concern was getting a job, and he was seeking training that would equip him to work as a cabinet maker. We summarized our raw impressions on a portable tape recorder on the way home:

> I have seen very few laconic stutterers—the kind that seem to fall asleep between blocks—and it always seems like role playing. I can't believe Joe is that indifferent to his stuttering. His blocks are very severe, at least 6.5 or maybe 7 on the Iowa Rating of Stuttering Severity scale, and they are complex. He has long fixations on a posture, a glazed look comes over his eyes, and a rapid tremor spreads over the right side of his face. When he really gets stuck, he makes a tongue-sucking noise, a sort of "tsk" to release the tonic fixation; one time toward the end of the interview, he made a spitting motion and sound as he attempted to release a fixed posture on a plosive.

This first contact with Joe, we discovered later, was of inestimable importance, as it is with most stutterers, in establishing a working clinical relationship. What had we done, what crucial episode had transpired? Several times we reviewed the events of that short encounter, but alas, we cannot identify that one critical factor; indeed much of what transpired appears exceedingly mundane. Perhaps it was not just a single aspect but a mixture of forces that ignited a spark between the clinician and client. Some of the following may have served as tinder: (1) The clinician demonstrated his interest by coming to the stutterer's home base. (2) The clinician is also a stutterer—we did mention this source of identification but we did not dwell on it. (3) We talked straight and tough to Joe, told him exactly what the institute entailed. Some clinicians think that a velvet-glove, Pollyanna approach is effective, but stutterers suspect this tactic, for they know deep inside that solving their problem will not be easy. (4) We invited him to take a chance, we extended a challenge which implied faith in his capabilities; everyone needs an open horizon to aim for in life's journey, and maybe we simply showed Joe the beckoning mirages ahead. Other features could be listed—we somehow revealed our competence even in that brief exchange, we showed that we could be trusted, and we verbalized for him the lack of hope we saw in his sad features. Later, when Joe was in therapy, we asked him to tell us the significance of that first meeting as he saw it. He pondered for a long time and finally said, "All the while you were talking about how hard it would be, you know, I kept thinking to myself, 'Hey, he believes I can do it!' " We agree with Gregory

(1969: 82) that "The expectation of help can be as strong a factor in bringing about changes on some dimensions of personality as therapy itself."

a day of testing and trial therapy

The brief interview at Hubbell provided only the dim outlines of Joe's stuttering problem. A more formal assessment was necessary; in order to plan therapy we must identify the specific facets of his speech disorder. Arrangements were made for vocational rehabilitation funds to provide air-travel expenses so Joe could spend a day for testing and trial therapy at the clinic.

We carefully analyzed Joe's moment of stuttering in a variety of speaking conditions (reading aloud, paraphrasing, conversation); the frequency and severity of stuttering were noted; adaptation and consistency were charted; paper-and-pencil tests designed to measure attitude, level of aspiration, and frustration were administered; we evaluated the client's laterality and diadochokinesis; a counselor probed for psychodynamic aspects; trial therapy was performed and video-taped for later analysis. In the late afternoon, two speech pathology majors took Joe hiking, treated him to a dormitory dinner, and then "rapped" in their room until we picked him up and drove him to the airport. Here is a report of our findings:

CLINICAL REPORT

Client: Dupreas, Joe　　　　　　　　Date: March 3, 1971
Birthdate: January 5, 1952　　　　　Examiners: G. Mistal
　　　　　　　　　　　　　　　　　　　　　　　　　 G. Hermann

Description of the stuttering pattern.　Predominantly fixative blocks, almost on every word (except a few stereotyped social ritual expressions or trite asides, which are generally uttered fluently) with little variation in frequency or severity in three types of talking—reading aloud, paraphrasing, and spontaneous conversation. Overall impression is of extreme tension as he moves slowly and deliberately from word to word. Careful scrutiny of the moment of stuttering revealed the following specific components:

Fixations of articulatory postures: silent plosives and affricatives, or audible prolongation on semivowels and fricatives; fixations may last as long as thirty seconds and be as brief as three seconds with an average duration of eight seconds; airflow shut off initially at lip or tongue-tip and gum-ridge valves, and as tension increases the locus of fixation shifts to the larynx; a fixation may be released with a surge of tension or with a deep breath and a retrial. If neither works and the tension increases, a tremor is noted.

Tremor seems to start at the right corner of his mouth, spreads rapidly down the right side of his face and neck; if the fixation is long (over five seconds), the tremor may extend into Joe's right arm to his index finger which is extended in a gesture that seems to say, "just a minute." He cannot tolerate the tremor for long and shifts to a glottal fry.

Glottal fry may extend for several seconds and be interrupted intermittently by phonemic prolongation; some phonemic prolongations may turn into rapid repetitive or clonic blocks; audible repetitions are the least acceptable form of disfluency to Joe and are terminated swiftly with release or escape behaviors (or he may revert to a silent fixation and begin the sequence again).

Release behaviors included in order of frequency of use: sudden surge of tension, often accompanied by postural shift; a tongue-sucking sound ("tsk"); sucking and lip-licking movements; a spitting motion which may or may not be accompanied by saliva. The latter three release devices are infrequently used to initiate a speech attempt or as transitions between fixations seemingly to keep his oral mechanism moving.

Expectation of stuttering is vivid. Joe read a passage silently, marking words on which he thought he would stutter if he read the same passage aloud; when he did read it aloud, his prediction was 93 percent accurate. He described his anticipation of stuttering in this manner: "I know I am going to have trouble getting the word out, and I feel inside like someone is going to jump on me." His posture is consonant with his report—his shoulders bend forward and sag down in a cowed, shrinking manner. (Note: reportedly, as a child, Joe was often struck by his father when Joe stuttered in Mr. Dupreas' presence.)

Avoidance behavior consists of starters ("um," "well," etc.), postponement (pretending to think what he intends to say); frequently giving up speech attempt or seducing the listener into completing the sentence. In group situations, Joe remains silent unless addressed directly and wears an ingratiating grin (an embarrassed smile which appears to be a nonverbal attempt to demonstrate his involvement with the conversation even though he is not directly participating). If persistently questioned he may resort to a sullen silence as if he is retreating to some private void. Eye contact is poor.

Poststuttering behavior includes the following overt features: he lowers his eyelids, feigns a relaxed or indifferent posture, and may spit silently several times (as if saying, "I just stuttered, but so what, I am still cool and it does not bother me"). Reports feeling "stupid" and "inferior" after stuttering.

Frequency and severity of stuttering.   Joe stutters on over 50 percent of the words in oral reading and over 60 percent in paraphrasing and spontaneous speech. The senior clinician and two student clinicians rated the client as "very severe" (value of 7 on scale running from 1=no stuttering, to 7) on the Iowa rating scale (Johnson, Darley, and Spriestersbach, 1963: 281). Elements included in the severity judgment were: frequency of stuttering; amount of tension present; duration of a moment of stuttering; complexity (number of features, or form-types) of the stuttering pattern; the peculiarity of the stuttering pattern (Darley, Aronson, and Brown, 1969); and the amount of avoidance and extent of covert features associated with the stuttering problem.

Adaptation and consistency. Joe read a short passage aloud five consecutive times while the examiner recorded stuttered words. The results are as follows: reading number one—eighteen stutterings; number two—sixteen stutterings; number three—sixteen stuttered words; number four—fifteen stutterings; on the fifth reading he stuttered thirteen times. His adaptation (see Johnson, Darley, and Spriestersbach, 1963: 269) was 27 percent. The severity of Joe's blocks showed a marked decline over the five readings. His moments of stuttering were very consistent (72 percent of the words stuttered in the first reading were also stuttered in reading number three). The client does not report any periods of speech fluency. He did reveal, however, that conversation with friends his own age is easier and that drinking tends to make him fluent.

Paper-and-pencil tests. Joe disliked this portion of the assessment. He said he does not like to read and that writing is difficult (his writing is characterized by irregular, jerky lines). He managed to complete three of four items:

On the Rosenzweig Picture Frustration Study Joe's responses were typically extrapunitive (expresses aggression outwardly toward the source of frustration). His responses were simple, direct, and sprinkled with curse words.

On the Cassel Test of Aspiration (see p. 72) Joe rather consistently set his goals at or slightly above his achievement level, indicating a tendency to predict future performance conservatively.

The Iowa Attitude Scale Toward Stuttering (Johnson and Ammons, 1944) was administered, and Joe obtained a score of 1.62, which represents an average, or moderate attitude, toward stuttering (Johnson, Darley, and Spriestersbach, 1963: 264).

An attempt was made late in the day to administer the Perceptions of Stuttering Inventory (Woolf, 1967), an instrument devised to assess three dimensions of stuttering behavior—struggle, avoidance, and expectancy—as perceived by the stutterer. From fragmentary responses (he failed to complete all sixty items), it was the examiner's impression that Joe would have obtained a symmetrical high-score profile—he perceives his stuttering to be severe.

Laterality and diadochokinesis. Joe is right-handed and right-sided on the basis of the examiner's observations and the client's responses to a laterality questionnaire. Diadochokinesis for the nonsense word *putukuh* was within normal limits. His motor behavior is slow, deliberate, almost rigid; it is difficult to discern if this is an affectation associated with his "cool male" image, a withdrawal because of the stuttering, or neurological impairment. Even though he makes a deliberate business out of lighting a cigarette, he looks as if he might drop it.

Psychological examination.   A highly skilled counselor who has worked jointly with the examiner in group therapy for stutterers, conducted an indepth interview with Joe and submitted this report:

> Joe appeared to have a good attitude about being able to profit from participating in the proposed summer institute, but he did admit that some earlier experiences in speech therapy were only partially successful.
>
> He is very self-conscious about his stuttering and is extremely sensitive about people feeling sorry for him. I would think that attempts to show empathy and concern for Joe should be handled carefully so that they are not misinterpreted as pity.
>
> Writing and thinking seemed to confuse him unduly, and he admitted to being easily tired with such activities. He prefers more practical activities. Joe exhibited a great deal of nervousness and confided that he trembles often. He appears to have a number of fears and doubts about himself, particularly about being accepted as a stutterer. Apparently he feels a lot of resentment and anger toward his father for not understanding and taking any interest. This would be an area to work on should Joe be involved in any encounter groups or personal counseling.

Additional psychological findings.   The rehabilitation counselor who referred Joe to us sent additional data compiled by a psychometrician. Here is a summary report of his findings:

> The Army General Classification Test indicates that Joe is functioning at the average level of intellectual ability (48th percentile). His basic skills in reading are at the eighth-grade level and his math skills are at the fourth-grade level. On the Purdue Pegboard he demonstrated slightly below average finger dexterity. The Kuder Preference Record shows high interest in the outdoors, mechanics, and music with lows in computation, clerical work, and literary interests.

Medical examination.   Joe was given a thorough physical examination by a local physician. He found a slight loss of visual acuity in the right eye, but otherwise Joe was physically normal.

Is there any meaning in the way a client goes about his stuttering? Some feign bewilderment, others an uneasy amusement; some whimper and moan, a few snarl and bare their nonfluent fangs. On first impression, Joe seems to present a great stone face to the world, but actually he is more like a badly frightened arctic hare, frozen, immobile. Apparently, he has been hurt by the very people who should have loved him; and to prevent the nagging ache, he retreated behind a Maginot Line of silence and nihilism. He covers up with machismo, a simulated indifference, beer-drinking, reckless driving, and rumbles.[7] Hopeless and helpless, he spits at the world in mock defiance (athletes

---

[7] It became evident later that much of this bravado was, in fact, self-destructive behavior. It just didn't matter, he told us, so he pressed down on the accelerator. One evening in early November, shortly before we first contacted him, Joe had walked out on a rickety bridge that spanned Bourgeois Bay and looked down at the dark waters. "What's the use," he thought; he could not find employment, his father denigrated him constantly, and he stuttered so severely he could not share his thoughts or feelings.

and junior high-school males frequently expectorate small quantities of saliva apparently to show defiance and reveal their maleness).

Trial therapy was performed with Joe. We employed one simple, direct goal: we practiced putting words back together again. The following routine was used (Van Riper, 1970):

1. He was to integrate the sound (air-voice-proper articulatory posture)
2. Then, he was to attempt to integrate the syllable, shaping for the second sound before saying the first
3. Finally, he was to utter the word slowly but with strong deliberate movements

Joe was reluctant at first, but we stuttered along with him, starting with his sticky blocks and then gradually changing to show him how to reintegrate the fractured sounds and syllables and utter the words with strong positive movements. We explained that there are many different ways to stutter and that we meant to show him how to speak without the tension and tremors. A faint flicker of hope showed in his sad eyes—he smelled the cheese at the end of the maze.

The student clinicians submitted this brief report:

> We noticed the machismo bit you mentioned: he dressed all in black, complete with a black leather vest, and pointed shoes; he told us about the beer, broads, and rumbles; he showed us a picture of a car he had "totaled." He said that three years ago he bought a set of weights and vowed that no one would give him any grief anymore—which is probably true, because he bench-pressed over 200 pounds! We feel this is mostly window-dressing. Several times he hesitantly asked if we thought he could be helped. He likes what he has seen so far, but he is afraid to take a chance. The outdoors turned him on, though, he really liked the hike. Joe mentioned his father and asked if the abuse he experienced as a child from him would show up on the psychological tests. Do we have any kind of case history?

a final meeting

We made one final trip to Hubbell to scrutinize the family home, interview Mr. and Mrs. Dupreas, and spend some time with Joe. The clinician casually sounded Joe out: what did he expect from therapy? Here is a brief summary report dictated on a portable recorder:

> Joe's expectations are low indeed. He wants to hope, but too many past failures and hurts weigh heavily. He feels so unworthy of positive regard that he suspects the motives or intelligence of the clinician. How can anyone possibly like him, he feels, when he knows he is so unlovable? There are some positive features, however. We discovered a common interest in the woods and waters of the North, and both of us have a deep and abiding affection for the Copper Country. Perhaps out of mutual affection for this area we can fashion the type of relationship he apparently needs to take a chance on making a shift in his speech.

We then interviewed Joe's parents in their home and prepared the following case-history summary:

Case-History Summary

Respondents: Mr./Mrs. Pierre Dupreas   Date: May 19, 1971

Address: 117 Allouez, Hubbell   Examiner: E.

Rapport: Mr. Dupreas left shortly after the interview commenced. He was alternately glib and baiting. In jest, but with heavy sarcasm, he said that Joe had had several years of speech therapy, but that "it wasn't worth a pitcher of warm spit." Mrs. Dupreas apologized for her husband's behavior and appeared to be open and honest in her comments.

Father: Pierre Dupreas, age fifty-one, mine foreman, born in Canada. Finished high school and came to the Copper Country in the late 1930s. Was never interested in children or family life. Spends most of his time with lodge brothers, playing cards, fishing, etc. Is a problem drinker and becomes abusive when intoxicated. Derides Joe continually about the length of his hair, his bad driving record, his chronic unemployment, and most of all about his stuttering. Frequently tells his son to "spit it out."

Mother: Leona Dupreas, age forty-four, born and raised in the Copper Country. Finished high school and practical nurse's training, but has not worked outside the home since having children. Reports that there is now little but economic convenience in the marriage. "You would think a man would notice when a marriage has been platonic for several years," she added. She defends Joe in family altercations. Impresses the interviewer as a warm, affectionate person who is concerned with Joe's welfare. Will be a key figure in his therapeutic reentry program.

Siblings: Two younger brothers, ages fourteen and nine. Reported to get along well with Joe.

Home: Middle-class neighborhood. Well-kept eight-room frame house. Modern furnishings.

Birth history: Full term, weighed eight pounds, eleven ounces. Prolonged, hard labor. Difficulty initiating breathing.

History of stuttering: Began to stutter at the age of eighteen months following hospitalization for a severe case of pneumonia. Had talked normally (one- and two-word sentences) for several months prior to the illness. Father applied pressure, including physical abuse, and stuttering got worse. Was teased at school and had several fights. Gradually became silent and sullen. At age sixteen Joe confronted his father and physically "shook him up" for attempting to slap him when blocking. Presently feels severely restricted by his stuttering. Stutters more severely to strangers; refuses to use the phone. Gains token group acceptance from his peers by buying beer and holding parties at his home.

Educational history: Attended parochial school from kindergarten through eighth grade. Graduated from public high school. Did very poorly in school. Disliked all classes except industrial arts. Refused to participate in oral work.

treatment plan

Several premises were considered when devising an outline of therapy for Joe:

1. We must be simple and direct in our approach.
2. We must stress action.
3. We must emphasize real situations as much as possible.
4. We must provide release of pent-up emotions and assist him in devising alternate plans to deal with stress points.
5. We must, most of all, create hope; we must create and maintain the expectation in Joe that he can and will get better.

We include below an outline of therapy (from Van Riper, 1970: 2–3); for a complete account of the intensive therapy program conducted with Joe and two other adult stutterers, see the Speech Foundation of America booklet by Starkweather (1972).

> The basic plan of therapy will consist of the following: whenever Joe stutters with any force or struggle or abnormality, he must stop, write the word on a piece of paper or card, and then follow this routine: (1) integrate the sound (air-voice-proper articulatory posture); (2) integrate the syllable, shaping for the second sound before saying the first; (3) say the word *slowly* but with strong deliberate movements. If he fails at any of these he must do the whole sequence until he is successful, *and he is not to continue until these three steps have been done correctly.* We must be completely consistent in preventing any reinforcement of old stuttering behaviors by having them lead to the consummation of communication. Note: (1) The only exception to this policy is when he stutters smoothly and easily on a word. Reward these. (2) He is not to complete the word in which he starts stuttering but to stop immediately. This is not a cancellation exercise but a *searching, integrating procedure.*
>
> 1. Begin the session by having him tell you of the activities and procedures used by the previous therapist with some evaluation of their possible effectiveness or difficulties. Don't use these same activities in your session; devise new ones to serve the same purpose.
> 2. Next have him read the words on his list of those he had trouble with, and lists of words you can obtain from various sources. He should practice saying them both in the old way and with the new, smooth, slow-motion stuttering alternately several times, with increasing speed and loudness; he should then put the new forms into a sentence and speak it in a loud, assertive voice, after pantomiming them and whispering them to get the motor feel of how they are produced.
> 3. He should enter at least one feared situation involving authority, time pressure, involved explanation, threat of interruption such as telephoning, requesting favors, and speaking to impatient listeners or strangers. Find out from him what kinds of situations would be useful here but have some set up for him. Have him verbalize his feelings beforehand, plan exactly the first sentence he will say, and after the situation is over, analyze his performance and reactions.
> 4. Have about five to ten minutes of reading, monologue, and conversation in which he has to use a lot of egocentric speech in which he talks about himself —his past, his future, his problems, his good and bad memories. Use reading materials that might help him to make comments. In doing this he is to fill his speech with tiny facsimiles of the new way of stuttering. Do the same when you speak to him.

5. Spend part of the day working on the proprioceptive monitoring of speech, using masking, DAF, electrolarynx, or any other method to block out sight and sound and to emphasize the feel and movement of speech.

Making a prognosis of success and failure in stuttering therapy is a little like predicting next season's fashions—even though the territory to be covered has finite limits, the possible variations make precise forecasting impossible. In the past decade, we have seen over two hundred adult stutterers, and for each client we made a private prognosis about the outcome of treatment. Our accuracy is only slightly better than 50 percent, which, interestingly enough, corresponds almost exactly with our ratio of therapeutic success. Some of our most disabled clients have made startling recoveries, often despite an awesome array of negative environmental factors. On the other hand, stutterers with an impressive number of personal advantages have failed to make a significant shift in their behavior. Even more confusing, many clinicians have been startled, as we have been, when a stutterer with whom we had only minimal success later returns and, talking easily, offers his thanks for our help. (For a fascinating account of success and failure in stuttering therapy, see the Speech Foundation booklet edited by Luper [1968]). But perhaps we have overstated the dangers of prophecy in clinical work with stutterers; there are, in fact, a number of considerations which therapists find useful in predicting a client's potential for treatment.

The following is an incomplete and heuristic list of factors which help in making prognoses. The items are presented in random order, for we at present have no data that would allow us to assign weight to them.

Severity.   Paradoxically, the more severe stutterers, other factors being equal (which they seldom are), seem to make better progress than do milder stutterers. Perhaps the reason is that contemporary therapy is especially designed for the more involved cases (Gregory, 1969). The only way they have to go is up; they have nothing to lose but their blocks. The mild stutterers, on the other hand, do get by, and it is difficult for them to relinquish their symptoms for the dubious sanctuary of "fluent stuttering."

Motivation.   You can lead a client to the therapy room, but you can't make him follow the plan of treatment. Motivation is, of course, a most significant variable in all types of therapy.

Timing.   A client's motivation for treatment is often related to crucial life experiences; stutterers who have reached a critical stage and feel blocked by their disordered speech, barred from job advancement, education, or marriage, and voluntarily seek therapy have a more favorable prognosis.

Age.   Adolescents, particularly between the ages of thirteen and sixteen, are especially resistant to therapy. Similarly, clients over forty tend to do poorly in treatment, probably because older individuals are more rigid, and somehow, they may have made an accommodation with stuttering.

Sex. Women seem to be more difficult to treat in stuttering therapy than men. Our own records show not a single therapeutic success with adolescent girls.

Type of stuttering. Predominantly repetitive stutterers make more rapid progress than do predominantly fixative stutterers; clients who feature escape reactions are easier to work with than chronic avoiders. Interiorized stutterers—especially those manifesting laryngeal blocking—are very resistant to therapy.

Organic or neurotic concomitants. Clients presenting organic complications (sensory impairment, motor slowness) or neurotic symptoms (compulsions and conversion symptoms) require more prolonged treatment and do less well than stutterers who do not have those characteristics.

Identification. The interpersonal relationship is crucial in stuttering therapy; the stutterer and clinician must come to share a common set of values, at least regarding the solution of the fluency problem. Clients who exhibit unusual life styles tend to see participation in therapy as an act of submission.

Prior therapy. It is far worse to have tried and failed than never to have tried at all. Clients with a history of therapeutic failure have a poor prognosis.

False fluency. Sudden, dramatic fluency early in treatment—we have even seen the phenomenon in trial therapy—is a poor prognostic sign. It rarely lasts and the client is often devastated upon the return of his symptoms. A rapid "flight to health" is generally attributed to suggestion.

The stutterer's environment. The prospects for successful treatment are enhanced by a supportive environment. Be wary of relatives or friends, however, who say when change is discussed, "But we love him just the way he is now, we don't notice the stuttering." Secondary gains—benefits from being a stutterer—are tough therapeutic competitors.

Inconsistency. Variability in the client's stuttering pattern and fluctuation in his self-concept (Van Riper, 1971) are good prognostic signs. Clients who exhibit cycles in the frequency and severity of their stuttering seem to make better progress than those who do not. Perhaps they can see the possibility for change.

Assets and liabilities. Except in cases of overcompensation, clients who have acknowledged expertise or talent in some area make better progress than individuals with an excess of liabilities.

Intensive therapy.   Token treatment is worse than no treatment at all. When intensive therapy (minimal daily contact of at least one hour) is available and the client can participate in a comprehensive program, the prospects for recovery are significantly more favorable.

PROJECTS AND QUESTIONS

1. Contrast and compare the classification systems of stuttering offered in the following references; separate them into two categories: types of stuttering at *onset* and in *adults*.

ANDREWS, G., and M. HARRIS. *The Syndrome of Stuttering.* Clinics in Developmental Medicine No. 17. London: William Heinemann Medical Books, Ltd., 1964. Pp. 31–32.

BLOODSTEIN, O. "The Development of Stuttering: I. Changes in Nine Basic Features." *Journal of Speech and Hearing Disorders,* 25 (1960): 219–37.

————. "The Development of Stuttering: II. Developmental Phases." *Journal of Speech and Hearing Disorders,* 25 (1960): 366–76.

————. "The Development of Stuttering: III. Theoretical and Clinical Implications." *Journal of Speech and Hearing Disorders,* 26 (1961): 67–82.

DOUGLASS, E., and B. QUARRINGTON. "The Differentiation of Interiorized and Exteriorized Secondary Stuttering." *Journal of Speech and Hearing Disorders,* 17 (1952): 377–85.

EISENSON, J. "A Perseverative Theory of Stuttering." In *Stuttering: A Symposium,* ed. J. Eisenson. New York: Harper & Row, Publishers, 1958. Pp. 246–59.

FRANSELLA, F. "The Stutterer as Subject or Object?" In *Stuttering and the Conditioning Therapies,* eds. B. Gray and G. England. Monterey, Calif.: Monterey Institute for Speech and Hearing, 1969.

FREUND, H. *Psychopathology and the Problems of Stuttering.* Springfield, Ill.: Charles C Thomas, 1966. Pp. 136–52.

GLASNER, P. "A Holistic Approach to the Problem of Stuttering in Young Children." In *Psychological and Psychiatric Aspects of Stuttering,* ed. D. Barbara. Springfield, Ill.: Charles C Thomas, 1962.

LUCHSINGER, R., and G. ARNOLD. *Voice-Speech-Language.* Belmont, Calif.: Wadsworth Publishing Company, 1965. Pp. 746–51.

PRINS, D., and E. LOHR. "Behavioral Dimensions of Stuttered Speech." *Journal of Speech and Hearing Research,* 15 (1972): 61–71.

QUARRINGTON, B., and E. DOUGLASS. "Audibility Avoidance in Nonvocalized Stutterers." *Journal of Speech and Hearing Disorders,* 25 (1960): 358–65.

ROBINSON, F. *Introduction to Stuttering.* Englewood Cliffs, N.J.: Prentice-Hall, Inc., 1964. Pp. 80–102.

VAN RIPER, C. *The Nature of Stuttering.* Englewood Cliffs, N.J.: Prentice-Hall, Inc., 1971. Pp. 101–17, 249–64.

WYATT, G. *Language Learning and Communication Disorders in Children.* New York: The Free Press, 1969. Pp. 300–301.

2. Can stuttering, as a clinical disorder, be defined in terms of speech phenomena alone? Review the definition of a speech defect in Chapter 1, and then see if you can characterize fluency breakdowns in terms of three facets.

3. What other environmental modifications (parental attitude and adjustments) would you seek in the case of Craig Ryan? Outline what you would say, for example, to the university girl who lives with the family.

4. Review the following two sources on the assessment of stutterers:

JOHNSON, W., *et al. Speech Handicapped School Children.* New York: Harper & Row, Publishers, 1967.

VAN RIPER, C., and L. GRUBER. *A Casebook in Stuttering.* New York: Harper & Row, Publishers, 1957.

5. Research the measurement of attitude toward stuttering. Here are two references to provide a beginning:

ERICKSON, R. "Assessing Communication Attitudes Among Stutterers." *Journal of Speech and Hearing Research,* 12 (1969): 711–24.

REESE, G. "An Attitude Test for Stutterers Based on the Semantic Differential." Unpublished Master's thesis, University of Colorado, 1963.

6. Is there such a thing as graphic stuttering? See Fagan, C., "Graphic Stuttering," *Psychological Monographs,* 43 (1932): 67–71.

7. Review the article by Yairi and Williams, "Reports of Parental Attitudes by Stuttering and by Nonstuttering Children," *Journal of Speech and Hearing Research,* 14 (1971): 596–604. How could the Children's Report of Parental Behavior Inventory be used therapeutically?

8. What are the least stress-producing topics for stutterers to discuss? See Moore, W., "Relations of Stuttering in Spontaneous Speech to Speech Content and to Adaptation," *Journal of Speech and Hearing Disorders,* 19 (1954): 208–16.

9. Van Riper (1971: 9) quotes Kluckhohn with emphatic finality regarding the universality of stuttering. See what an eminent anthropologist wrote in another publication: Kluckhohn, C., *Mirror For Man* (New York: Fawcett World Library, 1957), p. 155.

10. Below we have presented short sketches of clients coming for diagnosis. Within the limits possible before seeing the individual, what should you be prepared for in terms of the three goals of interviewing?

Randy is the only son (age five) of Mr. and Mrs. Neuman. Both parents are employed; father is a metallurgist, Mrs. Neuman owns and runs a small flower shop. The child began to stutter two months ago just before starting kindergarten. The family lives in an isolated area. The child has no playmates his own age.

Heino is a fourth grader (age ten) in a rural school. He has stuttered since childhood and is a poor student. His father is deceased, his mother works as a cook at the school. Two older siblings are both married. The child's teacher sent this note:

I certainly hope you can help this child. The last therapist told me that we might have to wait until Heino was older because he didn't seem to cooperate I tried to talk to him about his problem but he just answers all my question with "I don't know."

Harvey is a college freshman. He was referred to the clinic by his humani ties instructor because he refused to give an oral report. Harvey first ap peared at an evening open group therapy meeting that had been announced in the student newspaper. He spent most of his time trying to convince the other members that he was not a stutterer, and if he did stutter occasionally it did not bother him. He is very defensive and hostile.

11. Discuss the pros and cons of having an adult write an autobiography as par of the evaluation process.

12. Compare the assessment procedures employed by operant and two-facto clinicians.

13. Review the following article: King, S., "Aggression and Cardiovascular Re actions," *Journal of Abnormal and Social Psychology*, 50 (1955): 206–11 Can you see any application to the assessment of stutterers?

14. Is anxiety unitary or multiple in nature? Are there any implications fo stuttering? See Jackson, D., and R. Bloomberg, "Anxiety: Unitas or Multi plex," *Journal of Consulting Psychology*, 22 (1958): 225–27.

15. What is the relationship between mood and cyclical variations in the fre quency of stuttering? What implications might there be for prognosis? See

QUARRINGTON, B. "Cyclical Variations in Stuttering Frequency and Severity and Some Related Forms of Variation." *Canadian Journal of Psychology*, 10 (1956): 179–83.

SHEEHAN, J. "Cyclic Variation in Stuttering." *Journal of Abnormal Psychology* 74 (1969): 452–53.

16. What implications do the following articles have for the assessment of adul stutterers?

GUSTAVSON, C. "A Talisman and a Convalescence." *Quarterly Journal o Speech*, 30 (1944): 465–70.

LANYON, R. "The Measurement of Stuttering Severity." *Journal of Speech an Hearing Research*, 10 (1947): 836–43.

PRINS, D. "Personality, Stuttering Severity, and Age." *Journal of Speech an Hearing Research*, 15 (1972): 148–54.

SILVERMAN, F., and D. WILLIAMS. "Prediction of Stuttering by School-Age Stut terers." *Journal of Speech and Hearing Research*, 15 (1972): 189–93.

WERTHEIM, E. "A New Approach to the Classification and Measurement o Stuttering." *Journal of Speech and Hearing Disorders*, 37 (1972): 242–51.

YAIRI, E., and D. WILLIAMS. "Speech Clinicians' Stereotypes of Elementary School Boys Who Stutter." *Journal of Communication Disorders*, 3 (1970) 161–70.

17. Define or identify the following:

spontaneous recovery	Thematic Apperception Test
base rate	rhythmokinesis
MMPI	Bears' Questionnaire
Palmer Sweat Index	Purdue Questionnaire
Van Riper's equation of stuttering	superstutterer

BIBLIOGRAPHY

ANDREWS, G. and M. HARRIS (1964). *The Syndrome of Stuttering*. Clinics in Developmental Medicine No. 17. London: William Heinemann Medical Books Ltd.

BEECH, H. R. and F. FRANSELLA (1968). *Research and Experiment in Stuttering*. New York: Pergamon Press.

BLOCH, E. and L. GOODSTEIN (1971). "Functional Speech Disorders and Personality: A Decade of Research." *Journal of Speech and Hearing Disorders*, 36: 295–314.

BLOODSTEIN, O. (1969). *A Handbook of Stuttering*. Chicago: National Easter Seal Society for Crippled Children and Adults.

CASSEL, R. (1957). *The Cassel Group Level of Aspiration Test*. Beverly Hills, Calif.: Western Psychological Services.

CHAPMAN, M. (1959). *Self-Inventory*, 3rd ed. Minneapolis: Burgess.

COOPER, E. (1972). *The Cooper Chronicity Prediction Checklist for School-Age Stutterers*. University, Ala.: Cooper.

DARLEY, F., A. ARONSON, and J. BROWN (1969). "Differential Diagnostic Patterns of Dysarthria." *Journal of Speech and Hearing Research*, 12: 246–69.

DOUGLASS, E. and B. QUARRINGTON (1952). "The Differentiation of Interiorized and Exteriorized Secondary Stuttering." *Journal of Speech and Hearing Disorders*, 17: 377–85.

EMERICK, L. (1970). *Therapy for Young Stutterers*. Danville, Ill.: Interstate Printers and Publishers.

——— (1970). *With Slow and Halting Tongue*. Marquette, Mich.: Guelff.

EMERICK, L. and C. HAMRE (1972). *An Analysis of Stuttering*. Danville, Ill.: Interstate Printers and Publishers.

EMERICK, L. and A. TEIGLAND (1965). "Pediatricians and Speech Disorders." *Central States Speech Journal*, 16: 290–94.

FOX, D. and E. CONNELLY (1970). *Exiting the Circle*. Houston, Tex.: University of Houston.

FREUND, H. (1966). *Psychopathology and the Problem of Stuttering*. Springfield, Ill.: Charles C Thomas.

GAVIS, L. (1946). "Bombing Mission No. 15." *Journal of Abnormal and Social Psychology*, 41: 189–98.

GODLEE, R. (1917). *Lord Lister*. New York: The Macmillan Company.

GOVEN, P. and G. VETTE (1966). *A Manual for Stuttering Therapy*. Pittsburgh: Stanwix House.

GREGORY, H. (1969). *An Assessment of the Results of Stuttering Therapy* Evanston, Ill.: Northwestern University, Office of Education Research Report.

GRINKER, R. and J. SPIEGAL (1945). *War Neuroses*. Philadelphia: Blakistor Company.

HOFFER, E. (1969). *Working and Thinking on the Waterfront*. New York: Perennial Library.

JOHNSON, G. (1961). "Environmental Reorganization in Primary Stuttering." Unpublished manuscript.

JOHNSON, W. (1959). *Toward Understanding Stuttering*. Chicago: National Easter Seal Society for Crippled Children and Adults.

JOHNSON, W. and R. AMMONS (1944). "Studies in the Psychology of Stuttering: XVIII. The Construction and Application of a Test of Attitude Toward Stuttering." *Journal of Speech Disorders*, 9: 39–49.

JOHNSON, W., F. DARLEY, and D. SPRIESTERSBACH (1963). *Diagnostic Methods in Speech Pathology*. New York: Harper & Row, Publishers.

KINSTLER, D. (1961). "Covert and Overt Maternal Rejection in Stuttering." *Journal of Speech and Hearing Disorders*, 26: 145–55.

LASSERS, L. (1945). *Eight Keys to Normal Speech and Child Adjustment*. San Francisco: Lassers.

LEE, L. (1969). *The Northwestern Syntax Screening Test*. Evanston, Ill.: Northwestern University.

LUCHSINGER, R. and G. ARNOLD (1965). *Voice-Speech-Language*. Belmont, Calif.: Wadsworth Publishing Company.

LUPER, H., ed. (1968). *Stuttering: Successes and Failures in Therapy*. Memphis, Tenn.: Speech Foundation of America.

MARTYN, M., J. SHEEHAN, and K. SLUTZ (1969). "Incidence of Stuttering and Other Speech Disorders Among the Retarded." *American Journal of Mental Deficiency*, 74: 206–211.

MULDER, R. (1960). *Tangled Tongues*. Monmouth, Oreg.: Educational Materials Production.

MURPHY, A., ed. (1962). *Stuttering: Its Prevention*. Memphis, Tenn.: Speech Foundation of America.

PENNINGTON, R. (1955). *For Parents of a Child Beginning to Stutter*. Danville, Ill.: Interstate Printers and Publishers.

ROBINSON, F. (1960). *Children Who Stutter*. Oxford, Ohio: Miami University Press.

————— (1964). *Introduction to Stuttering.* Englewood Cliffs, N.J.: Prentice-Hall, Inc.

Rosenzweig, S., E. Fleming, and H. Clark (1947). "Revised Scoring Manual for the Rosenzweig Picture-Frustration Study." *Journal of Psychology,* 24: 165–208.

Sander, E. (1959). "Counselling Parents of Stuttering Children." *Journal of Speech and Hearing Disorders,* 24: 262–71.

Schuell, H. (1949). "Working with Parents of Stuttering Children." *Journal of Speech and Hearing Disorders,* 14: 251–54.

Shearer, W. and J. Williams (1965). "Self-Recovery from Stuttering." *Journal of Speech and Hearing Disorders,* 30: 288–90.

Sheehan, J. (1970). *Stuttering: Research and Therapy.* New York: Harper & Row, Publishers.

Sheehan, J., P. Cortese, and R. Hadley (1962). "Guilt, Shame, and Tension in Graphic Projections of Stuttering." *Journal of Speech and Hearing Disorders,* 27: 129–39.

Sheehan, J. and M. Martyn (1970). "Stuttering and Its Disappearance." *Journal of Speech and Hearing Research,* 13: 279–89.

Sheehan, J., M. Martyn, and K. Kilburn (1968). "Speech Disorders in Retardation." *American Journal of Mental Deficiency,* 73: 251–56.

Silverman, E. (1972). "Generality of Disfluency Data Collected from Preschoolers." *Journal of Speech and Hearing Research,* 15: 84–91.

Silverman, F. (1970). "Concern of Elementary-School Stutterers about Their Stuttering." *Journal of Speech and Hearing Disorders,* 35: 361–63.

Simpson, B. (1966). *Stuttering Therapy: A Guide for the Speech Clinician.* Danville, Ill.: Interstate Printers and Publishers.

Starkweather, C. W. (1972). *Stuttering: An Account of Intensive Demonstration Therapy.* Memphis, Tenn.: Speech Foundation of America.

Stennett, N. (1967). *A Workbook for Stuttering.* Chicago: King Company.

Van Riper, C. (1971). *The Nature of Stuttering.* Englewood Cliffs, N.J.: Prentice-Hall, Inc.

————— (1970). "A One-Week Stuttering Therapy Program." *Western Michigan University Journal of Speech Therapy,* 7: 2–3.

————— (1963). *Speech Correction: Principles and Methods.* Englewood Cliffs, N.J.: Prentice-Hall, Inc.

————— (1961). *Your Child's Speech Problems.* New York: Harper & Row, Publishers.

—————, ed. (1964). *Treatment of the Young Stutterer in the School.* Memphis, Tenn.: Speech Foundation of America.

Van Riper, C. and L. Gruber (1957) *A Casebook in Stuttering.* New York: Harper & Row, Publishers.

WEISS, D. (1964). *Cluttering*. Englewood Cliffs, N.J.: Prentice-Hall, Inc.

WILLIAMS, D. (1971). "Stuttering Therapy for Children." In L. Travis, ed., *Handbook of Speech Pathology*. New York: Appleton-Century-Crofts.

WINGATE, M. (1971). "The Fear of Stuttering." *Journal of the American Speech and Hearing Association*, 13: 3–5.

———— (1964). "Recovery from Stuttering." *Journal of Speech and Hearing Disorders*, 29: 312–21.

WOOLF, G. (1967). "The Assessment of Stuttering as Struggle, Avoidance, and Expectancy." *British Journal of Disorders of Communication*, 2: 158–71.

WYATT, E. (1969). *Language Learning and Communication Disorders in Children*. New York: The Free Press.

7

the assessment
of aphasia in adults

Aphasia is a disturbance in the very attribute that is so uniquely human, a person's ability to symbolize.[1] More specifically, aphasia is a syndrome of language impairment resulting from destruction of cortical tissue and is characterized by one or more of the following symptoms:

1. Disturbance in receiving and decoding symbolic materials via auditory, visual, or tactile channels. Although the individual can still hear and see, he has difficulty deciphering the learned associations of messages.
2. Disturbance in central processes of meaning, word selection, and message formulation.
3. Disturbance in expressing symbolic materials by means of speech, writing, or gesture.

Aphasia is not, however, simply a loss of words. It can generally be shown clinically, by the use of open-end sentences, oral opposites, or other forms of cueing, that even severe aphasics are capable of uttering words. The problem seems to be in *retrieving* words—that is, translating internal idiosyncratic

---

[1] Rarely is a client totally impaired in the use of language, and hence the term dysphasia may be more appropriate. Indeed, there is a rather wide range of disturbance extending from the mild impairment suffered by former President Eisenhower (1965) to the almost total loss of language described by McBride (1969). In keeping with traditional writing, however, we shall use the term aphasia to refer to this total range of impairment.

symbols into conventional language forms (Schuell, Jenkins, Jimenez-Pabon 1964; Eisenson, 1971).[2] The following description, written by a rehabilitated aphasic, is instructive:

> It was not alone that I found I could not speak; words tumbled over themselves in my mind, but I could not get them to my lips. When they came I had sometimes forgotten what I wanted to say. This division between meaning and words which normally are one, is one of the plagues of the stroke sufferer. It accounts for his apparent mental slowness. But worse than this difficulty was the lack of vocabulary with which to make people aware of what I thought, and the lack of means of expression which prevented them from understanding the matters that were uppermost in my mind. They could not grasp the physical stress that was shaking me; all its peculiar nature was hidden from them, along with the compound of aches, pains, and nervous sensations. This causes much of the ill feeling between stroke victims and the outer world. The victim is bewildered because he cannot explain his predicament: he tries to explain, but sputters and gives up in despair (Wint, 1965: 28).

In addition to the language impairment, the individual may also have difficulty in the mechanical production of speech sounds due to paralysis or weakness of the oral area. This is termed *dysarthria*. Another curious disorder *apraxia,* is sometimes associated with aphasia: it is a disturbance in voluntary muscle control but without paralysis or weakness; the individual seems to have lost the ability to do what he wishes. Clients with verbal apraxia seem to have somehow lost the automaticity of sound, syllable, and word sequencing.

> Apraxia is not unlike an exaggerated type of self-consciousness which affects many nonaphasic individuals while attempting to perform a complex psychomotor act under close scrutiny. The more attention they pay to how they are doing, the worse their performance. An apraxic may be observed to lick his lips while eating an ice-cream cone but a moment later be unable to duplicate the act upon command. In fact, the more volition involved in the execution of a particular act, the worse the apraxic's performance seems to be. Is apraxia a language-dependent disorder or simply a disturbance of skilled movements? (See Ettlinger, 1969; Aten, Johns, and Darley, 1971.)

Early students of aphasia concerned themselves with an elaborate taxonomy based upon symptomatology. There was a compulsion to name and classify every possible phenomenon, even to the last anosmia. A host of isolated subtypes of aphasia disturbance was identified, accorded an appropriately obscure Latin or Greek term, and localized to specific sites on the cortex. In

---

[2] The more common a word is, the more probable that it will be retained. For example, an aphasic may understand or use the words "kiss" or "rain" but not "osculation" or "precipitation," even though all four might have been in his premorbid vocabulary. Words more frequently used—such as special occupational vocabulary items—have a greater number of associations and hence greater probability of recognition or recall. See Project 1.

our judgment, the many classifications and recategorizations tend to confuse rather than clarify:[3]

More recently, theoretical models have been devised (Schuell, Jenkins, and Jimenez-Pabon, 1964; Wepman, *et al.*, 1960; Osgood and Miron, 1963) to account for the linguistic, neurological, and behavioral manifestations of brain injury. Although there is some controversy as to whether the language disturbance in aphasia is uni- or multidimensional (Jones and Wepman, 1961; Schuell and Jenkins, 1962), careful clinical assessment of patients fails to reveal subtypes with isolated linguistic deficits (Smith, 1971); in fact, aphasics typically show some degree of disturbance in all areas of language usage:

> Usually, in aphasia, the active linguistic processes, speaking and writing, show more impairment than the passive ones, listening and reading. Here *show* may be the important word; it may be that impairment is only more observable in the active modalities, although this is questionable. However, the same kind of linguistic impairment tends to be apparent in all modalities. Patients tend to write much as they talk; auditory and reading comprehension tend to break down at a somewhat similar level of difficulty in terms of word frequency and length of unit that can be grasped (Schuell, Jenkins, and Jimenez-Pabon, 1964: 104).

See also the work of Keenan (1968) and others (Schuell, *et al.*, 1969; Goodglass, Gleason, and Hyde, 1970; Eisenson, 1971).

With regard to evaluation of aphasic clients, it is more helpful to simply describe what the client can and cannot do with language. Instead of using esoteric labels, the clinician can delineate the client's ability to talk, listen, read, and write. However, the clinician should be familiar with the traditional terminology, for it tends to be used by members of the medical and paramedical professions (see Project 2).

In our zeal to identify the psycholinguistic dimensions of aphasia, it is possible to forget that brain injury is a grave health problem. In addition to the language impairment, the individual may present paralysis or paresis of the extremities (generally the right side, sometimes including the face), sensory abnormalities, and behavioral disturbances. There seems to be little, if any, relationship between these difficulties and the extent of the language impairment. Above all, the diagnostician must remember that aphasia is both a personal catastrophe and a family crisis, as Buck (1968) so eloquently points out.

DIFFERENTIAL DIAGNOSIS

The clinician is called upon occasionally to distinguish between aphasia and a number of other conditions involving abnormality in language. We include

---

[3] Despite the different terms employed, the various classification systems are essentially alike (Eisenson, 1971).

below a brief discussion of five disorders that might be confused with aphasia; laymen frequently misidentify aphasia as one of the first three listed, often with harmful consequences for the client. However, it should be kept in mind that impairment of symbolic functioning can coexist with any of these anomalies.

mental retardation

The most frequent interpretation of aphasia by laymen, in our clinical experience, is that the patient has become hopelessly retarded. Because of the stigma of brain damage, even educated persons have told friends or colleagues that their spouse has suffered a heart attack, rather than a stroke. Consider the impact of these impressions upon the aphasic:

> Mr. Vernon Nelson, a forty-three-year-old former teamster and self-educated amateur archeologist, resided in a grim nursing home surrounded by old people. Following a stroke almost a year before our consultation, his relatives insisted upon admitting him, claiming that he was senile and incapable of handling his affairs. Like many aphasics, Mr. Nelson on superficial observation, did seem infantile; he lacked expressive language, except for some automatic speech which he generally used inappropriately; he cried easily and appeared apathetic and withdrawn. He used one phrase over and over again: "I can't think." He, too, was convinced of his mental incapacity. On testing, we found that he indeed could think; he scored at the 90th percentile on a test of recognition vocabulary and showed good auditory comprehension for short, simple messages. It took a great deal of supportive counseling and demonstration therapy before he agreed to enter treatment; but once he did, Mr. Nelson made excellent progress. He later took a seasonal position as a receptionist in a local museum that featured an extensive collection of American Indian lore.

It is sobering to speculate how many untested and untreated aphasic individuals are languishing in nursing homes or occupying some dim corner in private residences on the mistaken premise that they are mentally defective.

psychosis

Although it is rather easy for the professional to distinguish aphasia from psychosis, it is understandable why laymen are often confused. The aphasic may say "yes" when he means "no," use obscenities and other antisocial language or gestures freely, laugh or cry often, lapse into euphoria, deny his symptoms, or withdraw into severe depression and despair. The distinguishing features of psychosis are, however, rather obvious: severe personality decomposition—not just frustration or emotional overflow when trying to comprehend or speak—and distortion of, or loss of contact with, reality. The vast majority of aphasic patients do not show evidence of mental deterioration or gross disturbances in processing reality.

Considering all the frustrations aphasics encounter, we have often wondered why they do not behave in a more abnormal manner than they do. Indeed their demeanor and social interaction, aside from the language impairment, are remarkably normal.

> Aphasic patients respond appropriately to situations and people, even when comprehension of language is impaired. Their behavior is reasonable and their responses are predictable within the framework of what is known about the organization of language. They do not present bizarre responses or bizarre behavior (Schuell, Jenkins, and Jimenez-Pabon, 1964: 323).

Nevertheless, some individuals with aphasia do experience psychotic episodes, particularly periods of severe depression. (See the book by Hodgins [1964] for a personal account of an involutional depression following aphasia.)

paralysis of tongue or vocal folds

Many relatives assume that the patient's language impairment stems from paralysis of the tongue or larynx. Even trained and experienced nurses will hand a pen to the adult aphasic and request that he write the message he cannot utter. Aphasia is a *breakdown of symbolic functioning*—the content (language) of messages is disturbed regardless of the modality attempted—while individuals with dysarthria or laryngeal paralysis present a disturbance in the mechanical production (speech) of language forms. Some clients will, of course, have difficulty with both aspects following a stroke or other type of brain injury.

voluntary or hysterical mutism

The clinician will see a certain number of persons who feign an inability to talk when no organic impairment exists, or who exaggerate a problem that does exist. A few individuals may be trying to work out a psychological conflict by unconsciously embracing speechlessness. This is called a conversion neurosis. Three features distinguish nonorganic mutism from aphasia. First, an aphasic almost always has difficulty with comprehending; the hysterically mute will generally understand everything said to him, even complex instructions. Secondly, the brain damaged patient will exhibit concern over his language barrier; the psychologically disturbed individual, on the other hand, doesn't seem to mind his inability to talk because his "impairment" is a solution to his anxiety. Finally, the hysterically mute will be too silent, too speechless. Even profoundly impaired aphasics exhibit some automatic speech such as swearing, counting, and ritual social language; many respond to open-ended statements ("The flag is red, white, and ———"), and some can even repeat words after the examiner.

language confusion

Persons suffering generalized brain damage manifest language aberrations which, on cursory appraisal, might be confused with aphasia:

> Delver Lespi, age fifty-seven, was referred to us for evaluation in a veterans' hospital. His medical record revealed a diagnosis of multiple brain lesions (lead inhalation), bilateral weakness of the lower extremities, and disorientation. When we examined him, Mr. Lespi was confused and disoriented. Although his message was inappropriate to the situation, his sentence structure was normal. He frequently interrupted the testing situation to relate, in a rambling, fragmented manner, some tale of his early years as a lumberman. In general, his responses were slow, occasionally bizarre; at times he would begin to answer a query, stop, stare into space, and then lapse into a one-sided conversation with someone from his past.

Additional material on the differential diagnosis of aphasia may be found in Darley (1964: 36–40) and Schuell, Jenkins, and Jimenez-Pabon (1964: 315–28). For detailed discussions of the nature of aphasia, consult the work of Wepman (1951), Schuell, Jenkins, and Jimenez-Pabon (1964) and others (Burr, 1964; Osgood and Miron, 1963; Buck, 1968; Sarno, 1972).

INCIDENCE AND ETIOLOGY

Aphasia is always caused by damage to the brain.[4] Brain damage, however, will not *always* result in aphasia. Automobile accidents in which head injury is incurred, infectious diseases (such as meningitis), tumors, or certain degenerative diseases are all possible sources of cortical damage and aphasia. The most frequent cause of aphasia, however, is a disturbance of the blood supply to the brain, commonly called a stroke. The cerebral vascular accident (CVA) is a relatively common illness that affects approximately a million persons each year. In the United States, stroke now stands in third place as a cause of death, outdistanced only by heart disease and cancer. No one knows precisely how many surviving stroke victims are left with language impairment; estimates suggest at least a quarter of a million or more individuals present some degree of aphasia that warrants treatment.

Information regarding the etiology of aphasia may be found in the following sources: Buchanan, 1957; Netter, 1958; Page *et al.*, 1961; Grinker and Sahs, 1966; Chusid and McDonald, 1967.

---

[4] Persons who suffer migraine headache, a condition that produces temporary cerebral edema, reportedly experience transient auditory aphasia (Hockaday and Whitty, 1969).

CASE EXAMPLE

In order to portray the nature and scope of the clinician's involvement in the evaluation of adults with language impairment, we now present an extensive case example. The account is chronological and delineates our role from the moment we were first alerted by the physician until a treatment plan was devised.

prologue

A series of events transpired prior to our entry into the case, and the following account was pieced together only after we began to work with the client—from limited fragments Mr. Tenhave could tell us, descriptions offered by his wife, and hospital records. Compare the following account with those by Hodgins (1964: 7) and Whitehouse (1968: 21):

Roy Tenhave arose abruptly at 11:30 p.m. soon after retiring, muttering something about an idea he must write down or he would surely forget it. His wife, familiar with her husband's late evening flashes of insight, turned over and dozed. Padding through the darkened house and into his study, Mr. Tenhave noticed that his right leg was somewhat stiff and felt a tingling and creeping numbness as if his limb were going to sleep. Turning on his desk lamp, he found his notebook and selected a pencil. Mr. Tenhave had been working on a manuscript dealing with bird migration in Upper Michigan, and just as he was drifting off to sleep, he had suddenly divined a novel way to illustrate flight routes. (Later, Mr. Tenhave could not recall the idea; that page of his notebook contained only an illegible scrawl.) As he bent over his desk and started to write, he felt dizzy and watched in curious fascination as the pencil slid slowly out of his hand. Then the room became a fuzzy blur, and he felt himself cascade over the swivel chair and crash to the floor in a grotesque heap. "This is silly," he thought; as he was struggling to arise, he discovered that his right arm and leg stubbornly refused to function. After several unsuccessful attempts to get up, he called for his wife—at least, he meant to call—but all he heard was a strange vowel sound, almost like an animal bleating. In that instant, Mr. Tenhave knew what was happening to him: he was having a stroke. Mrs. Tenhave immediately summoned the city ambulance and alerted her husband's physician, Dr. Roger Wilson, a specialist in internal medicine. In the emergency room, the resident physician worked swiftly to insure the patient could breathe easily, carefully measured his blood pressure, and administered antibiotics.

early intervention

We entered the case five days later, on January 25, when Dr. Wilson's nurse called and requested consultation. A note from Dr. Wilson followed:

Roy Tenhave, fifty-two-year-old high-school biology teacher, suffered a moderately severe CVA on January 19. Left cerebral hemisphere, clinically diagnosed as thromotic. Right hemiplegia: the leg is responding to physical therapy but, though it is early yet, the arm is doubtful. He may also have a visual field cut on the right—his responses are inconsistent. A neurological workup is being done, and the results will be in his record when you get to the hospital. He is having a great deal of difficulty communicating. I talked briefly with his wife, but she needs more information about aphasia.

We cannot overemphasize the critical importance of early intervention in the clinical management of aphasic clients; this position becomes obvious when we consider the broader definition of aphasia as a personal and family catastrophe (Buck, 1968). A little bit of early support and counseling is much more effective than a great deal of help later. By prompt involvement, we do not necessarily mean initiating language therapy, although if accomplished indirectly in the form of general stimulation, it is certainly a wise recommendation. Rather, we refer to the following: (1) Nurses and others who work with the patient should receive inservice training. Hospitals in smaller, isolated communities are not generally equipped or staffed to deal adequately with aphasic patients during the primary stage of recovery (Twamley and Emerick, 1970). (2) There should be information-sharing and planning conferences with professional team members—the physician, physical therapist, occupational therapist, social worker, and others concerned with the rehabilitation of the patient. (3) Supportive monologue interviews with the aphasic patient should be conducted to provide release of feelings and to reassure him that a professional worker is concerned and attempting to do something about his language problem. (4) Finally, family counseling is most important.

interview with Mrs. Tenhave

In order to adequately understand the aphasic patient, it is necessary to understand something about the people close to him, their prior relationships with him, their present fears and reactions, and their hopes for the future. Families are confronted with a crisis when an adult member is suddenly afflicted with a deadly, often mysterious illness that results in such profound physical and psychological alterations. A serious illness disrupts communication patterns, dissolves or shifts roles, and forces family members to assume unfamiliar responsibilities. The resolution of the crisis situation, the manner in which members reorganize the family structure, will have profound implications for the patient and the prospects for his rehabilitation. (Taylor and Myers, 1952). See Project 3.

As we planned our initial counseling session with Mrs. Tenhave, we reviewed the many difficulties with which the family of an aphasic must cope —often, unfortunately, without professional guidance (Derman and Manaster, 1967).

We arranged to meet Mrs. Tenhave in the speech clinic, assuming that she had become satiated with the aseptic atmosphere of the hospital during her prolonged vigil. On January 26, she arrived early for the interview, a petite, attractive woman in her late forties. She was well dressed and groomed but looked haggard and worn. Despite her subdued manner, however, we sensed almost immediately her basic strength of character.

We directed Mrs. Tenhave to a comfortable chair and offered her a cup of coffee. Recalling Derman and Manaster's (1967) advice that relatives of aphasics need information, reassurance, and an outlet for frustration, we invited her to tell us about her husband's illness. We began by acknowledging quietly that the past few days must have been very difficult for her. She seemed to welcome the opportunity to pour out some of her pent-up thoughts and fears:

> Yes, it certainly was a shock. Roy was perfectly well and then, suddenly, he was struck down like this. At first I was terrified that he was going to die; then, when I saw he was paralyzed and couldn't talk, I found myself praying that he would. That made me feel so terribly guilty—but an active life means so much to him. What will he be able to do now? If only I would have insisted that he see Dr. Wilson earlier when he had the dizzy spells and the tingling in his arm and leg; I just attributed it to arthritis and the fact that he had been working so hard on his bird migration manuscript. I feel so . . . so alone. No . . . (she raised her hand to politely reject our murmur of reassurance), I don't mean to play the little housewife in a quandary. I have taught elementary children for almost twenty years. I mean, Roy and I did so much together—hikes, I edited all his writing, went on field trips with his students, I even went hunting with him. Now I don't know what will happen. The doctor talks about brain damage . . . but will he be normal? What can I expect? What will he be able to do? Here I am feeling sorry for myself when I should be thinking about him. He must be so upset.

At this point Mrs. Tenhave began to weep softly. We gently suggested that it was good to let the tension and uncertainty come out, that we understood how she felt, and that it was certainly normal to have the feeling she reported. When she recovered her composure, Mrs. Tenhave was full of questions:

> Dr. Wilson said that Roy is aphasic. I looked that up in the dictionary and found it meant loss of power to use and understand speech. But how much can he understand? Can he write? I gave him a pencil the other day when he was trying to tell me something, and he just pointed to his right arm and shook his head. What can I do to help him? A colleague of mine at school gave me a child's first alphabet book and suggested I start teaching Roy with it. She said that it had helped her father when he had a stroke. When I tried it with Roy, he threw the book and knocked over a vase of flowers. He never was a violent man. He swears so much now and cries so easily. He was always such a reserved and quiet person and now he seems so exposed. Perhaps that's why he doesn't want to see any of his colleagues or students. They come to the hospital, but I can tell Roy is terribly embarrassed. How can I make his friends understand when I don't myself?

Mrs. Tenhave had much more to say during this initial interview; we have included only a portion to show some of the concerns she reported. In many respects, she was an unusually easy respondent. Often we have had to be much more directive and reassuring with less educated and perceptive spouses. By the end of the hour, she was eager to receive the information we provided:

> Aphasia is more than a disturbance in speech. It is an impairment of language that is coded and stored in the brain. When a person has a stroke, a portion of the brain dies. Initially, because of the swelling that occurs around the specific area of injury, the patient shows more disturbance in language and other respects than he will later. No one really knows how much recovery will take place spontaneously, or how long it will continue. Usually, however, spontaneous improvement occurs within the first three months after the stroke. The pamphlet I will give you at the end of our chat will explain this more fully.
>
> I wanted to mention a bit more about language. As you know from teaching elementary children to read, language is an elaborate system of symbols. The word "cow," for example, stands for, or is used as, a shorthand way of identifying a Holstein or Hereford. It would be impossible to run out in the pasture and lead in a furry, lactating quadruped every time we wanted to use the word "cow." We use symbols, as you know, in four basic ways—talking, listening, reading, and writing. Usually an aphasic patient has difficulty in all four areas, although he generally seems to have more trouble generating language—that is, speaking and writing. So, Mr. Tenhave's reluctance to write may not just be due to his paralyzed arm. Often people think that the aphasic person seems to understand everything spoken to him. But it usually can be shown that the patient indeed cannot understand everything but rather detects certain nonverbal cues or makes some socially proved gestures that give the impression of accurate listening. As Mr. Tenhave seems to, many aphasics have some oral expression that we can call automatic speech. They may be able to count, recite letters of the alphabet (and other items occuring in a series), swear, and repeat memorized prayers and poems. It is important to remember that this language is mostly involuntary, it does not involve the conscious search for and use of words. Some patients can even imitate words uttered by others. This, too, is not true language. Most aphasics have a low threshold of frustration—and a horde of frustrations! Small wonder that they cry or swear so frequently. Your husband does not have the usual verbal outlets to release pent-up feelings. What should you do when this happens? The best response is to acknowledge his feelings, let him know you understand, and then divert his attention to something else.

We advised Mrs. Tenhave to avoid the role of teacher with her husband; he needed her support and affection, not tutoring. We explained that children's books are insulting to aphasics who, even though severely retarded in language usage, retain an adult outlook. It is essential, we added, that people continue to deal with the aphasic on an adult level; it is infantilizing enough to be physically helpless, to have lost the power of speech, and to be utterly dependent upon others for satisfaction of all one's needs. Finally, we stressed the importance of maintaining lines of communication with her husband.[5]

---

[5] Human contact and stimulation appear to be vital deterrents to withdrawal and depression (Buck, 1968; Farrell, 1969; Knox, 1971).

Keep talking to him, even if the responses are negligible. In some cases, because the patient is more or less silent, the persons surrounding him cease to talk. They assume that because he does not verbalize, he does not want to hear conversation. It is obvious, of course, that no one should talk *about* Mr. Tenhave in his presence. Don't bombard him with questions that demand a response, for this will only serve to point up his lack of verbal ability and further frustrate him. Experiment with different ways to communicate with him—gestures, printed cards, anything (Eagleson, Vaughn, and Knudson, 1970). I plan to give your husband a brief screening test soon, and then we can get together again to discuss the best ways of communicating with him.

In order to further her understanding of Mr. Tenhave's problem, we loaned her a copy of a well-known pamphlet on aphasia (Taylor, 1958)[6] and promised we would meet at a later date to discuss its contents. Thinking she might need additional support, as well as an emotional outlet, we gave her the phone number of the wife of a former patient who had recently started a discussion group for relatives of adult aphasics.

the screening test

On January 28, we went to St. Luke's Hospital to make a preliminary appraisal of Mr. Tenhave's language problem. Although he had been in the hospital only eight days, his physical recovery, according to Dr. Wilson, had been remarkable. Mr. Tenhave now sat up in a chair twice daily for almost an hour, had regained bowel and bladder control, and seemed alert and responsive to his environment. We questioned the nurses on the floor, and they revealed that although he was still swearing and labile when he tried to communicate, he appeared to understand short, simple sentences, responded with a reliable "yes" or "no," and was using more words spontaneously. He also manifested considerable "reactive language"—words and short phrases that seemed to be prompted by the situation or a verbal stimulus but which he could not repeat voluntarily.

Checking Mr. Tenhave's medical file, we noted the neurologist's report:

This alert, oriented adult male suffered a CVA on 1/19/70. Expressive-receptive aphasia. Right hemiplegia. Babinski sign on the right. Gross motor functioning of involved leg is returning; arm and hand are doubtful. Electroencephalography revealed a focal lesion in the left parietal-temporal region. Site of lesion confirmed by brain scan and angiography. Right side astereognosis. Right homonymous hemianopsia.

This report told us several important things about the patient: the brain damage was apparently localized and was not widespread; the aphasia was probably not transitory since lesions in the region cited generally result in

---

[6] There are several excellent publications written for relatives of adult patients with aphasia (Horowitz, 1962; American Heart Association, 1965; Longerich, 1955; Boone, 1961; Peterson and Olsen, 1964).

more persistent language impairment; he could not identify objects by touch when they were placed in his right hand; and he could not see in the right field of vision. This last anomaly would require that we present testing materials from the patient's left side. (See Project 4 regarding the neurological examination.)

Administering the screening test.   An adult aphasic, especially during the primary stages of recovery, has little or no means of communication. He is, in a very real sense, isolated. Investigations in sensory deprivation have shown what a frightening and devastating experience isolation can be; in aphasia it can lead to profound depression and withdrawal as well as non-verbal habits that make subsequent therapy difficult. Therefore, by early testing, we must discover ways to establish bonds of communication with the client. In order to rapidly assess a client's language capacity, a short screening test was devised (Emerick and Coyne, 1972).[7]

This instrument is designed to swiftly evaluate a patient's language abilities prior to the administration of a more lengthy inventory. It assesses a patient's communicative abilities in two broad areas, *input* (or the evaluation of stimuli from an external source) and *output*, the generation of verbal responses. Although patients change rapidly during the first month following brain injury, it is important that the workers in the helping professions have some preliminary notion of the individual's communicative abilities so they can: (1) advise relatives about the best means of communicating with the patient; (2) assist other professional workers in the management of the patient; and (3) chart the patient's progress or lack of progress during the early stages of recovery (prognostically, of course, early improvement is a good sign).

When I entered his room, Mr. Tenhave was sitting up in bed, looking idly out the window; his right arm lay useless in his lap. Approaching from his left side, I extended my hand and introduced myself as a speech therapist. He pointed to his paralyzed arm and shook his head in a gesture of futility. I sat down next to his bed, opened the kit of testing materials, and immediately came to the point.

> I would like to find out in what ways you are having difficulty talking and understanding. I will ask you some questions and have you look at some pictures. Some of the tasks will be simple; others will be more difficult. Just answer the best you can. Okay?

I talked slowly and distinctly, pausing often and watching carefully for any signs of confusion. Mr. Tenhave looked curiously at the testing kit, pointed to

---

[7] Shortened versions of published language inventories may be used for early screening (Eisenson, 1954; Sklar, 1963; Taylor, 1963; Wepman and Jones, 1961; Schuell, 1957; Porch, 1967; Emerick, 1972). See also the work of Orgass and Poeck (1969) and Spellacy and Spreen (1969).

his mouth, and made a motion that seemed to say, "Let's get on with it." Testing need not be traumatic if the patient is approached in a friendly, humane, and adult manner. In fact, as Schuell, Jenkins, and Jimenez-Pabon (1964) point out, most aphasics expect that the clinician will want to determine what they can and cannot do with regard to language. We prefer not to refer to the tasks as "tests," but rather encourage the patient to explore his problem with us so we can determine where to begin helping him.

Rather than beginning directly with the items on the screening test, we decided to check Mr. Tenhave's auditory comprehension by using several verbal disparities (Snidecor, 1955). This procedure would allow him time to "tune-up" his input circuits and also permit us to check the reliability of his "yes" and "no" responses. Keeping in mind Buck's (1968) advice that it is important to provide links with a client's former life, and remembering that Mr. Tenhave was an accomplished ornithologist, we named several real birds and some imaginary ones, and asked him to indicate which were real by nodding or answering.

We then turned to the screening kit and, starting with the input tasks (why do we begin with the input portion?), moved through the various items. The completed test protocol form is included (Figure 8) in order to show the type of tasks employed and the patient's response to them. The total test took less than ten minutes to administer, but even that brief period of concentration left Mr. Tenhave somewhat fatigued.

As I thanked him and collected my things to leave, Mr. Tenhave seemed to be upset. He pointed to the testing kit and then his mouth; his eyes glistened with tears and his chin quivered slightly. Sitting down again beside his bed, I realized my error: aphasic patients need closure like any other client. Remembering that monologue interviews are often helpful in providing an outlet for language-impaired adults (Anders and Emerick, 1963), I began to verbalize his feelings, speaking slowly and carefully:

> This is tough for you. You have words inside and you can't seem to get them out. Some people talk down or too loudly; some talk too fast and don't give you a chance to understand. It's booming and buzzing; your own language is like a foreign one. You get mad and want to fight, but your arm and your leg are holding you back. You swear and sometimes can't stop crying. But it is going to get better. I am encouraged by how you did today. Oh, sure, the tasks were simple ones, but the point is, you could do them. You recognized false bird names; you matched pictures and words; you were even able to repeat some words when I provided the model. These are all good signs, especially so soon after the stroke. I also like the way you are able to tell when you do make a mistake. I am going to talk to Dr. Wilson and arrange to come back again.

During this brief monologue, Mr. Tenhave sighed, nodded, and appeared to relax considerably.

Before leaving the hospital, we wrote this short note to Dr. Wilson:

SCREENING TEST OF APHASIA

Test Protocol

by

Lon Emerick, Ph.D.
J. Michael Coyne, M.D.

| Roy O. Tenhave | January 4, 1918 | January 28, 1970 |
| patient | date of birth | date |

I. INPUT

   A. Auditory (to be answered "yes" or "no" or in some
       manner of signaling affirmative and negative)

      1. Disparities:

         a. Is your name Mr. (use incorrect name)   "yes"
         b. Are you in the hospital? "yes"--disgusted look
         c. Are you 20 years old? shook head "no," smiled
         d. Is this the year 19 "yes" "yes"
         e. Do you take a bath in a teacup? "no," emphati-
            cally, waved as if wishing to move to more
            difficult tasks.

      2. Commands (the patient is instructed to point to
         appropriate objects and pictures after hearing a
         verbal cue): Card I

         a. match +   f. bed   +
         b. coin   +   g. pencil +
         c. key   +   h. knife +   swift, certain
         d. pen   +   i. chair +   responses
         e. books +   j. hammer +

      3. Understanding multiple commands (avoid gestures
         that reveal the appropriate response):

         a. Put the key on the bed picked up the key--asked
            for repetition
         b. Put the pen on the table   +
         c. Put the coin in my hand put the coin on the table
         d. Put the match on the table   +

FIGURE 8   Screening Test Protocol: Mr. Tenhave.

B. Visual (matching tasks):

1. Matching identical objects (The objects--pens, keys, coins, and matches--are arrayed in random fashion on the table before the patient, and he is instructed to place like objects together.) The examiner can demonstrate if necessary.

_____+_____   _____+_____

all correct--swift
certain responses

_____+_____   _____+_____

2. Matching pictures and written words (the patient is instructed to place the word cards on the corresponding picture): Card I, Card Series Ia

a. books   +   d. car   +
b. pencil   +   e. bed   +   All correct
c. knife   +   f. hammer   +

II. OUTPUT

A. Automatic speech (have the patient perform the following tasks):

1. Count from 1 to 10 _____+_____
2. Say the letters of the alphabet stopped at "m," refused to continue
3. Repeat the days of the week when cued
4. Does the patient exhibit other forms of automatic language, for example, swearing? yes
5. Does the patient use gestures? points; expressive gestures (wave of dismissal; shoulder shrug); no complex pantomime

B. Simple repetition (have the patient repeat after the examiner):

1. Say "methodist episcopal"   "methdist piscopal"
2. Say "ah"   +
3. Say "puh"   +   no abnormality noted
4. Say "tuh"   +
5. Say "iuh"   +
6. Say "puh-tuh-kuh" several times _____ refused _____

FIGURE 8   (Continued)

C. Repetition of words (have the patient repeat after the examiner):

    1. car   "drive"   4. paper   "write"
    2. snow   "snow"   5. rake   "rake"
    3. clock "time"   6. leaves "rake"

    7. Winter is cold "it's winter" (looked out window)
    8. In fall the leaves turn many colors "leaves
        turn . . ."
    9. She had a face that launched a thousand ships
        "Troy!"

D. Open-end sentences (have the patient complete the sentences):

    1. You pound nails with a "wood, no, no, pound . . ."
    2. You chop wood with a "ah, ah, oh, shit, no, wood--
        chop--axe!"
    3. You read a "book"
    4. When you want to stop a car you step on the
        "pedal"
    5. Don't change horses in the middle of the "...shit"
    6. Don't put all your eggs in one (no response)

E. Spontaneous speech (the patient is asked to name objects that the examiner points to about the room):

    1. bed   "sleep"   4. light "lamp"
    2. table (no response) 5. door (no response)
    3. window "window"   6. chair "sit"

F. Self-formulated responses: (not tested)

    1. Is it good to get an education? Why or why not?
    2. What is democracy?
    3. What does it mean to say "one swallow doesn't make
        a summer?"

Comments: visual field cut; lots of struggle behavior; self-correction attempts noted. See attached report.

FIGURE 8 (Continued)

The results of the screening test are encouraging. Mr. Tenhave has good auditory recognition (pointing to objects and pictures when named) and his comprehension for auditory materials is good within his limited auditory memory span. His listening is accurate for simple, short messages. He seems to understand more than he really does because he is alert, well oriented, and he picks out a crucial word in a sentence. He has a good supply of automatic (counting, emotional language) and reactive speech. He frequently gives associations when asked to name objects or pictures; for example, he said "pedal" for "brake." His gestures are not more complex than his verbal output. We did not ask him to write at this time, but it is my impression that his language deficit cuts across all modalities. No dysarthria was observed, although he did "simplify" complex words such as "Methodist." He is making a great many attempts at self-correction. On balance, then, I would say that he has a good prognosis.

the case history

Language therapy for an adult aphasic has to be very personalized. Therefore, we need to know as much as possible about the individual when planning a program of treatment. What sort of person was he before the stroke? How did he meet his problems? What educational level did he achieve? What was his occupation? His avocations? What changes in his behavior, if any, have occurred following the brain injury? The style, pace, and content of therapy will be based upon the answers to these and many other questions.

Unfortunately, the aphasic patient himself is in no position to provide the kind of detailed information we seek. In some instances, official records (educational tests, military records) and personal documents (diaries, letters) are helpful. Usually, however, we must rely on the accuracy and veracity of informants who presumably are familiar with the patient. The most common method of assembling information about the language-impaired individual is a case-history form that is filled out by a spouse or other close relative. Ideally, the clinician also interviews the respondent to clarify any ambiguities in the written information and to permit additional questioning.

On the basis of our initial contact with Mrs. Tenhave, we decided that she would be a detailed and objective reporter. We therefore gave her an aphasia case-history form and simply requested that she answer the various queries to the best of her ability. The entire form follows (see Figure 9, pp. 234–37).

We then had a rather detailed description of the salient aspects of Mr. Tenhave's premorbid personality, health history, and social orientation. We knew a lot about the man he had been, but what impact had this sudden illness wrought? How much change could we expect, and in what areas? Would his responses to the language impairment and physical disabilities merely be an exaggeration of earlier behavior patterns?

There are only limited answers to these questions. We suspect, however, that the nature of the illness, the treatment the patient receives, and his interpretation of both these aspects (as well as premorbid factors) are all crucial in determining the impact of the problem upon the individual. Understand-

General Information

Name Roy O. Tenhave   Birthdate Jan. 4, 1918   Sex M

Address 211 Radisson   Phone 226-3801

Person filling out this form Mary Tenhave (wife)
                              (name and relationship to client)

Address -----   Phone ----- Date Feb. 3, 1970

Person(s) or agency who referred you to the Clinic
                  Dr. Roger Wilson

Personal and Family History

Marital status: single __ married X separated __
                 divorced __ widowed __ remarried __ .

Spouse's address _____ Phone _____

Children: Names: Addresses: Ages:

              Raymond   APO San Francisco   28
                         (in Viet Nam)

              _____   _____   _____

              _____   _____   _____

Grandchildren: Number -----   Ages _____

Father's Name: Ogden Tenhave   Living ____   Deceased x

If deceased, give cause of death heart disease

Mother's name: Bertha Trezona Tenhave Living ___ Deceased x

If deceased, give cause of death cancer

Medical Information

Date of injury (accident, illness, stroke) January 19, 1970

What caused the injury? C.V.A.

Was the client unconscious? Yes If yes, for how long?
    less than two hours

Was the client paralyzed? yes Describe right arm and leg

Did the client have convulsions? no Have they been
    controlled? _____

Does the client complain of dizziness, fainting spells,
headaches? did have several dizzy spells prior to the stroke

FIGURE 9   Aphasia Case History: Mr. Tenhave.

Does the client have any visual or hearing problems?
__Myopia, corrected__

Has the client been treated for other illnesses? _____
heart condition ___ stroke ___ others __Skin disorder__
__(herpes zoster), kidney stones, arthritis__

Name and address of physician __Dr. Roger Wilson, Ishpeming,__
__Michigan__

Has the patient been seen for any of the following services:

	DATE	PERSON/AGENCY	ADDRESS
Speech Therapy			
Psychological counseling or testing			
Vocational counseling			
Physical Therapy	Presently	St. Luke's Hospital	Marquette
Occupational Therapy			

Speech and Language Information

Describe what the client's speech was like at the onset of
the problem __couldn't say anything but "ah"__

How has it changed? __says some words__

Check the appropriate column as it applies to the patient
now. Add comments on the right if needed to qualify the
answers.

CAN	CANNOT		
x	____	Indicate meaning by gesture	some
____	x	Repeat words spoken by others	
x	____	Use one or a few words over and over	swearing
x	____	Use emotional speech (swear words); (count or use other words that occur in a series, days of week, prayers)	
x	____	Use some words spontaneously	bird names
____	x	Say short phrases	
____	x	Say short sentences	
x	____	Follow requests and understand directions	

FIGURE 9   (Continued)

___	_?_	Follow radio and television speech
_?_	___	Read signs with understanding
_?_	___	Read numbers with understanding
_x_	___	Read single words
___	_x_	Read newspapers, magazines
_?_	___	Tell time
___	_x_	Copy numbers, letters
___	_x_	Write name without assistance
___	_x_	Write single words
___	_x_	Write sentences, letters
___	_x_	Do simple arithmetic
___	_x_	Personal care (dressing, shaving, etc.)
___	_x_	Handle money

How did the client react when he discovered that speech was difficult? very frustrated

What was your reaction? thought it was temporary, then concerned

What do you do when the client cannot answer or when he tries to talk? try to give him a "yes - no"

How does the client react when he cannot say what he wants to? swears; tries to use signs or gestures; scribbles with left hand

How does the client respond to personal contacts other than family members (friends, associates)? he does not seem to want to see them--or have them see him like he is.

Personal and Social Information

A. Before the injury:

Where did the client spend his childhood? Upper Peninsula, White Pine, L'Anse

Where did he go to school? L'Anse, Michigan

How far did he go in school? M.A. degree, plus extra course work

What is his occupation? biology teacher
Did he like his work? yes, very much

FIGURE 9   (Continued)

236

How long has he worked at this job? 24 years

What other work has he done?

naturalist in summers at state parks (11 summers)
　　　　　　(give dates and length of time)

What is the client's native language? English

Does he speak any other? some Finn

What hobbies or special interests does he have? bird
study; photography; hiking and canoeing; hunting and
fishing

What did he like to read? all types--ecology, philosophy,
biographies

Which television programs did he enjoy? movies; news
programs

Did he do much writing (if so, what kind)? yes; pamphlets,
a science unit

Which hand did he prefer? right

Describe the client's personality A. Before the injury:

Nervousness not especially

Shyness basically a private person although he liked
small groups

Moods no   Getting along with others good

Meeting problems: gave up easily ___ kept on trying __x__
other he always tried to approach things rationally

B.　After the injury:

How has the client reacted to the injury? very frustrated.
I think he feels that his body is letting him down.

What seems to bother him the most? can't make himself
understood

What personality changes have you noted? he is so
emotional now

What is his attitude toward speech therapy? I don't know

Has the physician talked to you about the client's
speech difficulty? briefly

Any further information which may aid in the examination?
Roy always prided himself in his ability to think and
reason. He is a skilled naturalist, especially in the
area of ornithology. He is an expert in bird calls,
and he has written a widely used pamphlet on attracting
birds. He was an excellent teacher, and his students
seem to have great respect for his quiet strength and
wry humor.

FIGURE 9　　(Continued)

ably, the literature is limited in this area (see Project 5). Some workers refer to the aphasic's altered behavior patterns with handy labels, for example: "egocentricity," "catastrophic response," "concretism." It is often inferred that these nonlanguage "deviations" are a direct product of the brain damage. The designation of "organicity" then excuses the clinician from identifying any further the dynamics behind the labels.

We do not deny that many aphasics become obsessed with themselves and their situation, that they often respond emotionally to even seemingly minor barriers, or that they have difficulty dealing with abstractions. However, it is our position that *an aphasic's behavior is largely a product of his drastically altered life experience, not merely a result of damaged brain cells* (Wepman, 1951). Further, we contend that if the experience of being aphasic is carefully examined, the basis for many of the so-called nonlanguage deviations becomes evident. Let us consider briefly two important interrelated factors: isolation and infantilization.

The parallels between the experience of sensory (and perceptual) deprivation and aphasia are startling. It is surprising, then, that to the best of our knowledge, the results of research dealing with subjects' responses to isolation have not been applied to the situation of the adult aphasic. Consider this sampling of findings from sensory deprivation studies (Solomon, 1961; Zubek, 1969):

1. Subjects show regression in perception and cognition to more primitive modes.
2. Subjects manifest a marked reduction in motivation.
3. Subjects tend to create internal images, experience hallucinations.
4. Subjects, after adjusting to a severely restricted environment, may exhibit severe emotional reactions to increments in sensation.

Now, consider again the aphasic patients: there is an abrupt reduction in sensory stimulation; the sensory input they do receive may be severely distorted or lack variety; their physical activity is restricted; there are prolonged periods of enforced rest in quiet, darkened rooms. Several publications that describe the recovery of adults with aphasia stress the importance of continued stimulation, especially during the primary stage of recovery (Buck, 1968; Farrell, 1969; Knox, 1971).

The bland, dependent existence of the aphasic tends to be infantilizing. There are at least four overlapping factors responsible:

The nature of the disorder.   Aphasia generally has a very sudden onset; the individual has no chance to prepare himself for the experience. The illness destroys or alters drastically those attributes most critical to human functioning—communication, control of body functions, and physical ability. Abruptly, the person is stripped of his identity, and without identity an individual is without humanity.

The sick role. Minor illness is a socially acceptable excuse for the temporary abandonment of normal adult decorum and responsibilities. The gravely ill person, such as the aphasic adult, is exempted from all his former role requirements and demands—work, family responsibilities, and social obligations. Since he is not responsible for his condition (although one middle-aged aphasic patient who suffered a stroke while shoveling snow, an activity forbidden by his physician, was severely and continually blamed for his condition by his family), he cannot be held accountable for anything except being a "good patient." A good patient submits without question to the hospital routine and treatment program; he forfeits reliance upon his family and follows orders given by strangers; his existence is passive, and he is always in a horizontal posture; he must not complain about his lost roles or the rules of the institution.

The hospital routine. Another closely related source of regression is the hospital experience (Coser, 1956). Note the possibilities for infantilization in this vivid description of the hospital experience by Duff and Hollingshead (1968: 269):

> Between admission to and discharge from the hospital, the patients were subjected to orders of the staff. They were separated from their families. Their street clothes were shed. They were assigned beds, given numbers, and dressed in bedroom apparel. They had to permit strangers access to the most intimate parts of their bodies. Their diet was controlled, as were the hours of their days and nights, the people they saw, and the times they saw them. They were bathed, fed, and questioned; they were ordered or forbidden to do specific things. *As long as they were in the hospital they were not considered self-sufficient adults.* (Italics ours.)

In some hospitals, nurses and aides are instructed to call patients by their first names, apparently to simulate personal involvement. It is ludicrous and an insult to his dignity when a fifty-two-year-old biology teacher is referred to as "Roy" by a twenty-year-old student nurse. Consider, finally, the impact upon a seriously ill and profoundly frustrated patient of the determined cheerfulness and casual bonhomie which often seem to be the main features of nurses' professional character armor.

The style of interaction. But perhaps the most devastating and pervasive source of infantilization the aphasic experiences comes with the altered style of interaction—verbal and nonverbal—used with impaired individuals. Persons do not (indeed, often cannot) talk to the patient the same way they did before the language disturbance:

1. They talk more loudly, more precisely.
2. They ask simple, obvious questions.
3. They frequently answer their own queries.

4. They talk around the person to others.
5. They may talk about the person in his presence.
6. They may overrespond to his infrequent verbalizations or minor communicative successes.

Note that each instance is a typical (but even so, unfortunate) mode of communicating with a child.

Physically, the aphasic patient is often dependent upon others (Smith, 1967). His wife, or someone else close to him, must help him bathe, dress, perhaps even eat. It is easy to slip back into childhood when one is hovered over, insulated, and guarded.

> And I had seen so many begin to pack their lives in cotton wool, smother their impulses, hood their passions, and gradually retire from their manhood into a kind of spiritual and physical semi-invalidism. In this they are encouraged by wives and relatives, and it's such a sweet trap. Who doesn't like to be a center for concern? A kind of second childhood falls on so many men. They trade their violence for the promise of a small increase in life span. In effect, the head of the household *becomes the youngest child* (Steinbeck, 1961: 19). (Italics ours.)

But is all of this discussion relevant to the assessment of an adult aphasic patient? We think it is. Any information about the individual is important since it might bear upon the responses to the examiner and to the tests employed. What does it mean if a client fails to respond to a test item? A simple minus designation? A scoring category value of one? Rejection of the task? Fear of failure, anxiousness? Severe depression/Hostility? Auditory comprehension difficulty? Reduced auditory memory span? Perhaps a combination of any or all of these?

The point is that we must attempt to understand the person and what has happened to him as completely as possible; the more time spent in this regard, the better a diagnostician we become. Otherwise, it is dreadfully easy to be seduced by a particular diagnostic tool to the point that we come to see aphasia and the aphasic solely through a test. Indeed, if it is worth forty hours of study to acquire proficiency in scoring a patient's language responses according to a multidimensional scale (Porch, 1971), then certainly it is worth at least as much time trying to appreciate the impact of aphasia upon an individual's humanity. A patient is more than a neat array of carefully charted profiles, as significant and desirable as those measurements may be.

the language inventory

Mr. Tenhave was discharged from the hospital on February 16. He wore a brace on his lower right leg and walked with the aid of a tripod cane; his right arm was held up in a sling. Each day he returned to the hospital as an outpatient for physical and occupational therapy. Although he was using some voluntary speech, including a few short phrases, his attempts to communicate were still extremely frustrating.

In order to devise a plan of treatment for Mr. Tenhave, as well as to predict the probable course and outcome of treatment, we would need a comprehensive appraisal of his present language abilities: Where is he having difficulty? Which modalities are working best? How does he make his errors? Are there discernible patterns to his errors? To answer these and other questions, we had to administer a language inventory.

The clinician has several published tests of aphasia from which to choose (Eisenson, 1954; Wepman and Jones, 1961; Taylor, 1963; Sklar, 1963; Schuell, 1965; Porch, 1967; see also Project 6). Some diagnosticians prefer to select portions of many different tests and, in this eclectic manner, assemble a comprehensive battery. Eisenson (1971: 1236) describes the efforts of several workers from different countries to devise a composite international diagnostic instrument which hopefully would provide a common basis for understanding among aphasiologists. In the hands of a skilled and perceptive clinician who is thoroughly familiar with the materials, any of the tests cited above will provide a detailed description of an aphasic's language disturbance; as we pointed out in Chapter 3, a test is only a tool, a way to help the examiner make precise observations of a particular client.

To evaluate Mr. Tenhave, we selected an instrument of our own construction (Emerick, 1971). The Appraisal of Language Disturbance (ALD) was developed as a product of the senior author's clinical experience with aphasic patients in Veterans' Administration hospitals, private medical settings, and an active outpatient speech-and-hearing center.

> The ALD is a clinical tool designed to permit the clinician to make a systematic inventory of a patient's communicative abilities both in the modalities of input and output and the central integration processes. It enables the worker to make a careful appraisal of all possible linguistic transmission factors—gesture to oral, aural to gesture—delineated in the research of Wepman and his associates (Wepman, *et al.,* 1960; Jones and Wepman, 1961). In this manner, the clinician receives a precise description of the patient's capacity with respect to the various pathways for stimulation and response. In addition, tasks are arranged in an ascending order of linguistic complexity within each subtest assessing input and output factors; this permits the clinician to determine not only the nature of the dysfunction but also the extent of the problem. (The several open-end items included provide additional flexibility.) The ALD also includes a unit designed to assess central language processes and a final segment for evaluating areas of functioning peripheral to symbolic language such as tactile recognition, arithmetic abilities, and the oral area (Emerick, 1971: 1).

We arranged to administer the language inventory to Mr. Tenhave at an early morning appointment when he was most alert and rested. On March 3, we met Mr. Tenhave sitting impatiently in the clinic waiting room. Ushering him into a quiet, plainly furnished office, we offered him coffee and made him comfortable at a long table. The clinician positioned himself on the patient's left side. In order to give him time to adjust to the room and the communicative situation before starting the formal testing, we engaged Mr. Tenhave in casual conversation about the weather and the visitors to his bird-feeding station. We then carefully explained the purpose of testing and provided several examples of the types of tasks to be included. Mr. Tenhave nodded that he understood and motioned eagerly toward the testing materials.

We proceeded through the ten subtests in a casual manner, pausing often, commenting about specific items, and watching carefully for signs of fatigue. At one point Mr. Tenhave objected mildly to the wording of a particular sentence, and we reinforced his criticism; if a patient can criticize the test, he will not be threatened by it. The ALD is carefully designed to insure initial success by having the subject begin with simple items. We agree with Toubbeh (1969) that failure, especially at the beginning of the language testing, can be devastating; indeed it may inhibit the patient's ability to focus on all incoming stimuli. A portion (subtest I) of the ALD, containing Mr. Tenhave's responses, is included in Figure 10 to show the kind of tasks employed and to illustrate his responses. The total time consumed by testing, including the brief breaks and desultory conversation, was just over seventy-four minutes. We again chatted briefly with Mr. Tenhave at the end of the formal testing; we told him that although we would need to analyze the results carefully before starting therapy, we were encouraged by his responses.

The completed ALD provides a protocol that outlines the severity of a patient's language disturbance and the areas (modalities) of impairment. The test does not yield a classification system nor does it attempt to place aphasics into various categories. We agree with Buck (1968: 85) that "too often our diagnostic labels blind us to the true state of affairs and prevent further investigation." It is far more useful clinically to simply identify what the patient can and cannot do with language symbols. The ALD, however, does provide a summary form for collating data obtained from the patient on the ten subtests. Figure 11 shows the completed summary form for Mr. Tenhave.

The column on the left simply lists the ten subtests. Note the five columns enumerated 1 through 5 and labeled "rating." After administering the ALD we rated Mr. Tenhave's performance on each subtest utilizing the following crude scale:

1. All, or almost all, responses correct
2. Majority of responses correct
3. Approximately half the responses correct, half incorrect
4. Majority of responses incorrect
5. All, or almost all, responses incorrect

Thus, we have a summary profile of the patient's language abilities as manifested by his responses to the ten specific subtests.

It is also important to examine *how* the patient made his errors: Did

1. Aural to Oral

In this subtest the examiner provides auditory stimulation and the patient responds with oral language.

A. Automatic:

   1. ask patient his name *Roy*"
   2. ask patient to count to 10 (the examiner may provide some stimulation to get the patient started)
   3. ask patient letters of the alphabet
   4. ask patient days of the week

B. Imitative: the patient repeats the following words after the examiner; listen for articulation errors.

   1. cat   6. scissors
   2. hair   7. do you have a match
   3. paper   8. very few have freedom
   4. rock   9. judge not lest thee be judged
   5. leaves   10. six times six is thirty-six

C. Symbolic:

   1. oral opposites: have the patient supply the opposite orally.

      a. thin   d. fast
      b. man   e. living
      c. strong   f. anarchy *nR*

   2. open end sentences: have the patient finish the sentence orally.

      a. you sleep on a "*bed*"
      b. the boy picked up his bat and ball and went to play "*ball*"
      c. please get me a drink of "*milk*"
      d. a bird in the hand is worth two in the _____
      e. he who hesitates is *N.R.*

   3. definitions: have the patient supply the word orally.

      a. something to read *"book"*
      b. a farm animal that gives milk *"cow"*
      c. a white cylinder of tobacco *"don't smoke"*
      d. something that registers the passage of time *"watch"*
      e. a black drink brewed from ground beans *N.R.*

   4. disparities: have the patient attempt to point out what is wrong with the following sentences.

      a. They filled the car with catsup.
      b. He spread his bread with butter and nails.
      c. She wrote a letter with paper and peanut butter.
      d. A penny saved is a penny burned.
      e. No man is an Ireland. *smiled*

FIGURE 10   Subtest I of ALD Showing Mr. Tenhave's Responses.

ALD SUMMARY FORM

Lon L. Emerick, Ph.D.
Northern Michigan University

Transmission	Rating					Comments
	1	2	3	4	5	
I. Aural-Oral		x				limited by short auditory memory span
II. Aural-Visual	x					
III. Aural-Gesture	x					
IV. Aural-Graphic				x		used writing brace; spells phonetically
V. Gesture-Visual	x					
VI. Visual-Gesture	x					
VII. Visual-Oral			x			used association
VIII. Visual-Graphic			x			

IX. Central Language
    Comprehension   Rating: 1.5
    1. Matching   1 Peabody = 95%
    2. Sorting   2
    3. Manding   1

X. Related Factors   Rating:
    1. Tactile   5
    2. Arithmetic   1
    3. Oral Exam   1 normal

Observations: 1. Errors increase as length of material
                 increases.
              2. Mispronunciations are correctable by ear.
              3. Self-correction is evident.
              4. Visual field cut seems to have improved.

Roy Tenhave	71-493	March 3, 1970	E.
Patient	Number	Date	Examiner

FIGURE 11   ALD Summary Form for Roy Tenhave.

244

he seem to perseverate? At what level of complexity did his responses break down? Did he give synonyms or associations for words when asked to name pictures or objects? Mr. Tenhave, for example, when asked to name a picture of a dollar bill, said, "Put it . . . pocket . . . wallet. . . ." Obviously, his "error" is far better than a response of "soup" or "don't know." Was the patient attempting to correct his errors (Wepman, 1958)? Are his responses significantly delayed?

We summarized the test findings, together with our impressions and prognosis, in a detailed report:

Client: Roy Tenhave   *Date*: March 3, 1973

Test Findings. The Appraisal for Language Disturbance was administered and revealed the following information on each of the ten subtests:

I. *Aural-Oral* (client listens, responds with oral language). The client replied swiftly and accurately on tasks calling for automatic and imitative responses. His responses to symbolic items (oral opposites, open-end sentences, definitions) appear to be limited by reduced availability of less frequently used words. Auditory comprehension is good within the limits imposed by a reduced verbal retention span. Recognizes disparities easily.

II. *Aural to Visual* (client listens and points). Auditory recognition for objects, pictures, and simple written words is intact. Mr. Tenhave's responses were rapid and positive.

III. *Aural to Gesture* (client listens and makes appropriate gesture). The patient can follow commands (shake head, cough) with the appropriate gesture, point to body parts when named, and demonstrate complex gestures associated with writing, using a toothbrush, and throwing a ball.

IV. *Aural to Graphic* (client listens and writes). Mr. Tenhave was reluctant initially to attempt writing with his left hand; a Zaner-Bloser writing frame was offered, and he used it to complete the tasks.[8] Automatic items (his name, age) were accomplished easily. However, his attempts to write a series of dictated letters and numbers was limited by his reduced auditory memory span; he could retain three but not four or more digits or letters. No rotation of letters or confusion between them was noted. He missed over 50 percent of the total items included in this subtest. Several short words ("bird", "lamp") were written correctly, but in general his spelling tends to be done phonetically (e.g., "blu" for "blue," "nos" for "nose").

V. *Gesture to Visual* (clinician makes a gesture, client must select appropriate object, picture, or written word associated with the gesture). He responded accurately to each test item: he watched the clinician's gestures and selected the appropriate object, picture, and printed word from a series arrayed before him.

VI. *Visual to Gesture* (examiner shows an object, picture, or written word to the patient, and the patient makes a gesture typically associated with it). All items were done swiftly and correctly.

VII. *Visual to Oral* (client is presented a visual stimulus and is requested to read or name orally). Mr. Tenhave missed almost half of the items on this subtest. His oral vocabulary is reduced, and he frequently responded with words that were associated with the stimulus (e.g., "ring" for "bell," "eat" for "spoon,"

---

[8] The Zaner-Bloser Company, 612 N. Park Street, Columbus, Ohio.

"Ford" for "car"). His reading rate is very slow; he labored over the test sentences and paragraph, pausing often to reread portions. His comprehension for reading material was good, but again, it was limited by a reduced verbal retention span. No dysarthria or apraxia was noted. He tends to mispronounce or simplify longer words; however, when he is instructed to listen carefully and is given an auditory model, he corrects his errors readily.

VIII. *Visual to Graphic* (client is presented a visual stimulus and responds by copying or writing). Mr. Tenhave had considerable difficulty with this subtest, missing more than half the items. He was able to copy letters, numbers, and written words accurately. However, he was able to identify in writing only two of the ten objects and pictures presented. When shown a drawing depicting several features, he simply enumerated three items and, after a long pause, put down the marking pen in obvious disgust. (Note: at this point the testing was stopped and the examiner and client relaxed over coffee; a respite should have been given before beginning this subtest. His concentration was so intense that it was difficult to discern when he was getting fatigued. This will have to be taken into account in therapy with him.)

IX. *Central Language Comprehension* (in this subtest, the client is given various tasks—matching, sorting, object assembly, recognition vocabulary—which more directly assess the status of the client's central sorting and integrative functioning). Matching (objects to silhouettes, pictures to pictures, objects to pictures), object assembly, and manding presented no difficulty to Mr. Tenhave. He scored at the 95th percentile on the Peabody Picture Vocabulary Test (Dunn, 1958). His errors involved sorting: he arranged the circle and squares according to color initially (note: check to see if he has a type of colorblindness—he seemed to confuse green and blue. It is rather peculiar, though, for a skilled ornithologist to be colorblind) and when the request was made to recategorize them, he was unable to do so.

X. *Related Factors* (in this subtest, areas of functioning peripheral to symbolic language are examined—tactile recognition, arithmetic ability, and motor speech behavior). Tactile recognition in the right hand is totally absent; he made two errors with his left hand. Simple arithmetic problems presented no difficulty for Mr. Tenhave; he requested several repetitions of the short story problem, however, before he could successfully complete it. This reflected his reduced verbal retention span. Oral examination revealed normal functioning.[9]

Prognosis. Excellent prospects for recovery. The patient's auditory recognition is intact, and his comprehension is good; both are essential to a favorable response to therapy. Another favorable sign is Mr. Tenhave's ability to detect his errors and, when provided with an auditory model, correct them. A determined attitude augers well for his continued efforts during treatment.

plan of treatment

In order for therapy to be effective, it is essential to provide intensive (daily) sessions for adult aphasics, especially for patients like Mr. Tenhave who have such a favorable prognosis. Daily contact permits abundant stimula-

---

[9] Before starting therapy, Mr. Tenhave was given an audiometric evaluation; his hearing was within normal limits (see studies by Street, 1957; Miller, 1960; Needham and Black, 1970).

tion—a key factor in language therapy—and creates a momentum which can carry the patient (and clinician) over the inevitable reversals and plateaus. Token treatment, whereby the patient is seen for an hour two or three times per week, creates false hopes of recovery with little prospect for lasting change. Accordingly, a clinical team arranged to see Mr. Tenhave six days a week.

Before beginning therapy, the clinician met with three graduate students to form a team and discuss a plan of treatment for Mr. Tenhave. Each team member was familiar with the patient's case history and had studied the results of the language inventory. Additional information in the form of brief anecdotal reports from Dr. Wilson, the physical and occupational therapists, and Mrs. Tenhave were carefully examined and collated with existing data. We present now Team Memorandum No. 1, which outlines several general principles of therapy and then lists specific clinical activities:

Team Memo No. 1
Re: Mr. Roy Tenhave

i. general principles of therapy

A. Please refer to the client as "Mr. Tenhave" unless he specifically requests otherwise.

B. Start where he presently is; follow Van Riper's dictum (1972: 349), "Aphasia therapy consists of building bridges from the things the patient can do to those he cannot." Use the channels that are open (aural to visual, aural to gesture) to build up those that are not (aural to oral, visual to oral). For example, he can point to pictures on command—when he does, utter the word several times and invite him to model you.

C. Relate each session to the previous ones. We will hold a team planning session twice weekly to make sure we are all working on the same track.

D. Begin with easy tasks and end each session on a note of success.

E. Don't overload his system. Initially, plan to limit sorting, selecting, pointing tasks to three or four items. He is difficult to "read," but we must watch carefully for signs of fatigue or cumulative frustration; observe his face for signs of flushing or tearing, monitor closely for any increase in emotional expression, heavy sighing, or movements away from the work area.

F. Use social reinforcement, but keep it down to a minimum, since he seems to realize when he is doing well and that's rewarding enough.

G. When he makes errors, restimulate him rather than correct him (Schuell, Jenkins, and Jimenez-Pabon, 1964).

H. When talking with him, use short, simple sentences; keep the tempo of your speech slower than usual. But do not talk down to him or communicate in a childish fashion.

I. Take advantage of all possible clues when giving him a stimulus—auditory, gestural, written.

J. Plan to delay any writing activities until he expresses a need for them.

However, have him use a pencil for pointing activities so that he becomes accustomed to holding it with his left hand.

K. Prepare materials for him rather than using published items (this does not include bird books or other items related to his former occupation or avocations).

L. If he cannot provide a response to an item, or if he is blocked in his attempts to tell you something, follow this routine: restimulate or review the antecedents (identify the category from which he is trying to retrieve); translate (see Van Riper, 1972: 351); verbalize his frustration and indicate you will return to it later.

M. Keep in mind that we are not teaching him language—we are providing stimulation so that language processes will begin functioning again. We are attempting, in other words, to build a fire *within* the person, not under him. In order to chart progress as it occurs, we will reevaluate Mr. Tenhave weekly; these sessions will be video taped so that precise counts can be made.

ii. specific activities

A. First of all, we will want to make sure that he can handle emergencies and routine communications coming into the home. Mrs. Tenhave is reluctant to resume teaching until she is sure her husband could complete a phone call if he needed help, and handle incoming calls. Obtain a list of important phone numbers—the physician, police, fire department, and Mrs. Tenhave's school. Have him memorize an appropriate message in each instance (see Van Riper, 1972: 351) and then rehearse and role play (Schlanger and Schlanger, 1970).

B. General language stimulation: To stimulate language processes to work again, plan to sort, name, and discuss aspects of the following three topics:

1. Bird study. Point to the species named, identify the pictures presented, record visitors to his feeder; associate the name of the bird with its habitat, habits, nesting characteristics, migration. Listen to recordings of bird calls and associate them with pictures.

2. Photography. Outline developing procedures; go through the process with him; review slides.

3. Local history. Using the clinic's Polaroid camera, take pictures of local historical points—the sandstone courthouse, remains of the forge at Forestville on the Dead River, Chief Kawbawgam's grave, etc. Let him identify the sites, specify the dates, and encourage him to relate as much additional information as he can.

C. Specific stimulation: For the time being, we will limit specific language drill to improving his verbal retention span. Use materials from ornithology, local history, and famous quotations; have him point to three, then four and five items.

outcome of therapy

Mr. Tenhave made rapid progress. He enjoyed the therapy sessions with the students, and they in turn admired and respected him openly. Here is a portion of a therapy protocol written by one graduate clinician that illustrates vividly the impact of general language stimulation:

The spinoff from last Saturday's historical site photographing was fantastic. Mr. T. was waiting impatiently for me this morning. He had searched the family attic and found several old scrapbooks containing pictures and newspaper clippings. He had gone to the library Saturday afternoon and checked out a thick book about local history that he wants to read with the team. He already has found several discrepancies in their account of the Dead River, and he wants to interview several old-time residents to set the record straight—he even asked to borrow my cassette recorder!

Emotionally, the client made an excellent adjustment. After talking it over with his wife and the school superintendent, Mr. Tenhave decided to resign as a full-time biology teacher. Because of his unusual expertise, however, he was retained as a consultant in ornithology and environmental education.

For discussions of aphasia therapy, consult the following references: Wepman, 1951; Wepman, 1953; Longerich and Bordeaux, 1959; Stoicheff, 1960; Martin, 1962; Wepman and Morency, 1963; Schuell, Jenkins, and Jimenez-Pabon, 1964; Agranowitz and McKeown, 1964; Keenan, 1966; Smith, 1966; Boone, 1967; Keith and Darley, 1967; West and Ansberry, 1968; Engmann and Brookshire, 1970; Brookshire, 1971; Swinney and Taylor, 1971; Darley, 1972; Wepman, 1972.

PROGNOSIS

Selecting patients for treatment who have the best chance of recovery from aphasia is an unsettling task. Rather than abandon anyone, one's impulse is to attempt to work with every aphasic even though prospects for improvement in cases of severe language impairment are dim (Sarno, Silverman, and Sands, 1970). When there is little real progress, the patient's labors are like those of Sisyphus.

How then can the clinician identify aphasic clients with the best potential? A list of interrelated factors which we have found helpful for making a prognosis is presented below; however, we trust the reader's forecasting will be guided by three important maxims: (1) do not make a final prognosis on the basis of a single evaluation session—a period of trial therapy is always highly informative; (2) do not make a prognosis solely on the basis of a single measure of behavior—e.g., the client's performance on a language inventory; and (3) be sure you understand the value of predictors—they can be potent self-fulfilling prophecies.

1. *Auditory recognition.* Patients who make errors (even a few errors—two or three out of ten items—are significant) when identifying pictures or common objects named by the examiner have an unfavorable prognosis; an impairment at this level is apparently irreversible (Schuell, Jenkins, and Jimenez-Pabon, 1964).

2. *Comprehension.* Patients who have marked difficulty in comprehending

verbal messages make poor candidates for treatment. In fact, a reliable index of the severity of language impairment in aphasia is the degree of disturbance in comprehension (Smith, 1971).

3. *Self-monitoring.* Patients who are aware of their errors and attempt to correct them have a more favorable prognosis than those who do not. See the self-correction rating scale devised by Wepman (1958).

4. *Jargon.* The presence of jargon is a poor clinical sign, especially when it is coupled with lack of self-monitoring, euphoria, or denial (Cohn and Neumann, 1958).

Following a CVA, Carl Foreman, a fifty-seven-year-old attorney, was left with mild right hemiparesis and jargon aphasia. He talked constantly in long, involved, unintelligible sentences using appropriate gestures and exhibiting normal cadence and inflection; occasionally an intelligible word or epithet would appear in the stream of gibberish. Attempts to evaluate Mr. Foreman's comprehension were confounded by his incessant chatter—he simply would not listen. Following the advice of Lecours and Lhermitte (1969) we attempted to analyze the patient's jargon in an attempt to break his idiosyncratic code. It turned out to be a fool's errand. Although he seemed to use the same phonemes and phoneme distribution as in English speech, he was simply talking nonsense.

5. *Primary stage of recovery.* The more untoward events (infantilizing, isolation, withdrawal, exposure to negative attitudes) that occur during the first few months after the brain injury, the poorer the patient's motivation will be to undertake treatment.

6. *Time elapsed since onset.* The longer the time elapsed since onset of aphasia and the beginning of treatment, the poorer the prognosis. Habits of dependence, withdrawal, and possible secondary gains accruing from a nonverbal role tend to defeat therapeutic intervention.

7. *Family response.* Patients whose families provide supportive understanding and appropriate stimulation and permit the individual to regain his role within the family unit have a more favorable prognosis.

8. *Age.* Generally, the younger the patient the better are the prospects for recovery. Aphasics in or near retirement often lack the energy and motivation to persist in a treatment program. In addition, the older patients may have more widespread cerebral damage due to arteriosclerosis.

9. *Presence of other health problems.* In our clinical experience, aphasic patients presenting health problems in addition to the brain injury (such as diabetes, systemic vascular disease, or kidney disease) often do poorly in therapy.

10. *Premorbid personality.* The more outgoing, flexible individual generally responds better to treatment than does an inhibited, introverted person (Eisenson, 1949).

11. *Intelligence and education.* The more intelligent, better educated patients make better candidates for therapy. Although this is generally true, a few of our most highly educated clients were so vividly aware of the discrepancy between their premorbid abilities and their present condition, they simply withdrew in futility.

12. *Extent of the lesion.* The more extensive the brain injury, the poorer the prospects for recovery.

13. *Location of the lesion.* Damage occuring posterior to the Fissure of Ro-

lando, especially at the junction of the parietal temporal lobe, tends to result in more persistent aphasia (Penfield and Roberts, 1959).

14. *Physical disability.* We have observed good language recovery in aphasics with severe hemiplegia. Generally, however, those patients without paralysis, or with milder forms of paresis, made swifter and more complete improvement. Although we lack sufficient data to document this relationship, many of our aphasic patients have exhibited sudden spurts of progress in language as their physical condition improved.

The student will want to consult the following references for further information regarding prognosis in aphasia: Eisenson, 1949; Bourestom, 1967; Smith, 1971; Sarno, Silverman, and Sands, 1970; Culton, 1969.

PROJECTS AND QUESTIONS

1. The reduction of language in aphasia appears to be regular: the availability of words to the patient seems to follow their relative frequency of occurrence. What about specific occupational vocabularies? For example, will a limnologist retain the complex names of phytoplankton more readily than more common words? How does the concept of "saliency" figure in the probabilities of word retention? Do aphasics retain connotative meanings? How would you research the last question?

2. Traditional medical terminology: look up the meanings of the following terms:

alexia	anosmia	agraphia
amusia	agnosia	paraphasia
anomia	dysprosody	Gerstmann's syndrome
Broca's aphasia	prodromal	badinage
acalculia	Wernicke's aphasia	bradyphasia

3. The family's responses to aphasia: Why do some families draw together during a serious health crisis while others tend to become fragmented? What professional workers can assist families through the crisis period? Relate the problem of aphasia to the six basic functions of the family. Why would sexual relations be disrupted by aphasia and other sequelae of brain injury? Most of the literature assumes the husband is aphasic; can you identify any differences that might occur if it were the wife? Search for the answers to these questions in the references below:

ADLER, M. "Hemiplegia and the Social Structure." Unpublished Ph. D. dissertation, University of Pittsburgh, 1962.

ARTES, R. "A Study of Family Problems as Identified and Evaluated by the Wives of Stroke Patients." Unpublished Ph. D. dissertation, University of Iowa, 1967.

BIORN-HANSEN, V. "Social and Emotional Aspects of Aphasia." *Journal of Speech and Hearing Disorders*, 22 (1957): 53–59.

BUCK, M. *Dysphasia*. Englewood Cliffs, N.J.: Prentice-Hall, Inc., 1968.

Committee on Family Diagnosis and Treatment. *Casebook on Family Diagnosis and Treatment*. New York: Family Service Agency, 1965.

DE FOREST, R., ed. *Proceedings of the National Stroke Congress*. Springfield, Ill.: Charles C Thomas, 1966. P. 109.

DUFF, R., and A. HOLLINGSHEAD. *Sickness and Society*. New York: Harper & Row, Publishers, 1968. Pp. 25–340.

GARRETT, J., and E. LEVINE, *Psychological Practices with the Physically Disabled*. New York: Columbia University Press, 1962.

JACOBSON, M., and R. EICHORN. "Family Response to Heart Disease in the Husband-Father." *Journal of Marriage and Family*, 26 (1964): 166–73.

MABRY, J. "Medicine and the Family." *Journal of Marriage and Family*, 26 (1964): 160–65.

MALONE, R. "Expressed Attitudes of Families of Aphasics." *Journal of Speech and Hearing Disorders*, 34 (1969): 38–41.

McDANIEL, J. *Physical Disability and Human Behavior*. New York: Pergamon Press, 1969. Pp. 146–50.

PARAD, H., ed. *Crisis Intervention: Selected Readings*. New York: Family Service Association, 1965.

SCHUELL, H., J. JENKINS, and E. JIMENEZ-PABON. *Aphasia in Adults*. New York: Harper & Row, Publishers, 1964. Pp. 328–31.

4. The neurological examination and terminology: find definitions for the following terms in the references cited below.

Babinski	diaschisis	physiatrist
atherosclerosis	Ribot	papilledema
lumen	Minkowski	contusion
infarct	Pitrin	contrecoup
ischemia	atereognosis	hematoma
angiography	ventriculography	EEG
pneumoencephalography	synscope	EMG
fundus	little strokes	opthalmodynometry
Wada technique	petichial hemmorhage	caisson disease
geriatric strokes	echoencephalography	
brain scan	cerebraoscintogram	

ALVAREZ, W. *Little Strokes*. Philadelphia: J.B. Lippincott Co., 1966.

BOONE, D., and B. LANDES. "Left-Right Discrimination in Hemiplegic Patients." *Archives of Physical Medicine and Rehabilitation*, 49 (1968): 533–37.

CHUSID, J., and J. McDONALD. *Correlative Neuroanatomy*. Los Altos, Calif.: Lange Medical Publications, 1967.

COBB, S. *Foundations of Neuropsychiatry*. Baltimore: William and Wilkins, 1958.

FISCHER, C. "A Lacunar Stroke—The Dysarthria-Clumsy Hand Syndrome." *Neurology*, 17 (1967): 614–17.

GRINKER, R., and A. SAHS. *Neurology*. Springfield, Ill.: Charles C Thomas, 1966.

SHANKWEILER, D., K. HARRIS, and M. TAYLOR. "Electromyographic Studies of Articulation in Aphasia." *Archives of Physical Medicine and Rehabilitation*, 49 (1968): 1–8.

WEAVER, K. "Remote Sensing—New Eyes to See the World." *National Geographic Magazine*, 135 (1969): 47–73.

5. The experience of being aphasic: what can you learn about the problem of aphasia by consulting the references listed below? What impact does aphasia have upon the individual? Which is worse, denial or depression? Does the aphasic have a reduced threshold of frustration, or is he simply faced with more frustrations? What can you learn about the impact of aphasia by consulting biographies of famous stroke victims such as Louis Pasteur, Samuel Johnson, Woodrow Wilson, H. L. Mencken, Walt Whitman, R. L. Stevenson?

BAY, E. "The Lordat Case and Its Import on the Theory of Aphasia." *Cortex,* 5 (1969): 302–8.

BIXBY, L. "Comeback from a Brain Operation." *Harpers Magazine* (November, 1952), pp. 69–73.

BUCK, M. *Dysphasia.* Englewood Cliffs, N.J.: Prentice-Hall, Inc., 1968.

————. "The Language Disorders: A Personal and Professional Account of Aphasia." *Journal of Rehabilitation,* 29 (1963): 37–38.

COOLEY, C. *Social Aspects of Illness.* Philadelphia: W. B. Saunders Company, 1951.

EISENHOWER, D. *Waging Peace.* New York: Doubleday & Company, Inc., 1965. Pp. 227–28.

FARRELL, B. *Pat and Roald.* New York: Random House, Inc., 1969.

FRANK, S. "Patricia Neal: Suddenly I Wanted to Live." *Good Housekeeping* (July, 1967), p. 70.

HALL, W. "Return From Silence—A Personal Experience." *Journal of Speech and Hearing Disorders,* 26 (1961): 174–77.

HODGINS, E. *Episode: Report on the Accident in My Skull.* New York: Atheneum, 1964.

KNOX, D. *Portrait of Aphasia.* Detroit: Wayne State University Press, 1971.

MCBRIDE, C. *Silent Victory.* Chicago: Nelson-Hall, 1969.

RITCHIE, D. *Stroke: A Diary of Recovery.* New York: Doubleday & Company, Inc., 1961.

ROLNICK, M., and H. HOOPS. "Aphasia As Seen by the Aphasic." *Journal of Speech and Hearing Disorders,* 34 (1969): 48–53.

ROSE, R. "A Physician's Account of His Own Aphasia." *Journal of Speech and Hearing Disorders,* 13 (1948): 294–305.

SIES, L., and R. BUTLER. "A Personal Account of Dysphasia." *Journal of Speech and Hearing Disorders,* 28 (1963): 216–66.

SIMENON, GEORGES, *The Bells of Bicetre.* New York: Harcourt, Brace and World, 1964.

SOLOMON, P., et al. *Sensory Deprivation.* Cambridge, Mass.: Harvard University Press, 1961.

ULLMAN, M. *Behavioral Changes Following Stroke.* Springfield, Ill.: Charles C Thomas, 1962.

VAN ROSEN, R. *Comeback: The Story of My Stroke.* New York: Bobbs-Merrill Company, 1963.

WHITEHOUSE, E. *There's Always More.* Valley Forge, Pa.: The Judson Press, 1968.

WINT, G. *The Third Killer.* New York: Abelard-Schuman, 1965.

ZUBECK, J. *Sensory Deprivation: Fifteen Years of Research.* New York: Apple-ton-Century-Crofts, 1969.

6. Various methods of scoring responses are employed in the language inventories cited in this chapter. After consulting articles by Kaplan (1959), Schuell (1966), Sarno and Sands (1970), and Porch (1971), review the most widely used tests of aphasia in light of the questions posed below:

a. Which tests use plus-minus scoring? What rationale is offered for the efficacy of this method of scoring?

b. Which tests employ rating scales? How many categories are included? What might be the ideal number of steps in a rating scale—four, eight, sixteen? How might the concept of Occam's razor apply to the relative complexity of rating scales?

c. Which tests yield a numerical score to summarize the patient's responses? What is measurement? Are there levels of measurement? Do any tests of aphasia employ measurement levels more precise than nominal or ordinal? In terms of statistical procedure, is it permissible to perform arithmetical computation (adding, computing means) on ordinal data?

d. Which tests utilize psycholinguistic units for scoring responses?

e. The manuals of most aphasia tests present reliability data regarding the scoring system. Which include information on validity?

7. What is the concept of "glossomatics," and how might it relate to the appraisal of adult aphasics?

8. Can you outline an aphasia test based upon the Skinnerian language model?

9. Several observers report that aphasics cannot use symbols in a "second-hand" manner; that is, they cannot lie and they dream less frequently, if at all, than they did prior to the brain injury. How would you account for this?

10. What similarities can you identify, if any, between Schuell's five aphasics and Wepman's five categories of language impairment?

11. What is the significance of Diehl and England's (1958) article on imagery for the diagnosis of adult aphasics?

12. What applications might hyperoxygenation have for diagnosis and rehabilitation of adult aphasics (Jacobs *et al.,* 1969; Sarno, Sarno, and Diller, 1972)?

13. What language-related functions are subtended by the right hemisphere? Spatial relationships? Body schema? Stimulus equivalence? What characteristics identify patients with bilateral brain damage? The references listed below will provide a beginning for your search for answers to these questions.

BONKOWSKI, R. "Verbal and Extraverbal Components of Language as Related to Lateralized Brain Damage." *Journal of Speech and Hearing Research,* 10 (1967): 558–64.

FAGLIONI, P., H. SPINNLER, and L. A. VIGNOLO. "Contrasting Behavior of R. and L. Hemisphere Patients on a Discriminative and a Semantic Task of Auditory Recognition." *Cortex,* 5 (1969): 366–89.

HELAEN, H., and M. PIERCY. "Paroxysmal Dysphasia and Problems of Cerebral Dominance." *Journal of Neurology and Neuro Surgery,* 19 (1956): 194–201.

LaPointe, L., and G. Culton. "Visual-Spatial Neglect Subsequent to Brain Injury." *Journal of Speech and Hearing Disorders*, 34 (1969): 82–86.

Peck, L., L. Swisher, and M. Sarno. "Token Test Scores of Three Matched Patient Groups: Left Brain-Damaged With Aphasia; Right Brain-Damaged Without Aphasia; Non Brain-Damaged." *Cortex*, 5 (1969): 264–73.

14. See if you can devise a diagnostic instrument that evaluates syntactic (Parisi and Pizzamiglio, 1970) and semantic (Pizzamiglio and Appicciafuoco, 1971) comprehension.

BIBLIOGRAPHY

Agranowitz, A. and M. McKeown (1964). *Aphasia Handbook*. Springfield, Ill.: Charles C Thomas.

American Heart Association (1965). *Aphasia and the Family*. New York: American Heart Association.

Anders, J. and L. Emerick (1963). "Exploration on a New Frontier: The Social Worker in Speech Therapy." *Journal of Rehabilitation*, 29: 24–26.

Aten, J., D. Johns, and F. Darley (1971), "Auditory Perception of Sequenced Words in Apraxia of Speech." *Journal of Speech and Hearing Research*, 14: 131–43.

Boone, D. (1967). "A Plan for the Rehabilitation of Aphasic Patients." *Archives of Physical Medicine and Rehabilitation*, 48: 410–14.

———— (1961). *An Adult Has Aphasia*. Danville, Ill.: Interstate Printers and Publishers.

Bourestom, N. (1967). "Predictors of Long-term Recovery in Cerebral Vascular Disease." *Archives of Physical Medicine and Rehabilitation*, 48: 415–19.

Brookshire, R. (1971). "Effects of Delay of Reinforcement on Probability of Learning by Aphasic Subjects." *Journal of Speech and Hearing Research*, 14: 92–105.

Buchanan, A. (1957). *Functional Neuro-Anatomy*. Philadelphia: Lea and Febiger.

Buck, M. (1968). *Dysphasia*. Englewood Cliffs, N.J.: Prentice-Hall, Inc.

Burr, H., ed. (1964). *The Aphasic Adult*. Charlottesville, Va.: Wayside Press.

Chusid, J. and J. McDonald (1967). *Correlative Neuroanatomy*. Los Altos, Calif.: Lange Medical Publications.

Cohn, R. and M. Neumann (1958). "Jargon Aphasia." *Journal of Nervous and Mental Disorders*, 127: 381–99.

Coser, R. (1956). "A Home away from Home." *Social Problems*, 4: 3–17.

Culton, G. (1969). "Spontaneous Recovery from Aphasia." *Journal of Speech and Hearing Research*, 12: 825–32.

DARLEY, F. (1972). "The Efficacy of Language Rehabilitation in Aphasia." *Journal of Speech and Hearing Disorders*, 37: 3–21.

—— (1964). *Diagnosis and Appraisal of Communication Disorders.* Englewood Cliffs, N.J.: Prentice-Hall, Inc.

DERMAN, S. and A. MANASTER (1967). "Family Counseling with Relatives of Aphasic Patients." *Journal of the American Speech and Hearing Association*, 8: 175–77.

DIEHL, C. and N. ENGLAND (1958). "Mental Imagery." *Journal of Speech and Hearing Research*, 1: 268–74.

DUFF, R. and A. HOLLINGSHEAD (1958). *Sickness and Society.* New York: Harper & Row, Publishers.

DUNN, L. (1958). *The Peabody Picture Vocabulary Test.* Minneapolis: American Guidance Service, Inc.

EAGLESON, H., G. VAUGH, and A. KNUDSON (1970). "Hand Signals for Dysphasia." *Archives of Physical Medicine and Rehabilitation*, 51: 111–13.

EISENHOWER, D. (1965). *Waging Peace.* New York: Doubleday & Company, Inc.

EISENSON, J. (1971). "Aphasia in Adults: Basic Considerations." In *Handbook of Speech Pathology and Audiology*, ed. L. Travis. New York: Appleton-Century-Crofts.

—— (1954). *Examining for Aphasia.* New York: Psychological Corporation.

—— (1949). "Prognostic Factors Related to Language Rehabilitation in Aphasic Patients." *Journal of Speech and Hearing Disorders*, 14: 262–64.

EMERICK, L. (1971). *Appraisal of Language Disturbance.* Marquette, Mich.: Northern Michigan University.

—— and J. M. COYNE (1972). *Screening Test of Aphasia.* Danville, Ill.: Interstate Printers and Publishers.

ENGMANN, D. and R. BROOKSHIRE (1970). "Effects of Simultaneous and Successive Stimulus Presentation on Visual Discriminations by Aphasic Patients." *Journal of Speech and Hearing Research*, 13: 369–81.

ETTLINGER, G. (1969). "Apraxia Considered as a Disorder of Movements that Are Language-Dependent: Evidence from Cases of Brain Bisection." *Cortex*, 5: 285–89.

FARRELL, B. (1969). *Pat and Roald.* New York: Random House, Inc.

GOODGLASS, H., J. GLEASON, and M. HYDE (1970). "Some Dimensions of Auditory Language Comprehension in Aphasia." *Journal of Speech and Hearing Research*, 13: 595–606.

GRINKER, R. and A. SAHS (1966). *Neurology.* Springfield, Ill.: Charles C Thomas.

HOCKADAY, J. and C. WHITTY (1969). "Factors Determining the Electroencephalogram in Migraine: A Study of 560 Patients, According to Clinical Type of Migraine." *Brain*, 92: 769–88.

HODGINS, E. (1964). *Episode: Report on the Accident in My Skull.* New York: Atheneum.

HOLLAND, A. (1970). "Case Studies in Aphasia Rehabilitation Using Programmed Instruction." *Journal of Speech and Hearing Disorders*, 35: 377–90.

HOROWITZ, B. (1962). "An Open Letter to the Family of an Adult Patient with Aphasia." *Rehabilitation Literature*, 23: 141–44.

JACOBS, E. *et al.* (1969). "Hyperoxygenation Effect on Cognitive Functioning in the Aged." *New England Journal of Medicine,* 281: 753–57.

JONES, L. and J. WEPMAN (1961). "Dimensions of Language Performance in Aphasia." *Journal of Speech and Hearing Research*, 4: 220–32.

KAPLAN, L. (1959). "A Descriptive Continuum of Language Responses in Aphasia." *Journal of Speech and Hearing Disorders*, 24: 410-12.

KEITH, R. and F. DARLEY (1967). "The Use of a Specific Electric Board in Rehabilitation of the Aphasic Patient." *Journal of Speech and Hearing Disorders*, 32: 148–53.

KEENAN, J. (1966). "A Method of Eliciting Naming Behavior from Aphasic Patients." *Journal of Speech and Hearing Disorders,* 31: 261–66.

——— (1968). "The Nature of Receptive and Expressive Impairments in Aphasia." *Journal of Speech and Hearing Disorders*, 33: 20–25.

KNOX, D. (1971). *Portrait of Aphasia.* Detroit: Wayne State University Press.

LECOURS, A. and F. LHERMITTE (1969). "Phonemic Paraphasias: Linguistic and Tentative Hypotheses." *Cortex*, 5: 193–228.

LONGERICH, M. (1955). *Helping the Aphasic to Recover His Speech.* Los Angeles: College of Medical Evangelists.

——— (1958). *Manual for the Aphasic Patient.* New York: The Macmillan Company.

——— and J. BORDEAUX (1959.) *Aphasia Therapeutics.* New York: The Macmillan Company.

McBRIDE, C. (1969). *Silent Victory.* Chicago: Nelson-Hall.

MARTIN, B. (1962). *Communicative Aids for the Adult Aphasics.* Springfield, Ill.: Charles C Thomas.

MILLER, M. (1960). "Audiological Evaluation of Aphasic Patients." *Journal of Speech and Hearing Disorders*, 25: 333–39.

NEEDHAM, E. and J. BLACK (1970). "The Relative Ability of Aphasic Persons to Judge the Duration and Intensity of Pure Tones." *Journal of Speech and Hearing Research*, 13: 725–30.

NETTER, F. (1958). *The Nervous System.* New York: Ciba.

ORGASS, B. and K. POECK (1969). "Assessment of Aphasia by Psychometric Methods." *Cortex,* 5: 317–30.

OSGOOD, D. and M. MIRON (1963). *Approaches to the Study of Aphasia.* Urbana: University of Illinois Press.

PAGE, I. *et al.* (1961). *Strokes: How They Occur and What Can Be Done about Them.* New York: E. P. Dutton.

PARISI, D. and L. PIZZAMIGLIO (1970). "Syntactic Comprehension in Aphasia." *Cortex,* 6: 204–15.

PENFIELD, W. and L. ROBERTS (1959). *Speech and Brain Mechanisms.* Princeton, N. J.: Princeton University Press.

PETERSON, J. and A. OLSEN (1964). *Language Problems after a Stroke.* Minneapolis: American Rehabilitation Foundation.

PIZZAMIGLIO, L. and A. APPICCIAFUOCO (1971). "Semantic Comprehension in Aphasia." *Journal of Communication Disorders,* 3: 280–88.

PORCH, B. (1971). "Multidimensional Scoring in Aphasia Testing." *Journal of Speech and Hearing Research,* 14: 776–92.

——— (1967). *Porch Index of Communicative Ability.* Palo Alto, Calif.: Consulting Psychologists Press.

SARNO, M. (1972). *Aphasia: Selected Readings.* New York: Appleton-Century-Crofts.

——— and E. SANDS (1970). "An Objective Method for the Evaluation of Speech Therapy in Aphasia." *Archives of Physical Medicine and Rehabilitation,* 51: 49–54.

SARNO, M., J. SARNO, and L. DILLER (1972). "The Effect of Hyperbaric Oxygen on Communication Functions in Adults with Aphasia Secondary to Stroke." *Journal of Speech and Hearing Research,* 15: 42–48.

SARNO, M., M. SILVERMAN, and E. SANDS (1970). "Speech Therapy and Language Recovery in Severe Aphasia." *Journal of Speech and Hearing Disorders,* 13: 607–23.

SCHLANGER, P. and B. SCHLANGER (1970). "Adapting Role-Playing Activities with Aphasic Patients." *Journal of Speech and Hearing Disorders,* 35: 229–35.

SCHUELL, H. (1965). *The Minnesota Test for Differential Diagnosis of Aphasia.* Minneapolis: University of Minnesota Press.

——— (1966). "A Reevaluation of the Short Examination for Aphasia." *Journal of Speech and Hearing Disorders,* 31: 137–47.

——— (1957). "A Short Examination for Aphasia." *Neurology,* 7: 625–34.

——— and J. JENKINS (1962). "A Factor Analysis of the Minnesota Test for Differential Diagnosis of Aphasia." *Journal of Speech and Hearing Research,* 5: 349–69.

SCHUELL, H., J. JENKINS, and E. JIMENEZ-PABON (1964). *Aphasia in Adults.* New York: Harper & Row, Publishers.

SCHUELL, H. *et al.* (1969). "A Psycholinguistic Approach to the Study of Language Deficit in Aphasia." *Journal of Speech and Hearing Research,* 12: 794–806.

SKLAR, M. (1963). "Relation of Psychological and Language Test Scores and Autopsy Findings in Aphasia." *Journal of Speech and Hearing Research,* 6: 84–90.

SMITH, A. (1971). "Objective Indices of Severity of Chronic Aphasia in Stroke Patients." *Journal of Speech and Hearing Disorders,* 36: 167–207.

SMITH, B. (1966). "An Investigation by a Visiting Nurse Association of a Home Training Program for Adults with Speech and Language Problems Resulting from CVA and Other Chronic Diseases." Unpublished Master's thesis, University of Pittsburgh.

SMITH, G. (1967) *Care of the Patient With a Stroke.* New York: Springer Publishing Company.

SNIDECOR, J. (1955). "A Method of Disparities for Evaluating Aphasic Disturbance." *Journal of Nervous and Mental Disorders,* 122: 92–93.

SOLOMON, P. *et al.* (1961). *Sensory Deprivation.* Cambridge, Mass.: Harvard University Press.

SPELLACY, F. and O. SPREEN (1969). "A Short Form of the Token Test." *Cortex,* 5: 390–97.

STEINBECK, J. (1961). *Travels with Charley.* New York: The Viking Press.

STOICHEFF, M. (1960) "Motivating Instruction and Language Performance of Dysphasic Subjects." *Journal of Speech and Hearing Research,* 3: 75–85.

STREET, B. (1957). "Hearing Loss in Aphasia." *Journal of Speech and Hearing Disorders,* 22: 60–67.

SWINNEY, D. and O. TAYLOR (1971). "Short-term Memory Recognition Search in Aphasics." *Journal of Speech and Hearing Research,* 14: 578–88.

TAYLOR, M. (1963). *Functional Communication Profile.* New York: New York University Medical Center.

———— (1958). *Understanding Aphasia.* New York: Institute of Physical Medicine and Rehabilitation.

———— and J. MYERS (1952). "A Group Discussion Program with the Families of Aphasic Patients." *Journal of Speech and Hearing Disorders,* 17: 393–96.

TOUBBEH, J. (1969). "Clinical Observations on Adult Aphasia." *Journal of Communication Disorders,* 2: 57–68.

TWAMLEY, R. and L. EMERICK (1970). "The Nurses' Role in Aphasia." *Today's Speech,* 18: 30–33.

VAN RIPER, C. (1972). *Speech Correction: Principles and Methods,* 5th ed. Englewood Cliffs, N.J.: Prentice-Hall, Inc.

WEPMAN, J. (1972). "Aphasia Therapy: A New Look." *Journal of Speech and Hearing Disorders,* 37: 203–214.

———— (1953). "A Conceptual Model for the Processes Involved in Recovery from Aphasia." *Journal of Speech and Hearing Disorders,* 18: 4–13.

———— (1951). *Recovery from Aphasia.* New York: Ronald Press.

———— (1958). "The Relationship Between Self-Correction and Recovery from Aphasia." *Journal of Speech and Hearing Disorders,* 23: 302–5.

———— and L. JONES (1961). *Studies in Aphasia: An Approach to Testing.* Chicago: Education-Industry Service.

WEPMAN, J. and A. MORENCY (1963). "Filmstrips as an Adjunct to Language Therapy for Aphasia." *Journal of Speech and Hearing Disorders,* 28: 191–94.

WEPMAN, J. *et al.* (1960). "Studies in Aphasia: Background and Theoretical Formulations." *Journal of Speech and Hearing Disorders,* 25: 323–32.

WEST, R. and M. ANSBERRY (1968). *The Rehabilitation of Speech,* 4th ed. New York: Harper & Row, Publishers. Pp. 397–422.

WHITEHOUSE, E. (1968). *There's Always More.* Valley Forge. Pa.: The Judson Press.

WINT, G. (1965). *The Third Killer.* New York: Abelard-Schumann.

ZUBECK, J. (1969). *Sensory Deprivation: Fifteen Years of Research.* New York: Appleton-Century-Crofts.

8

voice disorders

Todd and Clyde grudgingly left their sixth-grade classroom for the semiweekly session with the speech clinician. Todd had been taking this same route twice each week for the past five years, and Clyde had a similar dismal record for lack of correction of a distorted /r/. For two years now speech therapy had become a burden, and several of their ploys to get dismissed had failed. It was not until this morning that the fail-proof method was to be employed. "I think I have it," said Clyde feigning the most hoarse voice he could muster. "We will both begin talking like this to the speech clinician, and she is sure to drop us from therapy and put us on the waiting list with all those other voice cases."

Contrived, yes. Inaccurate? We are not so sure. For reasons we shall soon enumerate, voice disorders are perplexing sources of failure for many speech clinicians. Although disordered voices represent but a small percentage of our total professional clientele,[1] any individual whom we cannot deal with efficiently is one too many.

definition of voice

The imprecision of labels, which is the bane of voice study, begins with

---

[1] Compare the incidence figures of Senturia and Wilson (1968) with those of Pronovost (1951).

261

the term "voice" itself. Some definitions restrict the term to the generation of sound at the level of the larynx, while others include the influence of the vocal tract upon the generated tone, and still others broaden the definition to ultimately include aspects of tonal generation, resonation, articulation, and prosody.

"It's good to hear your voice!" However, it is not just the voice, but also the words. Definitions reflect our point of view, and as such they tend to fit the circumstances of the moment. The laryngologist will listen to that same "voice" from a totally different perspective and hear only the signals of glottal malfunction. For our purposes voice refers to more than just the glottal tone, but not the total acoustic pattern, which includes articulatory, symbolic, and prosodic characteristics. Voice is the product of respiratory power, laryngeal valving and sound generation, vocal tract resonation, and alteration of tone; it is categorized into pitch, quality, and loudness. Our concern is with what the ear hears; but this is the end product of several interrelated systems, each having a specific influence.

As Van Riper and Irwin (1958) point out, voice is the carrier wave, while articulation is the message. The meaning and intent of a message are primarily matters of semantic choice, syntax, prosody, phone accuracy, and in certain instances (and more so in some languages) vocal characteristics. The effects of voice disorders go beyond drawing critical attention, causing personal concern, or interfering with communication. Indeed, in some instances the early identification of minimal changes in vocal quality may save a person's life. There are, of course, instances where the voice does indeed alter the content of a spoken message. The total lack of voice is a far more serious handicap than an altered phoneme or two.

The imprecise definitions and the subsequent insecurity of speech clinicians are both related to several factors:

1. The voice is the product of muscle functions that are not readily observed and are difficult to control directly. Whereas in articulation an individual can be told to elevate the tongue tip and the success of this action can be observed and measured, the voice clinician cannot request the client to bring his arytenoid cartilages together. There is a mystique which surrounds the unobservable, and much of voice rehabilitation has been "mystical."

2. The voice is indirectly influenced by several body systems, including the respiratory, phonatory, resonatory, endocrine, and neural. With so many systems functioning, it is often difficult to determine just which potential etiological factor is responsible for any given symptom.

3. There are contradictory points of view on the relative influence of the physical and psychic factors of vocal production. The voice is said to be a bellweather of the psychological state and is subject to insidious and hard-to-detect influences.

4. There is no clear concept of just what normal voice is, since the influences of culture, age, sex, role, and specific activity alter the expected vocal output. Under certain circumstances, nearly any voice variation could be termed "normal."

5. The various parameters of voice are subject to continuous and flowing change at the whim of the speaker. Whereas it would be considered aberrant for a speaker to abruptly alter his syntactical system or articulatory pattern, each of us continuously changes the pitch, loudness, and quality of his voice in keeping with the meaning of the spoken signal. Such instantaneous changes make pitch characteristics rather difficult to define precisely.

6. The listener's perceptions of vocal characteristics are mediated through other aspects of the speech signal. For example, Sherman (1954) pointed out that the perception of nasality is partially dependent on articulatory patterns.

7. In the literature concerning voice there has been a tendency to confuse perceptual and physical characteristics. To state that the "natural *pitch*" of the adult male is approximately 125 Hz encourages confusion and imprecision.

8. There is no clear idea of the compensatory capabilities of the vocal tract in voice production. It is not known if the resonators can and do mask phonatory differences in some individuals or, on the other hand, if an increased exhalatory effort results in a compensating function of the vocal folds which in turn causes minimal signal change.

9. The study of voice has been divided between the "scientists" and the "practitioners." "Voice scientists" and "experimental phoneticians" have provided the discipline with much of the hard data upon which to assess clinical behavior, but there have been precious few who have been willing to make clinical suggestions from the laboratory findings. Similarly, the flow of information has not been reciprocal; clinicians have been remiss in collecting clinical data which can hold up under the critical eyes of the researchers.

10. The versatility of the vocal mechanism is exemplified by the number of uses it is put to. Speaking, singing, shouting, crying, laughing, whispering, moaning, sobbing, sighing, burping, yodeling, snoring, coughing, sneezing, hiccuping, and ventriloquism—all involve some portion of the respiratory, phonatory, or resonatory systems.

With this set of factors in mind, then, there is little wonder that some clinicians are poorly prepared to deal with the disordered voice. University classes in voice disturbance typically dwell on descriptions of the problem, classification systems, research data, and the like but somehow find little time for thorough discussions of the actual clinical practice with the voice patient. The difficult voice cases are rare and are coveted by a few staff members or graduate students. Worthley (1969) found in a survey of over 400 public-school speech clinicians that they rate their training in voice disorders poorer than in any other area.

parameters of voice and vocal disturbance

Some systematic framework is necessary in order to conceptualize voice and voice disturbance as shown by Figure 12. The auditory characteristics of pitch, loudness, and quality constitute one dimension of our paradigm. All of these are perceptual attributes of the voice and relate generally to the fundamental frequency, amplitude, and complexity of the signal.

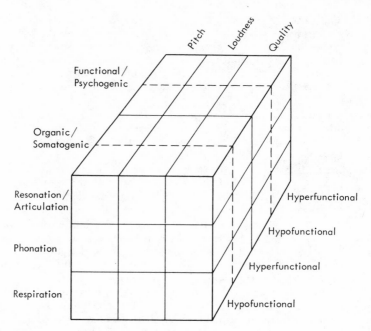

FIGURE 12   An Organizational Schema of Voice Disorders.

Pitch that is too high, too low, too invariant, or inappropriately variant for the speaker or the circumstances constitutes a voice disorder.

The loudness of the speaking voice is usually judged according to the speaking circumstance, the aberrant ranging from the total lack of voice (aphonia) to the inappropriately loud. Inappropriate loudness indicates a lack of control of the phonatory system.

For our purposes the term quality refers to the perceived pleasantness, or appeal, of the voice. This perception is linked both to the phonatory and resonatory characteristics of the speaker.

The physical systems that most directly influence the vocal production are the respiratory, phonatory, and resonatory-articulatory systems. Although these systems have the most direct impact on the voice signal, they are not the only systems that influence the voice.[2]

The respiratory system provides the motive force for voice production, and ultimately the resultant airstream becomes the vibrator that embodies all of the characteristics which the ear eventually senses. That the airstream is important to vocal production is not really the issue at this point, but there is some question as to the influence of the respiratory mechanism upon the various vocal characteristics. It appears that the respiratory mechanism must be capable of the following:

[2] Read Luchsinger and Arnold's (1965) account of the impact of the endocrine system on voice production.

1. Providing an adequate amount of air so that the speaker can sustain speech with ease to allow for natural phrasing and prosodic factors;
2. Providing adequate breath support so that the vibratory pattern can be established without undue laryngeal valving tension;
3. Providing adequate control of the flow of air so that the mechanism can, when necessary, either initiate or arrest the speech signal;
4. Providing an airstream that is not so indebted to active muscle contraction that it encourages unnecessary muscle tension in the respiratory and phonatory mechanisms;
5. Providing an airstream that is instantly available upon demand and able to be sustained somewhat constantly for a sufficient length of time.

The respiratory mechanism has been subject to a lot of misinformation. Early writings spoke of "breathing from the diaphragm," and stressed the "proper" inward movement of the abdomen during inhalation. Some clinicians still concentrate on the respiratory function when the disorder is clearly phonatory. If a tire loses air because of a leak in the air valve, one would not attempt to fix the leak by altering the pressure within the tire, one would attack the problem at the site of the breakdown.

A protracted discussion of the physiology of phonation is not within the scope of this text; however, some elements of laryngeal function are crucial in diagnostic evaluation. In order to be an efficient sound source, the larynx must perform a valving action upon the flow of air that establishes alternate, regular pressure changes within the body of air. In order to do this the vocal folds must:

(1) be capable of wide range valving actions, from keeping the passageway open and unrestricted to closed and totally restricted, and a wide variety of closures between those two points; (2) be able to valve fairly completely along their entire length; (3) be of approximately equal size and shape so that they can move in synchrony with one another; (4) close and open during phonation with just the right amount of firmness so that they are not subject to extremes of pressure during the closing phase; (5) be of appropriate size (length and mass) for the age and sex of the person; (6) be capable of natural movement that is free from superimposed and undue tension; and (7) be capable of small, subtle, instantaneous adjustments that must be made continuously to alter the various vocal characteristics. These adjustments must allow for a variety of cyclic variations in the potential time of glottal opening and closing. These range from the long closing time of the glottal fry to the short closing time of the falsetto voice.

The glottal tone is complex and rich in higher harmonics, but it is only through the resonant and damping effects of the vocal tract that the speech sounds achieve their identity. In order for the resonating chambers of the vocal tract to be efficient, they must be flexible in size, shape, texture, and relationship with one another. The effect of the resonators upon the laryngeal valve has been discussed by several writers (Curtis, 1968; Wendahl and Page, 1967), but the exact nature of this relationship has yet to be determined.

The term functional should imply more than the simple absence of measurable organic deviation; it should imply that the diagnostician has found some active agent of etiology and that that agent is nonorganic. We agree with Powers (1957) that the term functional has unfortunately come to mean diagnosis by default. We hope that the clinician will be encouraged to a more thorough search if he uses the more active definition of "functional." Voice disorders offer an interesting testing ground for the traditional organic-functional dichotomy. This separation does not stand up on almost any basis. Murphy (1964) points out the continuous nature of vocal-disorder etiologies, a concept with which we heartily agree.

Figure 12 identifies function/psychogenic and organic/somatogenic as clinically meaningful categories. The term functional refers to those disorders where the learned, psychic, or maladaptive behavior has resulted in faulty vocal production but not in physical alteration. If physical change has resulted from the functional cause, however, the proper designation is psychogenic. Similarly, if the original factor was physical or organic, then the term organic is justified; but if the physical difference results in behavioral change —i.e., emotional response or faulty compensatory adjustments—the term somatogenic is appropriate (Murphy, 1964).

The terms hyper- and hypofunctioning refer to an excess or insufficiency of laryngeal tension and, as such, could apply to a wide variety of organic or functional disorders.

The term voice disorder, then, refers to abnormal pitch, loudness, or vocal quality according to sex, age, status, temporary physiological state, purpose of the speaker, and elements of the speaking circumstance. Vocal disorders may be primarily organic or functional and may be affected by any of the primary systems of respiration, phonation, or resonance, as well as secondary systems that influence voice production such as the neurological and endocrine systems.

DIAGNOSTIC FORMAT

This chapter will not cover the anatomy and physiology of the mechanisms of vocal production. Moore (1971a), Zemlin (1968), Kaplan (1971), and others offer this information, and the student should study it carefully before undertaking voice diagnosis. We also cannot provide an elaborate description of each voice disorder type; this information is available to the student in several sources (Luchsinger and Arnold, 1965; Greene, 1964; and Boone, 1971). We shall not discuss pitch meters, sound spectrographs, respirometers, and the like. Most clinicians do not have a laboratory available and thus are forced to be inventive during the voice diagnosis. Hanley and Peters (1971) provide a complete discussion of the speech laboratory.

Our major focus will be on the actual thought, planning, preparation, and execution of voice diagnoses. Diagnosis is intended to define the parameters of the problem, determine the etiology, and outline a logical course of action.

the presenting complaint

The diagnostic process begins with a careful scrutiny of the original statement of the problem as provided by the referral source. Four perspectives guide our evaluation of this information: who, what, why, and when.

Who. It is important to know who presents the original complaint about the client's voice. We have found that the "best" source from a motivational standpoint is the client himself, but that any individual who might have a significant impact upon the client may be a satisfactory referral source. If the client and those around him do not consider his voice to be a problem, then in reality, there is none. With voice disorders, however, this may be dangerous because some minimal changes in voice quality may reflect anatomic changes. There is a circular pattern of cause and effect in voice disorders that is best treated early.

> Mrs. N. referred her husband to us with a pleading phone call. "He had his laryngectomy four months ago and the doctor says he will never talk again. Is there anything you can do?" For some unknown reason we resisted the urge to reassure Mrs. N. that her husband could indeed speak again, but we made an appointment for evaluation. When Mr. and Mrs. N. came into the office they had with them their newly purchased electrolarynx which was obtained at the insistence of their daughter. Much to our chagrin, it soon became evident why Mr. N. had been told he would not speak again. Not only had the surgeon removed the larynx, he had also excised the entire lingual structure. The fact that the referral came from the spouse rather than from our usually reliable laryngologist should have provided the first clue in this case. The truly interesting aspect is the daughter's naïveté and ignorance of the speaking process as shown by the purchase of that totally useless electrolarynx.

An amazing number of people do not consider voice characteristics to be in the realm of speech disorders. One high-school sophomore who spoke in a falsetto voice was referred to us by his English teacher, who stated, "I don't think this kid really has a speech problem, but I don't know who else to send him to." The typical response is "Oh, that's just Jimmy's voice, he's always sounded like that." The implication is that the characteristics that determine a person's voice are genetically determined and cannot be changed by training or practice.[3] When our screening process determines that an individual has a

---

[3] For an indication of the classroom teacher's efficacy in referral of children with voice disorders, see Diehl, C., and C. Stinnett, "Efficiency of Teacher Referrals in a School Speech-Testing Program," *Journal of Speech and Hearing Disorders*, 24 (1959): 34–36.

significant vocal deviation, we take particular pains to present this information to the individual so that he will not be tempted to use hidden and ill-defined factors to explain the problem.

What.   The description of the problem is important not only because it helps us to understand the problem better but also because it allows us to see the problem through the eyes (and ears) of another. When the statement comes from the person with whom we will be working, we listen not only to the actual words spoken, but also to the way in which they are presented. One of the best sources of information about the impact of the problem upon the individual is the way in which he describes it. Invariably, when interviewing the client we find it valuable to ask the following five questions: (1) "Describe your voice." Listen for the terms used, the factors which appear to alter the voice, other sources of variance in vocal characteristics, and subtle signs of concern. (2) "How do others react to your speaking voice?" Generally we attempt to judge this answer against reality as best we can. Very often the individual will respond that no one ever mentions his voice, and the diagnostician must take care not to reinforce such reactions, while on the other hand, not to strip the client of all his defenses. It is quite possible that there has been little environmental reaction and that the client is being quite honest in his reply, but we are concerned with the client's perception of other's reactions. Remember that you may be the first person to ask him such questions, and he should be given plenty of time to respond. (3) "How severe do you consider this problem to be?" Generally we give the client some sort of subjective rating scale upon which to judge. This is very useful baseline information and is directly related to the next question. (4) "How much does this problem bother you?" We have found that the degree of concern and the judgment of severity are not always directly related, but in any case we must know just how much this individual wishes to change his voice. The clinician must be careful in such discussions since the client may respond that he has no problem and he does not desire to change in the least. Although this is important diagnostic information, it is also important to the therapy process; and the diagnostician must be able to recover the initiative and put the client back on the track. (5) "What caused the problem?" Although generally the client claims ignorance, every once in a while we open a Pandora's box with this question.

> Following a rather benign discussion, Mrs. A. was finally asked just what caused her vocal hoarseness. Her response began cautiously enough, but soon she was describing her "second" visit to the state mental hospital (we had not known there was a "first" visit) and how the staff had resorted to electric shock treatments in an attempt to break the profound depression she was experiencing. From that point on, the discussion opened up and significant information was offered freely.

Murphy (1964: 92) presents a series of twenty questions to clarify the individual's self-concepts regarding his speaking voice. Such lists often provide a useful starting place for the diagnostician.

Why. The reasons for referral to the voice clinician may vary from an impending trip ("I just have to sound better than this by the first of August") to fears of serious medical problems. In evaluating the reasons for referral, it is important to keep in mind that a referral to a speech clinician is often seen as psychologically safer than referrals to medical doctors or psychiatrists. This points up the importance of secondary referrals.

When. Three things are of major concern here. First, it is important to know when, in the sequence of events of the problem, the referral was made. Is this a problem of long standing that has only recently become serious, or is it a relatively new phenomenon that has been detected early? Second, what is this person's age and maturational level? Whereas certain vocal changes are to be expected before puberty (Curry, 1949) and would thus be considered normal, a similar vocal quality at a later maturity level is serious. Third, does his problem appear in cycles? Does the client suffer from this vocal quality only during "hay fever" season? The time of year of the referral may provide some important diagnostic information.

historic data

A general case-history form is provided in Appendix A of this text and in several other texts (Johnson, Darley, and Spriestersbach, 1963; Berry and Eisenson, 1956). Our purpose is to identify those specific aspects within each of the historical subcategories that have particular relevance to voice diagnosis. Discussions of case-history evaluation tend to be rather sterile if the relevance of each aspect is not made clear. The reader is encouraged to complete the project outlined in Appendix A, since it is exactly that type of study which makes the bland discussion of routine diagnostic tasks come alive.

Family Data. Information regarding the parental occupation, number of siblings, history of family adjustment, other voice problems within the family, and general health pattern of the family tells us a great deal about the client's social and physical milieu. Generally, the following characteristics are considered danger signals: (1) too much or too little structure and organization to the home; (2) premium placed on verbal competition; (3) interparental friction; (4) unusual sibling competition; (5) history of voice disorders in others within the family; (6) poor parental adjustment; (7) history of extended or recurrent health problems within the family; and (8) general level of concern for physical and health problems within the family.

Onset of the problem. In many instances the nature of the onset of the voice problem will have great diagnostic significance. It is important to investigate not only the nature of the onset but the circumstances surrounding it. Physical or psychological trauma may have equally instant effects upon voice production. In some cases, extended questioning may be necessary because it is common for clients to repress uncomfortable incidents of the past. Unfortunately, physical trauma is often inextricably related to psychological trauma in a large number of cases; therefore, this information must be judged against all the other diagnostic data available. Just as the beauty of a painting is not appreciated through the microscope, individual bits of information only have meaning when viewed in broad perspective.

Although the abrupt onset of a vocal disorder is traumatic and startling, most voice disorders are of insidious origin. Many people cannot pinpoint the exact date of onset and tend to indicate when people first noticed or remarked about their voices. Since a gradual onset is not specific to organic or functional etiologies, the examiner must look to other data for final answers. Probably more important than the problem's rate of development is information on coincident factors such as the client's general health and emotional state.

Course of development. A careful description of the developmental stages of the voice disturbance may provide helpful diagnostic information. Not only are the developments themselves important, but also the sequence of events before and after.

Mrs. F. was seen in the speech-and-hearing clinic three times in three years, each time with a similar complaint. Vocal fatigue and hoarseness characterized this first-grade teacher's voice. Medical examinations had been negative on each of the first two occasions, but on the third visit small vocal nodules were noted. Looking over our records, it was noted that Mrs. F. had been to the clinic in late March of 1968, early April of 1969, and late April of 1970. After some further discussion with Mrs. F., we determined that she was not only suffering from vocal fatigue but from teaching fatigue as well.

The diagnostician is cautioned to observe for signs of medical problems, vocational stress periods, periods of particular personal stress, and other etiological influences that may affect the problem.

Social Adjusting. Assessment of the personality characteristics of the individual may assist the diagnostician in interpreting other information. Formal personality testing, briefly discussed in Chapter 3, is not within the jurisdiction of the speech clinician, but each clinician is expected to be perceptive and sensitive to clues about the client's basic adjustment to life. The concept that the voice is closely related to the individual's self-concept and reveals inner conflict has been carefully examined by several researchers. Moses (1954) and Rousey and Moriarty (1965) present interesting views of the interaction of the personality and voice production. This relationship is seen in a wide range of examples from the hypernasal whine of a college freshman giving his first speech in "Speech I" to the deep-seated symptoms of the psychotic. Classification of voice characteristics with specific personality types has not provided overwhelming evidence; but the personality and the voice interact in a complex fashion and this results in many symptomatic characteristics both permanent and temporary.

The danger in taking a purely symptomatic approach to voice disorders has already been implied. The following examples underscore the point.

Ted, a strapping six-foot high-school sophomore, presented himself to our office upon the referral of his English teacher. Ted knew that his voice was "too high" and stated that he desired to change it. Within the first session Ted was phonating at an appropriate pitch level, and the postpubescent falsetto voice appeared to be an easy challenge. Within three weeks Ted was speaking in controlled sentences at the proper pitch level, and our purely symptomatic approach appeared to be satisfactory. In fact Ted habituated to the proper pitch within the academic semester. This is not an unusual occurrence, however.

The following events, however, give reason to question the clinical approach. Ted was the younger of two sons and by far the "junior" in many respects. Ted's older brother was an excellent student, outstanding athlete, and class officer until he was killed in a hunting accident at the age of seventeen. Ted was twelve at the time of his brother's death, and his voice had already begun to change. Within a few weeks, however, Ted resorted to the falsetto voice and maintained that voice until he was seen for speech therapy some three years later. Early in our therapy Ted's mother was interviewed, and the tape recording of Ted's masculine voice was played. She immediately began to sob, relating that the voice was identical to that of the older brother. Fearful that we were forcing Ted to compete with the memory of his older brother, we nonetheless pressed our attack on his voice. By the end of the academic year Ted appeared delighted with his progress and had established a close relationship with the clinician. The following fall Ted called the clinician to set up a partridge hunting trip. We felt this would afford an excellent opportunity to test the carryover of the voice, and the trip took place as planned. Ted's voice had remained normal, although curiously, his speech contained several articulatory errors that had previously not existed. The startling event, however, was not his improved voice or speech. During our last walk down a tote road, Ted, who was a good distance behind, accidently discharged his gun and sprayed pellets in our direction. Ted responded by laughing hysterically to the point where he could not be controlled for some time. There are several interesting interpretations of this event, but the most disturbing is that Ted may well have been unconsciously displaying his hostility toward the person who forced him to employ a voice and role his psyche had previously rejected.

One of our most bizarre clients was a Mrs. K., a sharp-featured women in her mid-forties whose aphonia appeared to be linked to a tragic auto accident in which she was involved while transporting a group of young girls to a religious retreat. Two of the young girls had been seriously injured, and Mrs. K. had not uttered a sound since the event. Although severe chest and neck bruising had occurred, her physicians could not detect any specific organic etiology for the lack of voice. When we saw this woman, she had been without voice for several weeks. Mrs. K. displayed a high degree of tension and anxiety; she continuously moved about in her chair and maintained minimal eye contact with the male examiner. During the initial interview she was asked to clear her throat and cough, both of which she did with normal approximation of the folds.

The examiner requested that Mrs. K. provide him with a written autobiography, and the results were fascinating. Mrs. K. noted that her father had left the home when she was five years old. "My only recollection of him was that he punished my sister for lying about a date she had. He used very strange methods of punishment, and I was frightened to death of him." She then related that she had been an "exotic dancer" for some twenty years, although she felt that "men are no good!" She stated that her life took a dramatic turn when she was visited by a group of youths who were on a religious crusade. She ended up joining the group and heading a small band of young women who dedicated themselves to Christian conversion. It was at this point, "the high point" in her life as she wrote it, that Mrs. K. lost her voice. Mrs. K. regained her voice after several months of psychotherapy. When she returned to us for her last visit, she stated, "I can now fight for the liberation of women with greater understanding, since I have won the battle for my own personal liberation."

Vocation.   We are interested in the vocation of our voice client for two reasons. First, we must determine if the occupation demands a great deal of talking and if that talking is under adverse conditions. There is not only a boilermaker's ear but a boilermaker's voice as well. Not all teachers develop "teachers' nodules" however, and the vocation must be judged in relation to the person. Several writers have postulated that there is a personality type that develops vocal nodules (Jackson, 1941; Withers, 1961). We have found many of these people to be tense, energetic, high strung, and verbally aggressive. Place this type of person in an occupational setting that demands a great deal of speaking under tension, and a bit of poor judgment in choosing adaptive procedures, and the chances of finding an individual with vocal nodules are greatly enhanced.

A second factor in our evaluation of the vocation of an individual is the degree of satisfaction the person receives from his work. The task is not always easy, but clues may come from information on the person's interests, educational background, and qualifications, along with some measure of the rewards he receives from his work.

Health.   Realizing that the voice is influenced by many physiological systems, a complete medical history and examination are necessary in many instances. A history of the general health and physical development of the client should be obtained, along with information about specific illnesses, surgeries, and medication; the clinician should also obtain a familial health history and data concerning the general energy level and health-related habits such as smoking, drinking, and drug usage.[4] Luchsinger and Arnold (1965) present a particularly comprehensive discussion of vocal disorders of organic etiology.

[4] We recently questioned a rather elderly gentleman about his health during an initial interview. His amusing, if perplexing answer was: "My wife says I'm a hypochondriac, but that's compounded by the fact that I'm in very poor health."

Sherry was identified in the university speech-and-hearing screening program. Her voice was described as breathy, low in pitch and volume, expressionless, and with varying degrees of nasality. The case history revealed the following information: low metabolic rate, rapid fatigue, and body temperature generally below normal. Subsequent medical referral indicated specific muscle weakness and a medical diagnosis of myasthenia gravis. It should be noted that the speech clinician's alertness to the accummulation of medical danger signs in addition to the speech characteristics resulted in a proper referral and subsequent identification of the problem.

the evaluation process

The first step in the voice analysis involves simply listening to the client in an objective and yet analytical manner. We find it helpful to mentally rehearse the classifications of voice disorders while listening.

During the initial interview, Mr. B. was requested to recount the events which brought him to our office. While he was speaking, the following mental notes were taken: Volume appears adequate with good variety and inflection; only problem in this area appears to be his lack of projection at the end of particularly long phrases: this should be evaluated. Before he leaves I will take him into a classroom and have him speak to me as if he were addressing a large gathering. His pitch sounds high, but this is difficult to judge since there is good variety and a strange low-frequency component I can't identify. He is an animated speaker with a lively gesture system accompanying his speech. In fact he continues to move and gesture when he is listening, almost as if he were saying what I was saying right along with me. As I listen to his speech, however, it is not the pitch that bothers me—the predominant feature is the hoarse vocal quality. I hear a breathy escape during phonation and a strained rough sound. I feel like clearing my throat with every sentence he speaks (and my throat felt tense when he left). Particularly noticeable was the manner in which he initiated sound—almost as if the pressure build-up was so great the folds were blasted apart with unusual force. He also had an unconscious mannerism of clearing his throat abruptly upon initiation of a statement. I'll bet he is not even aware of this. There are no articulation or resonatory problems, but his phrase structure bothers me. He appears to run short of air at odd places and strains to continue talking until he gets to a natural juncture. This doesn't work all of the time, however, and often he just stops and begins with that coup de glotte vocal onset again. I really shouldn't bias myself with a prediction, but I'm betting on vocal nodules.

Respiration. The laboratory scientists have made clinicians appreciate the importance of the respiratory process in speech but have not provided any efficient and accessible means for measuring the variables of respiration. For this reason, and possibly others, speech clinicians have not paid enough attention to this function. Spirometers, pneumographs, and respirometers are not available to many public-school speech clinicians.

Our concern for the respiratory process involves both the vegetative processes and breathing for speech. There are six areas of concern for the diagnostician: air volume, respiratory type, respiratory rate and ratio, durational aspects, associated tension, and associated sounds.

AIR VOLUME. The maximum amount of air which can be exhaled following maximal inhalation is called vital capacity (Wood, 1971). The relationship of vital capacity to speech production is somewhat a matter of conjecture at this point. Vital capacity is apparently related to several factors such as body size, physical condition, and sex (Gray and Wise, 1959; Van Riper and Irwin, 1958). There is little or no research to vindicate those who have worked to increase the vital capacity of their voice clients. On the other hand, it is logical to assume that an individual with an extremely small amount of air available would find it difficult to sustain phonation and would resort to increased laryngeal tension and forcing to maintain normal or near-normal phrasing. It is probably not so much the volume of air as it is the individual's ability to control the airflow (Hardy, 1961).

Although we have made futile attempts to devise a mechanism that will adequately measure vital capacity, there appears to be no satisfactory substitute for the spirometer. Clinically we have found that a vital capacity insufficient for normal speech purposes was so obvious from normal observation that further formal testing was not necessary. Vital capacity measurements may be of particular concern in cases of emphysema, later stages of Parkinson's disease, and children with cerebral palsy.

RESPIRATION TYPE. The methods of respiration have been classically designated as clavicular, thoracic, and abdominal. The terms refer to the area of greatest excursion during inhalation. More precise and demanding categorizations have been proposed (Russell, 1931); however, there appears to be general agreement that respiratory type has little influence on vocal characteristics except in the case of extreme upper chest or clavicular breathing, which tends to encourage great laryngeal tension and insufficient intake of air volume.[5]

Observation appears to be the most satisfactory method of determining the type of respiratory process, although the enterprising public-school clinician may find that the science lab may have a kymograph, and such devices are easily altered for use as a pneumograph. Once again, our concern is not so much with the method employed in respiration as it is with the ease and efficiency of the operation.

While observing for the region of respiration, the clinician should also determine the coordination of the thoracic and abdominal regions. When the contraction of the thoracic muscles of inhalation coincides with the contraction of the abdominal muscles and the diaphragm, easy inhalation is impos-

---

[5] Diaphragmatic breathing has been a concept long held dear by many voice and elocution teachers. What is the function of the diaphragm during respiration? Is it possible to consciously control the contraction or relaxation of this muscle? What is a better term for diaphragmatic breathing? (See Van Riper and Irwin, 1958; Luchsinger and Arnold, 1965; and Cotes, 1965.)

sible, and the reverse of this situation results in the inability to control the exhalation of air. This pattern may result in an insufficiency of air or uneven phonatory patterns due to varying degrees of subglottic pressure. McDonald and Chance (1964) point out that this respiratory pattern is seen among cerebral-palsied individuals. We generally make an attempt to determine the degree of respiratory control while the client is engaged in the following activities: maintaining a slow, gradual inhalation; maintaining a slow, gradual exhalation; producing an isolated vowel for a few seconds duration; producing controlled phrases and sentences; panting; and speaking while engaged in some extraneous motor activity.

RESPIRATORY RATE RATIO. Vegetative respiratory rate varies considerably depending upon the age and activity level of the individual. A rate of thirty to forty per minute is not uncommon in the very young infant, but beyond one and one-half to two years of age the rate should have stabilized in the low twenties. With some children the extremely high respiratory rate appears to interfere with contextual speech development, just as most people find it difficult to carry on a conversation while jogging. The continual interruption of the speech for respiratory purposes makes flowing speech difficult.

While observing the respiratory rate, it may be helpful to make note of the rhythm of respiration as well. Inconsistency in the rhythm of breathing may indicate neuromusculature problems and is quite typical in some cerebral-palsied individuals.

Respiratory patterns are altered significantly during speech. The inhalatory phase is shorter in duration and generally the volume of air intake is greater, while the exhalation phase is more controlled and gradual, with pulses of air being released with each syllable. Whereas the ratio of inhalation to exhalation time is approximately equal in normal respiration, it now may vary around the ratio of 1 to 7. Just as too frequent inhalations may alter the flow of speech, so may inhalation patterns that take too long to accomplish. It is by no means an easy task to measure the temporal aspects of respiration without the aid of graphic representation. In those cases where there is some serious question regarding the respiratory ratio, it may be necessary to video- and audio-tape the person and make careful evaluation by using a stopwatch.

DURATION. The maximum duration of sustained exhalation reveals the respiratory mechanism's ability to regulate the exhalatory factors (rib recoil, muscle relaxation, lung tissue pressure, gravity) so as to provide a continuous flow of air without the intervening variable of vocal-fold interruption. This durational characteristic is obviously also related to vital capacity. Ptacek and Sanders (1963) obtained a low but positive correlation between this measure and maximum phonation time. These writers also determined that there is a much greater variability in exhalation time when phonation is employed than under unrestricted conditions, which indicates that the laryngeal interruption of the airstream has a significant influence upon the ability to control exhalation. Although Ptacek and Sanders provide data on this measure for various flow rates for young adults, no satisfactory normative information is available to aid the diagnostician. The measure is nonetheless useful in indicating the individual's ability to control flow rate while maintaining a steady airstream.

ASSOCIATED TENSION. Exhalation for speech purposes involves more than just the controlled relaxation of the inhalatory musculature. There is also a series of pulselike and sustained contractions of the thoracic and abdominal muscles. Although there is no clear experimental evidence to prove the point, we feel that there are some instances in which this process results in a musculature tension that has an overflow effect upon the laryngeal musculature. The resultant hypertension may result in faulty phonatory behavior. In examination we have found this is most evident upon sustained utterance; therefore, we have devised a series of run-on sentences which the individual utters without taking additional breaths. Several contaminating variables must be assessed, however, since once the person gets below his resting lung-volume level, additional musculature tension of both the respiratory and phonatory structures will be imperative in order to maintain sufficient subglottic pressure. What we are looking for is an inordinate amount of additional tension that can sometimes be "observed" by placing the fingers lightly on the individual's neck beside the thyroid cartilage.

ASSOCIATED SOUNDS. In the healthy structure the vegetative respiratory process is fairly silent. Unwanted noise upon inhalation or exhalation may be a critical sign of a wide variety of problems ranging from laryngeal polyps and enlarged adenoidal tissue to laryngeal webs, abductor paralysis, or various types of neoplasms. Inspiratory stridor should be medically investigated immediately.

Articulation/resonation. The juxtaposition of the terms articulation and resonation is common if confusing. We are far more familiar with the uses of the term articulation to refer not only to the alteration of the airstream through muscle contraction and structure movement but also the resultant effects of that movement upon sound production. The term resonation, however, has a vague and ill-defined quality to it. The texture of the cavities, the shape and relationship of those cavities, and the opening size all have some effect upon sound production, but the exact nature of these factors is not clear to most clinicians. Most unresolved of all is the question of the resonators' influence upon the so-called phonatory vocal characteristics. How much influence do the resonators have on vocal-fold action, and what effect do the resonating chambers have upon the perceived quality of the voice?[6]

---

[6] Hoops (1960) defines two types of "quality"—vocal and speech sound quality. How do these concepts relate to the present discussion?

Auditory skills. Routine testing for auditory acuity is suggested for all voice cases. We often go beyond simple acuity measures to evaluate the individual's ability to discriminate various speech characteristics. It is generally most appropriate to include discrimination of pitch, loudness, and quality differences, but be sure to evaluate the individual's ability to identify his own voice characteristics (see Project 8).

> Dan was ten years old when we first evaluated him. Referred by his classroom teacher as having a "monotonous" voice with a strange, harsh quality, we planned the following sequence of measures to measure his auditory discrimination abilities. (1) Following a hearing test we used the audiometer to see if Dan could determine the louder of two tones presented continuously. Pure tones were presented for three-second durations, followed by a two-second time lapse and a second tone 5 db louder or softer. Since this was a rather easy and possibly not too relevant task, we also used the live-voice circuit and gave Dan sentences with one word emphasized. His task was to select the word that sounded "louder" in each sentence. (This procedure ended up being a better therapy than diagnostic technique.) (2) In order to determine Dan's ability to discriminate among various pitch levels, we used a toy xylophone and had him replicate with the xylophone the various pitch patterns we presented to him. This was followed by some more vocal gymnastics on our part, with the examiner humming various inflectional patterns and Dan indicating the direction of the inflection by pointing either up or down. This same task later involved phrases and sentences and eventually, several directional changes within the same utterance. Finally, we concluded by having Dan determine the acceptability of a given utterance by ranking its adequacy on a seven-point scale. The examiner then attempted to imitate Dan's inflexible voice (without the quality distortion) and introduced sentences spoken with a moderate and maximum amount of vocal variety. (3) The examiner was put to the test when he tried to evaluate Dan's ability to discriminate various vocal qualities. A series of phrases was recorded on blank language master cards, and Dan was asked to categorize them into the following groups: normal, nasal, hoarse, and breathy. We used "hoarseness" in order to replicate Dan's own voice quality. Following this task, Dan was asked to tape-record a series of phrases which we then imitated, varying our degree of imitation from normal to close approximations of his voice. Upon playback Dan was asked to determine how close in quality the two voices were.

Motor skills. Some voice disorder types require an examination of general motor skills. The general procedures as described in Chapter 3 are sufficient, although it may be well to pursue this testing further to determine the client's general strength, stamina, and ability to sustain motor activity. The oral mechanism must be examined in certain cases of resonatory vocal disturbances. Oral-sensory discrimination skills as well as velopharyngeal functioning and basic reflexes should be investigated (see Chapter 5).

Evaluation of the vocal end product. It is generally advisable to evaluate each of the vocal characteristics—pitch, loudness, and quality—no matter which dimension is the primary contributor to the vocal disorder. The following discussion parcels the evaluation process into these three primary categories, although we generally try to evaluate as many aspects of vocal production at one time as possible.

LOUDNESS.   Disorders of loudness are sometimes in the ear of the beholder.

> Within a span of five weeks, Mrs. W., a diminutive, proper, and somewhat elderly seventh-grade language arts teacher referred six young girls to the speech clinician because, "They speak in such soft voices no one in the room can hear them." Our initial evaluation of the girls indicated that they were rather shy and reserved but apparently were able to speak up when necessary. Suspecting that this "epidemic" was peculiar to Mrs. W.'s classes, we sent out a notice inviting any teacher in the school who might wish to have his hearing tested to come to our office on any of the following Wednesday afternoons of the month. Sure enough, Mrs. W. was one of our first customers. Unfortunately amplification did little to aid her, but we did suggest preferential seating for those students with whom she had difficulty. The girls' "voice problems" soon disappeared.

Although some of the following measurement techniques are rather subjective, we have found them to be helpful when we analyze individuals with vocal disorders:

> Determine the normal conversational loudness level of the individual under a variety of speaking situations. First, open the conversation with your client seated a few feet away and gradually move back until you are ten to fifteen feet away. In order to determine his ability to adapt his voice to the speaking circumstance, you may wish to then provide a background noise such as a radio or tape-recorded conversation. Generally, we are listening to the loudness level at this point, but we also observe such factors as undue tension, pitch, quality change, and inability to alter with the circumstance.
>
> The ability to project the voice can be evaluated by bringing the client into a large lecture room or an auditorium. We try to make the procedure rather formal in order to put the speaker under a degree of tension.

> The ability to vary loudness with changes in meaning can be evaluated by using vocal variety drills such as those in the drillbooks of Fairbanks (1960) or Hanley and Thurman (1970). We generally ask the client to read "with feeling" sentences such as the following:
>
> Get out of here, get out of here!
> I don't know, I said I don't know!
> Wash your hands, Billy!
> I need more money Dad, I'm broke!
> Where did she go, I can't find her?
> Will you cut that out!

> The ability to produce isolated vowel sounds is examined under a variety of conditions. First, the examiner must generally determine if the client can produce front and back and high, mid, and low vowels at various loudness levels.

We listen for steadiness of tone, improved volume with changes in the resonant characteristics of the vowel, and ability to project without concomitant changes in other variables such as quality or pitch. We also determine the ability to produce a steady, unwavering tone at various loudness levels. The maximum duration of phonation of vowels is apparently related to a number of variables such as the vowel used, the frequency level, the sound-pressure level, and others (Michel and Wendahl, 1971). This variable involves both the respiratory capacity of the individual and his ability to coordinate respiration with the sound-generating mechanism of the larynx. Restricted ranges appear to be primarily related to laryngeal pathology, coordination of onset of phonation and exhalation, and vital capacity. Although there is an interesting discrepancy in the literature between the minimum length of time an individual should be able to phonate an isolated vowel, clinically we become concerned when the client cannot sustain the vowel beyond fifteen seconds.[7]

PITCH. Pitch is a perceptual phenomenon that correlates directly with the valving rate of the vocal folds. Obviously the pitch level of most voices varies continuously and flowingly, and for this reason it is sometimes difficult to measure it precisely. As the clinician attempts to formulate a diagnostic format to evaluate pitch characteristics, he must be concerned with several factors. First, there is probably a most efficient pitch level for each speaking voice. Second, each voice has a range of pitch variation. Third, there is a pitch level around which each speaker speaks during his contextual speech, and this level may or may not coincide with his most efficient pitch level. Fourth, several factors have a direct influence upon the pitch level of a given voice.

Optimal Pitch. The concept of optimal performance is attractive—indeed, it is enticing. The term implies maximum output with minimum effort, and we always expect an optimum performance from everything from our car to our golf swing. As voice clinicians we are concerned not only with the acoustic end product and its appropriateness, but with the vocal mechanism's operating efficiency as well. Performance at nonoptimal levels implies greater constriction and strain of the vocal mechanism with greater potential for abuse.

The term optimal pitch is somewhat of a contradiction in terms since optimal refers to the physical workings of the voice mechanism and pitch refers to the perceptual characteristics. Optimum frequency level would be a more accurate term. We will use the concept of optimal performance to mean optimal physical performance as measured through perceptual means.

The determination of optimal pitch is by no means precise. Several method have been described in the literature; and generally, when pitch level is of paramount concern, we use a combination of measures. The following is an abstract of the notes taken during an evaluation of a thirty-three-year-old male with vocal nodules.

---

[7] Compare the norms stated by Van Riper (1954), Fairbanks (1960), and Luchsinger and Arnold (1965).

A total pitch range was determined by first having Mr. N. clear his throat—phonation terminating in the /a/ vowel and then, using that tone as the starting point, phonating down the scale to the lowest tone possible. After he reached this point, he began back up the scale to the highest tone possible. He had some difficulty with this, but he produced an average of sixteen tones. Using the $\frac{1}{4}$ range suggested by Pronovost (1942) as a criterion for optimal pitch, it is interesting to note that Mr. N. could sing down four notes from that original starting point, indicating that the throat-clearing may have produced almost optimal pitch. Following Murphy's (1964) suggestions, we attempted to determine optimal pitch by having the client produce loud audible sighs. We found that we had to listen only to the onset of the sighs because the client tended to lower the pitch during the sound. We also had him cough and attempt to hold the tone of the cough at a constant pitch level. This appeared quite variable, but it seemed to agree with the other findings. We tape-recorded Mr. N.'s attempts to hum up and down the scale, but neither of us could hear a "more predominant" sound at any pitch level. The idea that the optimal pitch is more resonant and pronounced is theoretically valid, but we couldn't make it work. Similarly, we attempted to measure the increase in energy by placing our fingers on the client's face and nose while he hummed up and down the scale. Apparently we have an elephant's touch, since we were unable to detect any prominent area of resonation. All of this was complicated by the fact that Mr. N. couldn't carry a tune, but the overall conclusion from these several techniques was that Mr. N. should be speaking at a pitch level approximately four tones above his lowest tone.

Pitch range. The pitch range is determined in relation to the tests for optimal pitch level. Information about the client's pitch range tells us something about the health, flexibility, and control of his respiratory and laryngeal structures. Many clients will have great difficulty humming up and down the musical scale, and consequently they usually display pitch levels in conversational speech that are above or below the one displayed in testing. It may be helpful to have the person produce the highest and lowest tones possible; by using a pitch pipe or piano, the examiner can then calculate the total range (see Fairbanks, 1960: 122–26).

Habitual pitch. The pitch level around which a person's voice varies in contextual speech is termed his habitual pitch level. Obviously this level will vary from circumstance to circumstance, but our main concern is the chronic use of a pitch level too high or to low for the individual vocal mechanism. Once again this process is probably best done through instrumental analysis of the vocal signal; however, it is possible to train the ear to listen to the client's running speech and identify his fundamental pitch level. Probably the best method of doing this is to tape-record the client and concentrate on the pitch level while listening. Make every attempt to disregard content. Match the pitch level your ear hears on a pitch pipe. The client should be totally unaware of the fact that you are recording for the purposes of evaluating pitch level, because this may affect his performance.

Boone (1971) suggests taking a tape-recorded sample and stopping the recorder a number of times on the playback and determining the pitch level by matching it with a pitch pipe. The process then results in a modal pitch level, which is the level most frequently occurring in the sample, and this is usually interpreted as the habitual pitch.

Influencing Factors. Mass, effective valving length, and tension of the vocal folds are among the physical variables that influence pitch level; however, our concern at this point is with the variables that affect these three conditions and thus modify pitch.

The following evaluation techniques are used to determine the degree of pitch control, as well as the factors that influence the pitch level:

1. Ability to carry a tune
2. Ability to follow inflectional changes
3. Ability to produce a given pitch
4. Ability to match pitch change with meaning
5. Ability to maintain a steady pitch level for ten seconds
6. Ability to speak at three or more distinct pitch levels
7. Influence on pitch of changes in loudness
8. Influence on pitch of changes in vocal quality
9. Influence on pitch of physical exertion
10. Influence on pitch of distraction, encouragement, or hostility
11. Influence on pitch of posture changes
12. Influence on pitch of pressure on larynx, change in head position, or abdominal pressure
13. Influence on pitch of "aggressively" chewing gum while speaking
14. Influence on pitch of trial relaxation techniques
15. Influence on pitch of exaggerated articulation
16. Influence on pitch of verbal suggestion
17. Influence on pitch of alterations in vocal attack varying from breathy to gradual to abrupt.

QUALITY. The most difficult vocal characteristic to evaluate is quality. Involving both phonatory and resonatory characteristics, quality is that component of the voice which gives primary distinction to a given speaker's voice when pitch and loudness are excluded from judgment. Quality variations are essentially limitless but become of concern to the speech clinician when the variations take on an unpleasant and distracting character or are the precursors of physical abnormality. The variables of pitch and loudness can be scaled according to both physical and perceptual attributes, but the quality variable is still fairly dependent upon an array of subjective terms.[8]

The diagnostician must give the quality a label and describe it, deter-

---

[8] For a discussion of the various terms used to describe vocal qualities, the reader is directed to the writings of Moore (1971a: 5–11), Murphy (1964: 62–74), and Perkins (1971a: 279–88).

mine the impact of various variables, and identify associated characteristics of the individual's speech signal.

DESCRIPTION. Since quality disorders may be either phonatory or resonatory, one of the first tasks is to make this differential determination. Following this determination, it is useful to label the quality for purposes of communication as well as conceptualization. Since there is some agreement on the meaning of the terms hoarseness, harshness, breathiness, hypernasality, and denasality (see Moore, 1971), we feel fairly confident in using them.

The following is an example of our efforts to describe the vocal quality of a young client:

> Fred's voice is classified as hoarse in quality with associated components of glottal fry and breathiness. The glottal fry is transient and increases in severity at the end of phrases. Breath escape was evident throughout the phonatory period. Laryngeal tension, or constriction, was evidenced in excessive forcing and a general strained character to the voice. The quality disorder deserves a five on our seven-point severity scale.

Impact of Related Variables. During this portion of the evaluation the examiner determines what effects various behaviors have upon vocal quality. We generally use the same kinds of examinations as were described previously for pitch analysis.

The following conclusions were made following the examination of a young lady whose mild degree of hypernasality we had attributed to functional causes:

> Mrs. V.'s hypernasality was significantly reduced or eliminated under the following conditions: when she was asked to shout or speak with great force as if to a large gathering; when speaking while squeezing a rubber ball or attempting to lift the table; when overarticulating; and when attempting abrupt glottal attack. The common denominator appears to be increased muscle tone. Increased hypernasality was noted when Mrs. V. was speaking at a higher-than-normal pitch and when the examiner cross-examined her in a hostile manner to induce a feeling of threat. It is a positive sign that the client is able to voluntarily modify her voice quality under controlled conditions.

Associated Characteristics. Three additional characteristics are investigated. The nature of the glottal attack in contextual speech is determined. This is sometimes a rather difficult attribute to identify, so we generally also have the person produce a series of vowels and consonants. We also listen for the method of phonatory termination, since we have heard several speakers who terminate phonation with an abrupt grunting sound.

Second, we investigate the degree of laryngeal constriction, or tension, in phonation. Many vocal-quality disorders are directly related to laryngeal hyperfunction. We depend primarily upon four measures to determine the degree of vocal tension: observation, primarily for visible signs of strain;

auditory cues that indicate a greater-than-normal degree of laryngeal valving; placing the hand lightly on the neck while the individual is speaking; individual self-report on the degree and locus of tension within the speaking mechanism.

The third associated characteristic we investigate is the general communicative skill of the individual, which includes articulation, prosody characteristics, and language level.

> Mr. G. was a prospering insurance executive. He was fifty-four years old, married, and had three grown children. Our introduction to Mr. G. followed a referral note from a local laryngologist who stated: "You are going to enjoy working with this fellow. He has a unique and bizarre vocal quality which I can't describe. We have done a thorough laryngeal exam and find no pathology. Let me know what you think!" During the initial interview we obtained the following information. Mr. G. began to have some difficulty with his voice about eighteen years ago, and it had gradually become more severe over that time. No particular incident was associated with the onset, and Mr. G. stated that he felt he had no serious psychological problems. In fact, three years prior to our seeing him, his family physician had referred him for psychiatric counseling. "We met twice every week for six months, and he finally said I was sound as a dollar. He claimed there was something neurologically wrong with me. How about that? The medical doctors say I'm emotionally sick, and the psychiatrist says I'm physically sick—sounds like buck-passing to me." (The psychiatrist sent the following information upon our request: "Mr. G. appeared to me to be a highly controlled, relatively stable individual. He is a bit prone to depression and worry, but I found no evidence that his voice problem was related to any psychoneurotic condition.")
>
> Mr. G.'s voice was characterized by an irregular stoppage with a strained or strangled quality, relatively low monotonous pitch with some slight degree of harshness. He continuously cleared his throat in an abrupt manner, and his face contorted slightly during aphonic moments. The voice was like one subtype of spastic (or spasmodic) dysphonia. Once the voice quality was described and identified, it was our task to add any data we could in order to determine the etiology. We suspected both neurological and psychiatric factors. In analyzing the vocal quality, the following information was secured:
>
> 1. Mr. G. is able to prolong the /a/ vowel for six seconds, the /u/ for seven seconds, and the /i/ for five seconds.
> 2. The vowel sounds were intermittent in voicing, and showed some signs of tremor; and some air escaped during nonphonated periods, although the cessation of sound appeared to be related more to an increase in laryngeal pressure than to an abduction of the vocal folds.
> 3. Mr. G. was able to sustain nonphonated exhalation for seventeen seconds.
> 4. Examination for pitch range was incomplete because the client was unable to vary his pitch in the lower ranges. However, we discovered at that time that Mr. G. was able to phonate without any symptoms at the higher levels. He stated that he can sing in a high pitch quite well, and this was evident upon examination.
> 5. The disorder was noted to be quite variable; it improved noticeably when the client made casual comments ("oh, sure, I see, uh, uh") during the conversation.

6. When the examiner placed his fingers firmly on the side of the larynx and pushed with some force, the client was able to speak with hardly any symptoms. This same voice improvement was noted when the examiner placed his fingers lightly on the side of the larynx, or up to the neck but never touching the neck surface. This suggests that the improvement was due to suggestion rather than some anatomic change. This procedure was repeated on two different occasions with similar results.

7. Changes in the posture of the head did not affect the vocal quality.

8. Three methods of vocal attack were investigated: abrupt, gradual, and breathy. Mr. G. produced significantly improved voice with the gradual attack method but stated that he felt his voice was better with the abrupt attack method.

9. Alterations in pitch had a significant influence upon the voice. Higher pitch produced improved vocal quality. Upon later retests of this same phenomenon, it was found that there were still some symptoms in the higher pitch range but not as much as in the lower levels.

10. Vocal quality deteriorated during physical exertion, although the patient is an ardent jogger and stated that his voice is quite good when he is jogging and talking.

11. Exaggerated chewing and speaking produced some remission in symptom.

12. Mr. G. was asked to read a given passage four times and each time the vocal interruption occurred almost at the same place.

The following signs appeared to point to some sort of psychological etiology:

1. Variability from one pitch level to another
2. Symptoms disappeared during certain types of utterance
3. Consistency in place of interruption
4. The impact of suggestion as exemplified by the hand placed upon the neck
5. The general attitude of the client—he was cooperative to a fault and yet did not follow up on suggestions. He appeared somewhat blasé about his problem, even though it made communication nearly impossible. Several factors also indicated the need for neurological examination:

   a. The gradual onset of the problem
   b. The lack of identifiable problems in life adjustment
   c. The lack of any major symptom of psychological disturbance

Mr. G. refused to see a neurologist as suggested, and one year of speech therapy netted minimal improvement.[9]

---

[9] Spastic dysphonia is one of the most perplexing and fascinating vocal disturbances. Compare the findings of the following authors:

Aronson, A., J. Brown, E. Litin, and J. Pearson. "Spastic Dysphonia. I. Voice, Neurologic, and Psychiatric Aspects." *Journal of Speech and Hearing Disorders*, 33 (1968): 203–18.

——. "Spastic Dysphonia. II. Comparison with Essential (Voice) Tremor and Other Neurologic and Psychogenic Dysphonias." *Journal of Speech and Hearing Disorders*, 33 (1968): 219–31.

Robe, E., J. Brunlik, and P. Moore. "A Study of Spastic Dysphonia: Neurologic and Electroencephalographic Abnormalities." *Laryngoscope*, 70 (1960): 219–45.

Heaver, L. "Spastic Dysphonia: A Psychosomatic Voice Disorder." In *Psychological and Psychiatric Aspects of Speech and Hearing*, ed. D. Barbara. Springfield, Ill.: Charles C Thomas, 1960.

prognosis

There are several aspects to prognosis. First, there is the question of spontaneous remission of the presenting symptoms. Will this individual display an improvement in vocal quality without intervening voice therapy? Second, how much improvement can be expected following the prescribed clinical program? To what degree is the voice therapy as projected going to be effective? Third, how permanent are the gains shown in therapy going to be? Is the vocal quality of such a nature that continuous therapy will be necessary to maintain the optimal vocal performance? Finally, would some other clinical procedure be of greater benefit to the client?

We shall discuss a variety of factors that we have found to have prognostic value in voice cases. Some of the variables are directly observable and subject to quantification, while others are much more subjective. The factors appear to fall into three broad categories: characteristics of the disorder, of the person, and of the environment. They include:

1. Duration of the problem. Generally disorders of long standing have greater resistance to clinical treatment.
2. Etiological factors. Two factors are relevant here: first, is the cause of the problem identifiable? Second, is the cause of the problem alterable? And if so, is the type of habilitating service required available?
3. Degree of secondary psychological components. Generally, the greater the degree of physiological disturbance the poorer the prognosis.
4. Variability and general flexibility of the voice. Are there periods when the symptom seems to improve? Can the individual vary the pitch, loudness, and quality of his voice?
5. Ability of the individual to imitate various vocal characteristics.
6. Auditory skills. Ability of the client to hear his vocal disturbance and to discriminate it from other voices.
7. Impact, or degree, of the disability. The greater the impact of the voice difference upon the individual, the better the chances for cooperation. We have found this to be a real problem in children with vocal nodules, and have found that the "Weight Watchers" concepts of group pressure and encouragement are very helpful.
8. Cooperation of the family and environment.
9. Extrinsic motivational factors. Are there some factors in environment that reinforce this pattern and encourage its continuance?

DIAGNOSIS OF THE LARYNGECTOMEE

Working with the laryngectomized patient is a most rewarding professional experience. Laryngectomees develop a loyalty to one another and to their speech clinician that is unmatched by any other group of speech-handicapped individuals. There are approximately 35,000 to 40,000 laryngectomees in the United States as of 1973, with an additional three to four thousand new patients each year. Although many laryngectomees never find their way to a speech clinician, those who do provide a challenge which we have found to be worth the effort in every respect.

The exact nature of the diagnostic evaluation will vary depending upon when the client is seen. The preoperative evaluation will be markedly different from that of an individual who has been struggling to learn esophageal speech for some time. There are, however, three primary goals of the diagnostic process with the laryngectomee: to provide information, support, and release; to determine the speech potential; and to provide therapy direction.

providing information, support, and release

A preoperative visit by a speech clinician, skilled esophageal speaker, or both has potential for great value or harm. Even the most skilled clinician may find that he has done his client a disservice if the client simply is not emotionally or physically capable of dealing with the issues of this first meeting. Probably the physician is best qualified to make such judgments, and most speech clinicians depend upon the referral of the physician before working with the laryngectomee. The clinician must remember that he is dealing with an individual who is facing a trauma unparalled in his lifetime. Fears of death, loss of communication, loss of job and earning power, and social and marital adjustments plague him. The first confrontation is no social chat and may well demand all of the professional proficiency the clinician can muster. We have found on more than one occasion that the patient was not capable of dealing rationally with the topic immediately before surgery, and we terminated the discussion with assurance that we would be seeing them soon following their recovery.

One of the major goals of our first meeting with a laryngectomee is to provide some information about his operation and the implications for speech. Every attempt should be made to present a clear discussion of the anatomical changes. Charts and diagrams often are helpful. We generally use a demonstration tape of excellent esophageal speech or, if possible, have an exemplary esophageal speaker accompany us on this first visit. We stress that excellent esophageal speech is the major goal, but it is not the only one. Several options are discussed such as the electrolarynx, the Asai technique (with the physician's approval), and written communication.[10] Although there is still some controversy over the use of the electrolarynx, it is clearly the "treatment of choice" in some cases. We have found, however, that it is

---

[10] The Asai technique (see Miller, 1969) involves a series of three surgical techniques in which the patient's pharynx and trachea are connected by the neoglottis. Respiratory air provides the force for phonation, although the stoma must be blocked with finger pressure.

not always a particularly successful technique immediately after the operation, since the sublingual and cervical tissues tend to be extremely firm, which makes it difficult to get the generated tone into the resonating cavities.

Although further information is sometimes provided in this first discussion, generally, it is best to deal with related problems after surgery, or as they arise. Many times even the discussion of the anticipated communication problem has little impact until after the patient has experienced muteness. Nearly every laryngectomee can recall the first time when he opened his mouth to say something only to be reminded of his plight.

Providing adequate information to the family can have far-reaching clinical implications. The spouse must understand the anatomy of the operation as well as the patient himself. The wife of one of our laryngectomees told of walking into her husband's room just in time to find a well-meaning friend attempting to feed the patient through his stoma.

Very often clinicians stress what the laryngectomee will be unable to do; and although this information is important, we feel that it is also important to stress to the family what the patient will be *able* to do. We generally attempt to have a frank discussion with the spouse about the typical reactions of the family. If a pattern can be identified before it develops, it may be easier to control. The tendency to dominate the silent mate (or parent) must be controlled, as must the inclinations to infantilize, overindulge, and pity. Very often we have to warn the family not to shout at the patient. Almost as if by instinct many people find themselves shouting at the laryngectomee as if he were deaf rather than voiceless. One of our laryngectomee friends had a sign posted at the foot of his hospital bed stating, "My hearing is fine—it's my voice that I've lost!" Many families readily admit to a feeling of repulsion because of the physical changes. Interestingly, this is easily conveyed to the laryngectomee, since many are extremely sensitive about their operation. The silent mate is often excluded from conversation and decision-making in many families. Some laryngectomees have reported feeling that there was a conspiratorial mood in their house after the operation. The clinician must be sensitive to the fact that the spouse will have fears of his own. The fear of death, reduced income, new responsibilities, social changes, and changes in all facets of marital relationships may be topics for discussion. The student is encouraged to reread Chapter 2 in preparation for that first conference.

One of the primary purposes of the clinician's first visit with the laryngectomee and his family is to let them know that he understands their feelings. The laryngectomized speech instructors we have worked with feel that they are more effective than speech clinicians in this area. "You can tell me how much you understand my feelings all you want, but unless I see that stoma shield on your neck I know darn well you don't really understand," stated one of our most astute friends. It is expected that the clinician will be warm, sincere, and insightful, but we resist the temptation to dictate any specific attitude beyond this because each patient will require a somewhat different approach.

Some need to be dealt with gently, others straightforwardly and frankly. (We have several laryngectomee clients who learned to whistle soon after we told them that whistling was one of the things they could never do again.) Find the level and type of interaction your client responds to best and use it.[11]

determining the potential for speech

A thorough case history is helpful with the laryngectomee, but two facets are particularly crucial. It is important to know the extent of the surgery, the degree of involvement of related structures such as the tongue or pharynx, general health of the client, and the medical prognosis. The second crucial area is the individual's vocation and interests. We find it most helpful to plan our clinical work around the client's interests and activities. One of our laryngectomees learned to produce esophageal sound while practicing his golf swing in our office, while another first produced the sound while slamming his cards on the table and exclaiming "gin."

It may also be necessary to examine the client's oral anatomy. Generally we evaluate the tongue, lip, and jaw mobility as well as the oral discrimination skills. Some information about the previous articulation, speech, and language pattern of the client is helpful, but this is not always available.

If the client has already begun to learn esophageal speech, some measure of his current performance level will be helpful. Wepman and his colleagues (1953) provide an objective measurement device. Berlin (1963: 42) presents the following guidelines:

1. Ability to phonate reliably on demand
2. Maintenance of a short latency between inflation of the esophagus and vocalization
3. Maintenance of an adequate duration of phonation
4. Ability to sustain phonation during articulation

Careful analysis should be made of the client's method of air intake and associated mannerisms. It is generally easier to prevent poor speaking habits than to correct them.

An assessment of the hearing acuity and auditory discrimination skills may prove helpful. Since a high percentage of laryngectomees are males above the age of fifty-five, it is common to find a degree of hearing loss. A moderate-to-severe hearing loss may make the learning process more difficult but not impossible.

No formal intelligence test is suggested for the laryngectomee client, but

[11] The following booklets may be helpful in your early work with the laryngectomee:
Lauder, E. *Self-Help for the Laryngectomee*. 1115 Whisper Hollow, San Antonio, Texas 78230. ($3.50)
Waldrop, W. and M. Gould. *Your New Voice*. Available free from a local American Cancer Society office.

we do find it useful to assess the client's general understanding of our instructions. Generally, it is helpful to ask the client to rephrase your instructions to him, giving you some idea of his ability to understand and your ability to communicate. Similarly, the emotional state of your client should be appraised, although this is no time to administer formal tests, label, or judge. It would be difficult to know exactly what "normal" should be for such a client. Your task is to take note of the general tendencies and use this information for your work.

It is sometimes helpful to know something about the pre- and postsurgical habits of the client. Cigarette smoking and alcohol present two typical problems for these individuals. Although the sudden inability to smoke may contribute to further psychological upheaval, we have found that many previously heavy smokers claim almost no desire for cigarettes after the operation. This is a curious phenomenon and may be tied to the fact that inhalation smoking is obviously no longer possible, and the psyche has accepted this state of affairs with little struggle.

trial therapy and therapy direction

Once we have determined the performance level of the client, we must identify the most efficient method of air intake and sound production. We almost always begin by proving to the client that he can still make several speech sounds. At this same time we emphasize methods for building up oral pressure for the voiceless consonants. This process serves to motivate the client by showing him that he can still make sounds while also stressing articulatory precision, oral pressure, and separation of breathing and speech. The plosive injection method of air intake has proven most successful for us and is used almost exclusively in our first session. We accept any port in a storm, however, and generally begin by having the client produce esophageal sound by any method he can. If this initial attempt is not successful, every available method of air intake and sound production is tried. It is relatively important that the client make some esophageal sound during that first session! Very often we even accept a "volunteer" (burp) as proof that something must be working to get air into the esophagus.

Little has been said in this discussion about the need to motivate the laryngectomee. Success in sound production is the best inspiration, and we have abandoned an earlier practice of pep talks, lectures, and cheer-leading in favor of direction, success, and reinforcement. A few intelligible words spoken by the client do more than our most eloquent speeches.

CLEFT PALATE

There is no such thing as cleft-palate speech. Granted, typical speech and language patterns can be identified within the cleft-palate population, but the clinician must be encouraged to assess the total communication ability of the child rather than analyzing a few identifying aspects. *Cleft palate is an etiological category, not a symptomatic denotation.* It is with some reservation, then, that we discuss "cleft palate" diagnosis, since we are actually diagnosing the child's oral communication skills, not his physical state. We cannot, however, simply select portions of the total diagnostic process and apply them to the cleft-palate child, since there are specific considerations unique to these children.

In cleft-palate diagnosis the speech clinician is a member of a team. The "cleft-palate team" (see Wells, 1971: 143–75) is a well-accepted clinical entity, and in many communities represents the ultimate in interdisciplinary cooperation. The speech clinician is expected to inform the team members about the child's speech and language adequacy, assess other rehabilitation efforts upon the child's speech, and predict the effects of contemplated rehabilitative procedures. In addition he is also to serve as a primary agent for change in the child's speech development. The dramatic growth in the development of surgical and other rehabilitative procedures for the cleft-palate child during the two decades from 1950 to 1970 (see Morley, 1967) has been encouraging. What is needed now, however, is not only new knowledge, but also a general dissemination of present knowledge to those responsible for the rehabilitation of the cleft-palate child. The cleft-palate teams throughout the world serve this second function nobly.

diagnosis

The routine case-history data may need to be augmented for the cleft-palate child. Knowledge of the type of cleft the child was born with (see Harkins and others, 1962) as well as a description of the surgical, prosthodontic, orthodontic, and other rehabilitative procedures performed would be helpful. Some statement of the child's current medical status and plans for his future will also help direct the evaluative process.

Critical listening. Although the initial interaction between clinician and child should be free and relatively unstructured, the clinician has a most demanding task. Once the child is interacting and conversing in a spontaneous manner, the clinician must apply his critical listening abilities to assess the child's total communicative effectiveness. The first task involves systematically shifting perceptual sets from one aspect of the child's speech to another. First, the clinician should listen for the degree of nasality and the type. Although trained judges are able to identify nasality fairly adequately, the clinician may wish to tape-record the child and play the tape backwards (see Sherman, 1954; Spriestersbach, 1955) to isolate the nasality from the articulation. After noting the degree of nasality or denasality, preferably on some scaling device, the clinician should listen to the general articulatory pattern without recording actual errors. What influence does the articulation pattern have on the total judgment of the child's speech? Is there an obvious preponderance of a particular type of error (glottal stops, pharyngeal fricatives)? Does the articulation appear to alter with differing communication situations, rates, stress patterns? Next, he should listen to the language of the child, and check for appropriate word choice, sentence complexity and structure, and other grammatical aspects. The rate and rhythm of the child's speech should be evaluated. Lass and Noll (1970) found that cleft-palate speakers used a slower rate of speech. How does one judge the child's speaking rate? What other vocal quality characteristics are evident? Finally, what particular mannerisms attract your attention? Is there a facial grimace, constriction of the nares, or any other behavior which detracts from the child's total effectiveness? At this same time we generally note several particularly appealing characteristics of the individual. It is important not to fabricate, but to select the positive attributes. Later in the therapy process we will want to accentuate the positive, and now is the time to get started.

Articulation testing. Standard articulation-testing procedures may be satisfactory for cleft-palate children, but there are several special considerations.

First, the examiner must ask himself a critical question. Why would a child with a cleft palate have articulation problems? Certainly all of the functional, perceptual, and sensory factors which affect the normal child could be active, but what other factors unique to these children may be investigated? Most important are the degree of velopharyngeal closure and the resultant airflow and intraoral pressure.[12] The deviant geography of the oral cavity may also contribute to this problem, which is also complicated by the fact that the oral structure may well have undergone several architectual changes within the first few years of life. The diagnostician must keep in mind that this child has been trying to produce "standard" sounds with a nonstandard structure, and under these conditions he may have made unique compensatory adjustments. He may have increased the airflow in order to build up adequate oral pressure, or minimized it to lessen nasal escape. It is entirely possible that the habits developed before the final surgical adjustments may persist, even though he can now make the correct articulatory movements.

During articulation testing with cleft-palate children the following deserve particular attention:

1. Certain sounds have a higher probability for error than others. Be sure to listen carefully for the affricates, fricatives, and plosives. Modify the test to get a thorough sample of them.

---

[12] Subtelny and others (1970) noted a significant decrease (50 percent) in articulation errors following pharyngeal flap surgery. What indicators would you use to determine the need for such an operation? Look into the following: (1) type of articulation errors, (2) degree of nasality and nasal escape of air associated with velopharyngeal closure, and (3) intraoral breath pressure. Do you agree with the premise put forward by Alley (1965)?

2. Since articulation involves dynamic and overlapping movements, be sure to test for articulation errors with isolated sounds, sound groupings, words, and context testing. Make a careful analysis of blend production. Why would the dynamic nature of articulation be a more important consideration in cleft-palate children?

3. Certain types of errors, not often found with other children, are common among the cleft-palate population. Listen for glottal stops as substitutions for plosives and pharyngeal fricatives and distortions involving nasal escape of air.

4. Group the sounds in error according to manner of production. This may give you a clue to the nature of the problem.

5. Listen for alterations in articulation accuracy with variations in rate and force of speaking.

6. Listen for weak consonants with a light articulatory contact and inadequate plosive pressure.

7. Stimulability testing may be most efficient if it includes stimulability for the acoustic characteristics and the articulatory placement of the stimulus sound. Jacobs and others (1970) developed the Miami Imitative Ability Test to test stimulability.

8. It is imperative to analyze the dynamics of the articulation errors in cleft-palate children. What specific anatomical adjustments is this child making in order to produce this sound? Make a careful kinetic analysis. It should come as no surprise that these children are selecting improper places and manners of production for very good reasons; normal methods simply result in too much nasality and nasal escape. It is important to listen to the sound production in its various phases. What happens as the pressure builds up in the implosion stage of plosive production? Is there nasal escape or facial contortion?

Nasal resonance. Resonatory voice disorders are generally described as variations of two types: hyper- and hyponasality. Hypernasality is generally the results of inadequate velopharyngeal closure, which in turn may be related to functional factors such as tension and fatigue or organic factors such as bulbar polio or cleft palate. Listener evaluation of the nasality of a speaking voice is apparently related to such factors as articulation adequacy as well as the actual resonant characteristics (Lintz and Sherman, 1961). Although there is some controversy, trained judges can reliably measure nasality by playing tape-recorded stimuli backwards (Spriestersbach, 1955).

Many clinicians at one time felt that tongue carriage, oral opening, and articulatory precision were the primary factors in nasal quality and saw velopharyngeal closure as only a subordinate factor. (No doubt, some clinicians felt that they had more direct control over such factors as articulation and tongue carriage.) Now, however, it is evident that velopharyngeal closure is absolutely necessary to produce speech that is not hypernasal, although the exact nature of the relationship has not been determined.

Once the examiner has identified nasality in the voice, he must first determine the variations of nasality within the vowels. A careful study of vowel production may indicate a general pattern—i.e, low vowels are more nasal than high (Lintz and Sherman, 1961). Exaggerated articulation, force, light contact speech, strongly stimulated speech, and rate and tension variations—all will influence nasality.

Velopharyngeal closure. Velopharyngeal closure not only determines the ultimate degree of nasality in the speaking voice, but also articulatory accuracy. The child must be able to *dynamically* close and open the velopharyngeal port to produce intelligible speech, and the assessment of this ability has been a source of concern and consternation for speech clinicians for some time. Objective measurements through X-ray procedures are not always possible, and the clinician must find some way to evaluate this crucial function. The oral manometer measures intraoral breath pressure, which is related to the ability of the velar port to close; however, this action is rather static and may not be related to actual speech production. Morris (1966) indicates the need to supplement manometric results with other diagnostic information. A similar complaint could be made of measures using blowing, as McWilliams and Bradley (1965) point out; speech may require a type of velopharyngeal action other than blowing.

Examination of the oral mechanism may be helpful but is very susceptible to error. We attempt to observe the movement of the pharyngeal walls and velum during production of the /a/ vowels as well as the length, width, and mobility of the palate and the general size of the oropharynx.

Fox and Johns (1970) describe a technique for measuring static closure whereby the child is required to maintain intraoral pressure by puffing up his cheeks. If this is accomplished, then he is asked to stick his tongue out and then puff up his cheeks. The examiner holds the child's nostrils while this is done to aid in impounding pressure. If no air escapes when the nostrils are released, it is assumed that velopharyngeal closure is adequate. (Why would it be necessary to have the child stick his tongue out while puffing up his cheeks?)

Morris, Spriestersbach, and Darley (1961) developed the Iowa Pressure Articulation Test to measure velopharyngeal closure. The test includes primarily fricative, plosive, and affricate productions and compares favorably with more objective tests such as X-ray and oral pressure techniques. Evaluating the efficiency of velopharyngeal closure through articulation testing also appears to be a clinically valuable tool. In fact, Shelton and others (1965: 42) concluded that "articulation testing appears to provide a better test of palatopharyngeal adequacy for speech than do simple measures of nasal air escape or oral breath pressure."

Some cleft-palate children may be able to achieve adequate velopharyngeal closure during single-word productions but find the exact and rapid velar adjustments required for contextual speech impossible. Therefore, the comparison of articulation proficiency between single words and connected speech may provide an estimate of velopharyngeal competence. Van Demark (1964) devised a stimulated sentence articulation test which contains at least twenty examples of fricatives, stop-plosives, glides, nasal semivowels, and blends. The test is presented below with the test consonants italicized. Errors of the stop-plosives and fricatives as well as a predominance of distortion due to excessive nasal emission may indicate inadequate velopharyngeal closure.

1. *Most boys like to play football.*
2. *Do you have a brother or sister?*
3. *Ted had a dog with white feet.*
4. *We shouldn't play in the street.*
5. *Playing in the snow is fun.*
6. *Nick's grandmother lives in the city.*
7. *We go swimming on a very hot day.*
8. *I like ice cream.*
9. *Tom has ham and eggs for breakfast.*
10. *We went to town yesterday.*
11. *Can you count to nine?*
12. *Do you want to take my new cap?*
13. *Do you know the name of my doll?*

Oral mechanism. Obviously, examination of the oral mechanism is especially important in the cleft-palate child. The alveolar ridge is the contact point for 70 to 80 percent of the consonant sounds of contextual speech. Special note should be made of the contour and evenness of the ridge and the dental structure and occlusion. Berry (1949) postulated a higher incidence of lingual anomalies among the cleft-palate population; however, this thesis has been questioned by several authorities. Van Demark and Van Demark (1967) found that judges could not differentiate the articulation patterns of cleft-palate children from children with functional articulation disorders. This finding, among others, appears to substantiate the contention that lingual function in the cleft-palate population is similar to that of the normal population. However, the clinician must still examine the functioning of the oral structures. Marks (1968) indicated that cleft-palate children have a higher incidence of tongue-thrusting than the normal population; and Hochberg and Kabcenell (1967) found inferior oral stereognosis abilities among cleft-palate individuals. These factors should be evaluated with care during the oral examination.

Auditory acuity. The high incidence of auditory acuity problems among cleft-palate children has been well documented (Loeb, 1964; Sataloff and Fraser, 1952). For this reason it is absolutely essential that every cleft-palate child have a hearing examination at least once each year. These examinations should include both air- and bone-conduction testing and should be a part of every speech diagnosis.

Psychological and social adjustment. Although it has been frequently hypothesized that cleft-palate children have more adjustment problems than normal children, this thesis has not been substantiated by research (Phipps, 1965). The difference of opinion between clinicians and researchers may reflect the former's lack of confidence in the child to overcome gross physical differences or the latter's lack of research sophistication. There is no final answer to this, and each diagnostic session with a cleft-palate individual should include an evaluation of his adjusting characteristics. We have found it equally profitable to investigate the parental and family adjustment, since environmental reaction is often directly linked with the child's self-concepts.

Language assessment. Several researchers have documented the existence of a language deficit among cleft-palate children (Nation, 1970; Smith and McWilliams, 1968; Morris, 1962). The clinician should examine the child's traditional language abilities and pay particular attention to his expressive skills.

The diagnostic evaluation of a cleft-palate child should be comprehensive, and cover more than just certain aspects of speech. The speech clinician, as a member of the diagnostic team, must evaluate a large number of behaviors, but his responsibility does not end there. Following a careful evaluation, he must be able to accurately and concisely communicate his findings both orally and in writing. (In chapter 9 we will discuss the report-writing process.)

PROJECTS AND QUESTIONS

1. Devise a voice analysis checklist that employs each of the vowels of the "vowel diagram" as syllable-releasers, syllable-arresters, and in isolation.
2. Vowels are sometimes classified as front-central-back, high-med-low, tense-lax, and open-closed. How might you incorporate these categorizations into your voice analysis?
3. What do Michel and Wendahl (1971) mean by the terms jitter and shimmer?
4. What relevance to voice diagnosis would the following historical data have?
   a. Polio at age five
   b. Exceedingly slow metabolic rate
   c. History of drug abuse
   d. Problems of dry skin and hair
   e. Pain when swallowing
5. How does Moore (1971a) use the term compliance in vocal-fold movement? How might vocal-fold compliance be altered in the healthy mechanism, and how would those changes affect the voice?
6. When the laryngologist finds the site of the phonatory problem, he may have to identify any of the following factors: nodules, polyps, papillomas, edema, inflamation, laryngeal web, congenitally small larynx, contact ulcer, paralysis, ankylosis. Define each of these terms.
7. Michel and Wendahl (1971) suggest that sustained exhalation can be measured by having the individual blow through a straw, placing the tip of the

straw just below the surface of a glass of water. The purpose of the test is to determine duration of exhalation, but does it involve other variables? What are the advantages and disadvantages of this technique?

8. Why do most speech clinicians routinely administer a hearing test to individuals with voice disorders? Categorize your responses under the headings: general precautions, therapeutic implications, and coincident variables.

9. Determine your own "natural pitch level" using the technique described by Fairbanks (1960: 122–26).

10. F. Wilson and his associates have devised a scaling profile device for voice disorders which discards the traditional subjective labels of vocal quality. This method uses numbered scales to judge pitch, laryngeal valving, and resonation (nasality). A training tape recording, "Voice Disorders in Children," is available for $6.00 upon request to the Division of Speech Pathology, Department of Otolaryngology, The Jewish Hospital of St. Louis, 216 South Kingshighway, St. Louis, Missouri 63110. The reader is encouraged to obtain this demonstration tape and study the rating scale.

11. Perkins (1971a) uses the terms pitch, loudness, voicing, constriction, mode, and focus in his discussion of voice disorders. What does he mean by these terms?

12. The abilities to produce esophageal voice and to use the electrolarynx are important to clinical success with the laryngectomee. Be sure you have developed both skills before your first meeting with a laryngectomized client.

BIBLIOGRAPHY

ALLEY, N. (1965). "The Use of Speech Aid Prosthesis as a Diagnostic Tool." *Cleft Palate Journal*, 2: 291–92.

ARONSON, A., J. BROWN, E. LITIN, and J. PEARSON (1968). "Spastic Dysphonia: I. Voice, Neurologic, and Psychiatric Aspects." *Journal of Speech and Hearing Disorders*, 33: 203–218.

———— (1968). "Spastic Dysphonia: II. Comparison with Essential (Voice) Tremor and Other Neurologic and Psychogenic Dysphonias." *Journal of Speech and Hearing Disorders*, 33: 219–31.

BERLIN, C. (1963). "Clinical Management of Esophageal Speech: I. Methodology and Curves of Skill Acquisition." *Journal of Speech and Hearing Disorders*, 28: 42–51.

BERRY, M. (1949). "Lingual Anomalies Associated with Palatal Clefts." *Journal of Speech and Hearing Disorders*, 14: 359–62.

———— and J. EISENSON (1956). *Speech Disorders*. New York: Appleton-Century-Crofts.

BOONE, D. (1971). *The Voice and Voice Therapy*. Englewood Cliffs, N.J.: Prentice-Hall, Inc.

BRACKETT, I. (1971). "Parameters of Voice Quality." In *Handbook of Speech Pathology and Audiology,* ed. L. Travis. New York: Appleton-Century-Crofts. Pp. 441–63.

BRADFORD, L., A BROOKS, and R. SHELTON (1964). "Clinical Judgment of Hypernasality in Cleft-Palate Children." *Cleft Palate Journal,* 1: 329–35.

CHASE, R. (1960). "An Objective Evaluation of Palatopharyngeal Competence." *Plastic and Reconstructive Surgery,* 26: 23–39.

COTES, J. (1965). *Lung Function.* Philadelphia: F. A. Davis Company.

CURRY, E. (1949). "Hoarseness and Voice Change in Male Adolescents." *Journal of Speech and Hearing Disorders,* 14: 23–24.

CURTIS, J. (1968). "Acoustics of Speech Production and Nasalization." In *Cleft Palate and Communication,* eds. D. Spriestersbach and D. Sherman. New York: Academic Press. Pp. 27–60.

DARLEY, F. (1964). *Diagnosis and Appraisal of Communication Disorders.* Englewood Cliffs, N.J.: Prentice-Hall, Inc.

DIEDRICH, W. and K. YOUNGSTROM (1966). *Alaryngeal Speech.* Springfield, Ill.: Charles C Thomas.

DIEHL, C. and C. STINNETT (1959). "Efficiency of Teacher Referrals in a School Speech Testing Program." *Journal of Speech and Hearing Disorders,* 24: 34–36.

FAIRBANKS, G. (1960). *Voice and Articulation Drillbook,* 2nd ed. New York: Harper & Row, Publishers.

Fox, D. and D. JOHNS (1970). "Predicting Velopharyngeal Closure with a Modified Tongue-Anchor Technique." *Journal of Speech and Hearing Disorders,* 35: 248–51.

GRAY, G. and C. WISE (1959). *The Bases of Speech,* 3rd ed. New York: Harper & Row, Publishers.

GREEN, M. (1964). *The Voice and Its Disorders.* Philadelphia: J. B. Lippincott Co.

HANLEY, T. and R. PETERS (1971). "The Speech and Hearing Laboratory." In *Handbook of Speech Pathology and Audiology,* ed. L. Travis, New York: Appleton-Century-Crofts. Pp. 75–140.

HANLEY, T. and W. THURMAN (1970). *Developing Vocal Skills,* 2nd ed. New York: Holt, Rinehart & Winston, Inc.

HARDY, J. (1961). "Intraoral Breath Pressure in Cerebral Palsy." *Journal of Speech and Hearing Disorders,* 26: 309–19.

HARKINS, C., B. ASA, R. HARDING, J. LONGACRE, and R. SNODGRASS (1962). "A Classification of Cleft Lip and Cleft Palate." *Plastic and Reconstructive Surgery,* 29: 31–39.

HEAVER, L. (1960). "Spastic Dysphonia: A Psychosomatic Voice Disorder." In

Psychological and Psychiatric Aspects of Speech and Hearing, ed. D. Barbara. Springfield, Ill.: Charles C Thomas. Pp. 250–63.

HOCHBERG, I. and J. KABCENELL (1967). "Oral Stereognosis in Normal and Cleft Palate Individuals." *Cleft Palate Journal*, 4: 47–57.

HOOPS, R. (1960). *Speech Science*. Springfield, Ill.: Charles C Thomas.

JACKSON, C. (1941). "Vocal Nodules." *American Laryngological Association*, 63: 185.

JACOBS, R., B. PHILIPS, and R. HARRISON (1970). "A Stimulability Test for Cleft-Palate Children." *Journal of Speech and Hearing Disorders*, 35: 354–60.

JOHNSON, W., F. DARLEY, and D. SPRIESTERSBACH (1963). *Diagnostic Methods in Speech Pathology*. New York: Harper & Row, Publishers.

KAPLAN, H. (1971). *Anatomy and Physiology of Speech*, 2nd ed. New York: McGraw-Hill Book Company.

LASS, N. and J. NOLL (1970). "A Comparative Study of Rate Characteristics in Cleft-Palate and Noncleft-Palate Speakers." *Cleft Palate Journal*, 7: 275–83.

LAUDER, E. (1971). *Self-Help for the Laryngectomee*. San Antonio, Tex.: Edmund Lauder.

LINTZ, L. and D. SHERMAN (1961). "Phonetic Elements and Perception of Nasality." *Journal of Speech and Hearing Research*, 4: 381–96.

LOEB, W. (1964). "Speech, Hearing, and the Cleft Palate." *Archives of Otolaryngology*, 79: 4–14.

LUCHSINGER, R. and G. ARNOLD (1965). *Voice-Speech-Language*. Belmont, Calif.: Wadsworth Publishing Company, Inc.

MARKS, C. (1968). "Tongue-Thrusting and Interdentalization of Speech Sounds Among Cleft-Palate and Noncleft-Palate Subjects." *Cleft Palate Journal*, 5: 48–56.

MCDONALD, E. and B. CHANCE, JR. (1964). *Cerebral Palsy*. Englewood Cliffs, N.J.: Prentice-Hall, Inc.

MCWILLIAMS, B. and D. BRADLEY (1965). "Ratings of Velopharyngeal Closure During Blowing and Speech." *Cleft Palate Journal*, 2: 46–55.

MCWILLIAMS, B., R. MUSGRAVE, and P. CROZIER (1968). "The Influence of Head Position Upon Velopharyngeal Closure." *Cleft Palate Journal*, 5: 117–24.

MICHEL, J. and R. WENDAHL (1971). "Correlates of Voice Production." In *Handbook of Speech Pathology and Audiology*, ed. L. Travis. New York: Appleton-Century-Crofts. Pp. 465–79.

MILLER, A. (1969). "First Experiences with the Asai Technique for Vocal Rehabilitation After Total Laryngectomy." In *Speech Rehabilitation of the Laryngectomized*, ed. J. Snidecor. Springfield, Ill.: Charles C Thomas. Pp. 50–57.

MOORE, G. (1971a). *Organic Voice Disorders*. Englewood Cliffs, N.J.: Prentice-Hall, Inc.

—— (1971b). "Voice Disorders Organically Based." In *Handbook of Speech Pathology and Audiology*, ed. L. Travis. New York: Appleton-Century-Crofts. Pp. 535–69.

MORLEY, M. (1967). *Cleft Palate and Speech*, 6th ed. Baltimore: Williams and Wilkins.

MORRIS, H. (1962). "Communication Skills of Children with Cleft Lips and Palates." *Journal of Speech and Hearing Research*, 5: 79–90.

—— (1966). "The Oral Manometer as a Diagnostic Tool in Clinical Speech Pathology." *Journal of Speech and Hearing Disorders*, 31: 362–69.

——, D. SPRIESTERSBACH, and F. DARLEY (1961). "An Articulation Test for Assessing Competency of Velopharyngeal Closure." *Journal of Speech and Hearing Research*, 4: 48–55.

MOSES, P. (1954). *The Voice of Neurosis*. New York: Grune & Stratton.

MURPHY, A. (1964). *Functional Voice Disorders*. Englewood Cliffs, N.J.: Prentice-Hall, Inc.

MYSAK, E. (1966). "Phonatory and Resonatory Problems." In *Speech Pathology: An International Study of the Science*, eds. R. Rieber and R. Brubaker. Amsterdam: North-Holland Publishing Company. Pp. 150–81.

NATION, J. (1970). "Vocabulary Comprehension and Usage in Preschool Cleft-Palate and Normal Children." *Cleft Palate Journal*, 7: 639–44.

NOLL, J. (1970). "Articulatory Assessment." In *Speech and the Dentofacial Complex: The State of the Art*, ed. R. Wertz. ASHA Reports No. 5. Washington D.C.: American Speech and Hearing Association. Pp. 283–98.

PERKINS, W. (1971a). *Speech Pathology An Applied Behavioral Science*. St. Louis: C. V. Mosby Company.

—— (1971b). "Vocal Function: Assessment and Therapy." In *Handbook of Speech Pathology and Audiology*, ed. L. Travis. New York: Appleton-Century-Crofts. Pp. 505–534.

PHILIPS, B. and R. HARRISON (1969). "Language Skills of Preschool Cleft-Palate Children." *Cleft Palate Journal*, 6: 108–119.

PHIPPS, G. (1965). "Psychosocial Aspects of Cleft Palate." In *Proceedings of the Conference: Communicative Problems in Cleft Palate*, ed. D. Green. ASHA Reports No. 1. Washington, D.C.: The American Speech and Hearing Association. Pp. 103–110.

POWERS, M. (1957). "Functional Disorders of Articulation—Symptomatology and Etiology." In *Handbook of Speech Pathology*, ed. L. Travis. New York: Appleton-Century-Crofts.

PRONOVOST, W. (1942). "An Experimental Study of Methods for Determining Natural and Habitual Pitch." *Speech Monographs*, 9: 111–23.

———— (1951). "A Survey of Services for the Speech and Hearing Handicapped in New England." *Journal of Speech and Hearing Disorders,* 16: 148–56.

PTACEK, P. and E. SANDERS (1963). "Breathiness and Phonation Length." *Journal of Speech and Hearing Disorders,* 28: 267–72.

ROBE, E., J. BRUNLIK, and P. MOORE (1960). "A Study of Spastic Dysphonia: Neurologic and Electroencephalographic Abnormalities." *Laryngoscope,* 70: 219–45.

ROUSEY, C. and A. MORIARTY (1965). *Diagnostic Implications of Speech Sounds.* Springfield, Ill.: Charles C Thomas.

RUSSELL, G. (1931). *Speech and Voice.* New York: The Macmillan Company.

SATALOFF, J. and M. FRASER (1952). "Hearing Loss in Children with Cleft Palates." *Archives of Otolaryngology,* 55: 61–64.

SENTURIA, B. and F. WILSON (1968). "Otorhinolaryngic Findings in Children with Voice Disorders." *Annals of Otology, Rhinology, and Laryngology,* 77: 1027–45.

SHELTON, R., A. BROOKS, and K. YOUNGSTROM (1965). "Clinical Assessment of Palatopharyngeal Closure." *Journal of Speech and Hearing Disorders,* 30: 37–43.

SHELTON, R., E. HAHN, and H. MORRIS (1968). "Diagnosis and Therapy." In *Cleft Palate and Communication,* eds. D. Spriestersbach and D. Sherman. New York: Academic Press. Pp. 225–68.

SHERMAN, D. (1954). "The Merits of Backward Playing of Connected Speech in the Scaling of Voice Quality Disorders." *Journal of Speech and Hearing Disorders,* 19: 312–21.

SMITH, R. and B. McWILLIAMS (1968). "Psycholinguistic Abilities of Children with Clefts." *Cleft Palate Journal,* 5: 238–49.

SNIDECOR, J. (1969). *Speech Rehabilitation of the Laryngectomized.* Springfield, Ill.: Charles C Thomas.

SPRIESTERSBACH, D. (1955). "Assessing Nasal Quality in Cleft-Palate Speech of Children." *Journal of Speech and Hearing Disorders,* 20: 266–70.

———— and G. POWERS (1959). "Articulation Skills, Velopharyngeal Closure, and Oral Breath Pressure of Children with Cleft Palates." *Journal of Speech and Hearing Research,* 2: 318–25.

SUBTELNY, J., R. McCORMACK, J. CURTIN, J. SUBTELNY, and K. MUSGRAVE (1970). "Speech, Intraoral Air Pressure, Nasal Airflow—Before and After Pharyngeal Flap Surgery." *Cleft Palate Journal,* 7: 68–90.

VAN DEMARK, D. (1966). "A Factor Analysis of the Speech of Children with Cleft Palate." *Cleft Palate Journal,* 3: 159–70.

———— (1964). "Misarticulations and Listener Judgments of the Speech of Individuals with Cleft Palates." *Cleft Palate Journal,* 1: 232–45.

—— and A. VAN DEMARK (1967). "Misarticulations of Cleft-Palate Children Achieving Velopharyngeal Closure and Children with Functional Speech Problems." *Cleft Palate Journal*, 4: 31–37.

VAN RIPER, C. (1963). *Speech Correction Principles and Methods*, 4th ed. Englewood Cliffs, N.J.: Prentice-Hall, Inc.

—— and J. IRWIN (1958). *Voice and Articulation*. Englewood Cliffs, N.J.: Prentice-Hall, Inc.

WALDROP, W. and M. GOULD (1956). *Your New Voice*. New York: American Cancer Society.

WELLS, C. (1971). *Cleft Palate and Its Associated Speech Disorders*. New York: McGraw-Hill Book Company.

WENDAHL, R. and L. PAGE (1967). "Glottal Wave Periods in CVC Environments." *Journal of Acoustical Society of America*, 42: 1208.

WEPMAN, J., J. MACGAHAN, J. RICKARD, and N. SHELTON (1953). "The Objective Measurement of Progressive Esophageal Speech Development." *Journal of Speech and Hearing Disorders*, 18: 247–51.

WESTLAKE, H. and D. RUTHERFORD (1966). *Cleft Palate*. Englewood Cliffs, N.J.: Prentice-Hall, Inc.

WITHERS, B. (1961). "Vocal Nodules." *Eye, Ear, Nose, and Throat Monthly*, 40: 35–38.

WOOD, K. (1971). "Terminology and Nomenclature." In *Handbook of Speech Pathology and Audiology*, ed L. Travis. New York: Appleton-Century-Crofts. Pp. 3–26.

WORTHLEY, W. (1969). "The Report of a Survey for the Speech Clinician." Mimeographed manuscript.

ZEMLIN, W. (1968). *Speech and Hearing Science: Anatomy and Physiology*. Englewood Cliffs, N.J.: Prentice-Hall, Inc.

9

the
diagnostic report

A final and most important facet of the diagnostician's role is the preparation of an examination report. The clinical situation, test procedures, results, impressions, and recommendations must now be organized and committed to paper. The raw data are of limited value to the clinician or other workers until they are assembled in a clear, precise, and orderly fashion.

A diagnostic report, then, is a written record that summarizes the relevant information we have obtained (and *how* we obtained it) in our professional interaction with a client. It serves the following three purposes: (1) it acts as a guide for further services to the client (it provides a clear statement of where the client is now so that we can document change or lack of change); (2) it communicates our findings to other professional workers; and (3) it serves as a document for research purposes. The importance of the first function should be obvious; intelligent clinical plans evolve naturally from carefully prepared reports. The second purpose of diagnostic reports is to answer questions about clients so that other professionals can provide appropriate services. In addition to transmitting necessary information, a carefully prepared examination report will tend also to establish the credibility of the clinician in the eyes of other workers. Although the diagnostician may be highly skilled in testing and interviewing, his competence may be evaluated largely by his written communications.

FORMAT

There are several ways to organize a diagnostic report (McDearmon, 1961; Huber, 1961; Hammond and Allen, 1953; Johnson, Darley, and Spriestersbach, 1963; Irwin, 1965; Rees, Herbert, and Coates, 1969; Sanders, 1972; Hood, 1972). Since reports will vary somewhat depending upon the intended reader, no single detailed schema is appropriate for all circumstances. However, we have found the following generic format (see Figure 13) quite effective and recommend it to the beginning clinician. It contains four major sections:

Routine information. In this first section we present basic identifying information—the client's name, address, date of birth, telephone number, parent's name where relevant, and, of course, the date of the examination. An undated report is useless. In addition to these routine data, we generally identify the referral source (parent, teacher, physician) and include a succinct statement of the presenting problem. In some cases the reason for referral may be stated in the client's (or his parent's) own words, always indicated by quotation marks.

Test results. The results of the various tests and examinations are delineated in this section. The name of each test, an explanation of what it does, and the results obtained should be included. The information is simply presented and not interpreted at this point.

Clinical impressions. In this section we summarize our impressions of the individual and his communication impairment. What type of speech or language problem does he have? How severe is it? What caused it? What factors seem to be perpetuating it? What impact has it had upon the client and his family? How much does it interfere with his everyday functioning? What are the prospects for treatment? Although we can offer interpretations here, we must still be able to support our impressions with information obtained during the interview or testing. Speculations based upon clinical experience, such as similarity between the client and other cases the diagnostician has examined, should be clearly labeled as such. A brief resume of the salient features from the case history may also be included in this section.

Recommendations. This is perhaps the most crucial portion of the report. We must now translate our findings into appropriate suggestions or directions that will help the client solve his communication and related problems. Do we recommend further speech and language evaluations? Is a medical referral necessary? Is treatment indicated? By whom, when, and what

Diagnostic Report Worksheet

I. Routine Information

Name: _____

Date: _____ Birthdate: _____

Address: _____

Telephone: _____ Parents' Name: _____

Referral Source: _____

Brief Resume of Problem: _____

_____

II. Test Results:

III. Clinical Impressions:

IV. Recommendations:

_____
Clinician

_____
Supervisor

FIGURE 13 Diagnostic Report Worksheet.

direction should it take? The task is, then, to crystallize all the disparate interaction we have had with the individual, collate all the data, and then provide a flexible blueprint for further action. We must attempt to answer the question, "What happens now, where do we go from here?"

Here is an example of a diagnostic report illustrating the format just described. It was prepared by a graduate student for the school nurse and the child's classroom teacher:

i. routine information

Name: Bengston, Amy   *Date*: September 11, 1969
Address: 1927 Germfask Avenue,   *Parent*: Paul Bengston
         Granite Harbor, Michigan   *Phone*: 226–1749
Birthdate: August 2, 1960   *School*: Campus Demonstration School

Amy Bengston, nine years old, was referred to the speech clinic for speech evaluation by the school nurse and the child's third-grade classroom teacher. The referral note stated: "Amy has a skin disease that has resulted in contraction and dwindling of her tongue and lower lip causing her to lisp noticeably."

ii. test results

A picture test of articulation was administered (Amy named pictures of common objects) and revealed two sound errors: the /s/ and /z/ sounds are lateralized in the initial (*s*un, *S*anta), medial (ba*s*ket, whi*s*tle), and final (gla*ss*, grape*s*) positions. The air escapes over both sides of her tongue on /s/ and /z/, creating a "slushy" sound; this is termed a lateral lisp. A very slight lateral emission was also noted on the /sh/ sound.

The sound distortions were only partially stimulable: when the examiner made a standard /s/ and /z/, told Amy to watch and listen carefully and then imitate her sound production, she was able to alter her errors only slightly. She did, however, reduce the lateral escape of air.

A test of vocal phonics (analyzing words into their component sounds and synthesizing sounds into words) was given, and the child missed only one of twenty items. Amy also exhibited superior ability on a task of auditory discrimination (distinguishing like and unlike syllable pairs). She readily detected her sound errors when they were simulated by the examiner.

A screening test was administered and revealed that Amy has normal hearing at all test frequencies.

Amy's oral structure was examined and revealed: partial open bite and jumbled lower incisors; massive scar tissue and atrophy of left side of the tongue; the tongue is displaced toward the left side of the oral cavity. The lower lip is atrophied on the left side; and at a state of rest, her mouth is displaced downward at the left corner. Despite the structural abnormality, however, Amy is able to move her tongue tip up to and beyond the gum ridge behind the upper incisors, and she performed within normal limits on a test of oral diadochokinesis (she repeated the nonsense word "puh-tuh-kuh" 4.2 times per second).

Further, when the examiner touched Amy's tongue (the tip and anterior portion to the right of the midline), Amy was able to correctly identify the precise location of stimulation.

iii. clinical impressions

Amy presents a moderately severe lateral lisp on the sibilant sounds /s/ and /z/. Although it is difficult to determine at this time, the structural abnormality in the oral area may have been a causal factor; the articulatory defects are maintained now by habit strength. The child is reportedly a "good student," but in her teacher's opinion, the lisp is interfering with Amy's school performance (oral reading) and social adjustment (she has received considerable teasing). Amy is aware of her speech disorder and confided to the examiner that she would like to be able to "talk better."

The parents are also concerned about the child's speech, but ambivalent regarding therapy. Mrs. Bengston feels that another focus of attention on the oral area might heighten Amy's sensitivity about her appearance; plastic surgery is planned but, according to the parents, must be delayed until Amy has acquired more facial growth. The dermatologist is confident that the skin disorder is stabilized, although the child must be seen for frequent examinations. There are six siblings ranging in age from an eleven-month-old brother to a twelve-year-old sister. Amy is "very close" to her ten-year-old brother who, according to the parents' report, also lisps. The remainder of the case history is unremarkable.

Prospects for success in therapy appear good on the basis of excellent auditory functioning, partial stimulability, and, despite the scarring and atrophy, normal function of the oral apparatus. In addition, Amy related well to the examiner, exhibited an interest in the diagnostic tasks, and expressed positive motivation for treatment.

iv. recommendations

The first recommendation is to examine the older brother to determine the similarity between his speech pattern and Amy's articulation errors. It may be possible to work with them together, thus taking the direct focus away from Amy; or, if they identify as strongly as Mrs. Bengston reports, just the older child can be enrolled for treatment on the premise that Amy will follow his speech change.[1]

Second, steps should be taken to reduce the teasing Amy is receiving from her classmates. It may be possible to identify the ring leaders and discuss the matter with them; another plan would be to present the problem to the entire class in Amy's absence. The clinician assigned to Amy will also try to desensitize her to teasing.

It is also recommended that the school and the speech-clinic personnel meet jointly with Mr. and Mrs. Bengston to discuss the importance of therapy, outline a plan of treatment, and offer reassurance.

---

[1] Mason, Amy's older brother and close companion, did have an almost identical lateral lisp on the /s/ and /z/ sounds. We worked directly with him and included Amy only in nonthreatening listening activities. Interestingly, when Mason's lisp improved, so did Amy's.

Finally, it would be helpful to have a medical report regarding the skin disorder (through the school nurse).

(signed) M. Kelly
Graduate Speech Clinician

We also like to send a brief cover letter with each report. Here is the note that accompanied the diagnostic summary on Amy Bengston:

Mrs. Ruth Jenson, R. N.
Mrs. Julie Remmer
Campus Demonstration School

Dear Mrs. Jenson and Remmer:
Thank you for referring Amy Bengston to the speech clinic. We did a rather detailed evaluation of her speech and the results are summarized in the attached report. We would be most happy to discuss the findings and the treatment program with you.
Sincerely,

(signed) M. Kelly
Graduate Speech Clinician

STYLE

An extended discussion of prose style for report writing is not possible within the scope of this text. The reader will want to consult several of the following sources for more definitive statements about common modes of report writing (Hammond and Allen, 1953; Huber, 1961; Jerger, 1962; Johnson, Darley and Spriestersbach, 1963; Moore, 1969; Good, 1970). In the interest of brevity, then, we shall simply enumerate several principles of style which we have found useful:

1. Make your presentation straightforward and objective, using a topical outline. It is often helpful to write for a specific reader; picture the reader in your mind—a classroom teacher, physician, speech clinician—and then simply tell him the story of what you observed and recommend regarding a particular client. When in doubt about the reader's level of understanding, it is better to err in the direction of simplicity.

2. Use an impersonal style. Some clinicians use the first person when writing diagnostic reports, but in our view, it is preferable to keep the "I" out of it; a reference to the "clinician" or the "examiner" is more in keeping with professional reports. This style also tends to encourage objectivity.

3. Edit the report carefully to make certain that spelling, grammar, and punctuation are accurate. Errors, even trivial ones, undermine the confidence of the reader in the diagnostician. Remember, competence is judged to a great extent by the precision of your reporting.

4. Watch your semantics. Be wary of overused or nebulous words such as

"good," "beautiful," "cute," etc. Avoid pet expressions or stereotyped ways of phrasing information. One clinician used the phrase "in terms of" thirteen times in a two-page diagnostic report. Another laced his reports with currently popular words like "input," "interface," and "counterproductive." Avoid superlatives unless they are clearly indicated.

5. Avoid preparing an "Aunt Fanny" report (Sunberg and Tyler, 1962), a bland written statement that could represent anyone or is so filled with qualifications ("perhaps," "apparently," "tends to") that it reveals nothing—nothing, that is, except a timid diagnostician.

6. Make the report "tight." Don't leave gaps where it is possible to read between the lines. If findings in certain areas are unremarkable, always state this explicitly. Don't leave the reader to guess whether you investigated all possible aspects.

Turn back now to the illustrative diagnostic report and examine it closely for any important omissions. For example, should the examiner have asked *when* the skin disorder began and then related this to the possible etiology of the lisp? What about the child's capacity to learn? Should this area have been investigated?

7. A diagnostic report is no place to display your learning or to parade a large vocabulary. Pedantic reports are misunderstood or unread.

8. Stay close to the data until you wish to draw the observations together and make some interpretations. For example, tell the reader which sounds were in error instead of simply stating that the child sounds infantile.

THE WRITING PROCESS

Many students have a lot of difficulty writing. Most of them have found the task onerous, and a few are threatened and overwhelmed by the prospect of a blank sheet of paper in the typewriter. It has been our experience, however, that rather than a writing *deficiency* most of these students have a writing *bias*—they do not think they can do it. There are, of course, no quick and simple solutions, but we offer the following suggestions that have proven helpful to more than one beginning report-writer.

Write on a daily basis. Each night—before retiring, for example—sit down and write a descriptive paragraph concerning something that happened that day. At first it may be halting and difficult; as in any new task, your writing "muscle" will be sore. Don't wait for an inspiration, for that magic moment when, suddenly, it will *come* to you. You *go* to it. At the end of a week, review the writing you have done—edit, revise, ask yourself what you meant by each word or phrase. The best way to learn to write, in our opinion, is to write.

Get the message out and revise it later. A common error that some beginning writers make is to attempt to produce perfect writing in the initial draft. It doesn't matter how it looks at this point; you can always edit or have someone help you edit. When you meet barriers or mental blocks, jump over them and go on with the rest of the report. When you come back to it later, you will find that your mind has filled in the blank spots.

It is helpful to have someone read and comment on the initial draft of your report. Although it is difficult to submit one's prose for dissection, ask the reader to be frank and honest in his editing. So many times a phrase that seems clear to the writer who conceived it, is vague or obscure to an objective reader.

PROJECTS AND QUESTIONS

1. Abstract the following articles:

ENGLISH, R. and LILYWHITE, H. "A Semantic Approach to Clinical Reporting in Speech Pathology." *Journal of the American Speech and Hearing Association,* 5 (1963): 647–50.

MOORE, M. "Pathological Writing." *Journal of the American Speech and Hearing Association,* 11 (1969): 535–38.

2. In our clinical routine, we typically have a client sign two similar forms—one which permits us to obtain information about him from other sources and another which allows us to send information about him to referral agencies. Are such forms legal? We asked several other university speech-and-hearing clinics about this; all used forms of this type but were uncertain about their legal status. Design two brief forms—one for release of information and one for obtaining information.

3. Several authors have described the agony and ecstasy involved in learning the craft of writing. The account in the following reference is especially lucid: S. OLSON, *Open Horizons* (New York: Alfred A. Knopf, Inc., 1969), pp. 173–91.

BIBLIOGRAPHY

GOOD, R. (1970). "The Written Language of Rehabilitation Medicine: Meanings and Usages." *Archives of Physical Medicine and Rehabilitation,* 51: 29–36.

HAMMOND, K. and ALLEN, J. (1953). *Writing Clinical Reports.* Englewood Cliffs, N.J.: Prentice-Hall, Inc.

HOOD, S. (1972). "Format for Writing Diagnostic Reports." Unpublished paper. Bowling Green, Ohio: Bowling Green State University.

HUBER, J. (1961). *Report Writing in Psychology and Psychiatry.* New York: Harper & Row, Publishers.

IRWIN, R. (1965). *Speech and Hearing Therapy.* Pittsburgh: Stanwix House.

ERGER, J. (1962). "Scientific Writing Can Be Readable." *Journal of the American Speech and Hearing Association,* 4: 101–4.

JOHNSON, W., DARLEY, F., and SPRIESTERSBACH, D. (1963). *Diagnostic Methods in Speech Pathology.* New York: Harper & Row, Publishers.

MCDEARMON, J. (1961). *Handbook for Clinicians.* Pullman, Wash.: Washington State University Press.

MOORE, M. (1969). "Pathological Writing." *Journal of the American Speech and Hearing Association,* 11: 535–38.

REES, M., HERBERT, E., and COATES, N. (1969). "Development of a Standard Case Record Form." *Journal of Speech and Hearing Disorders,* 34: 68–81.

SANDERS, L. (1972). *Evaluation of Speech and Language Disorders in Children.* Danville, Ill.: Interstate Printers & Publishers.

SUNBERG, N. and TYLER, L. (1962). Clinical Psychology. New York: Appleton-Century-Crofts.

appendix a:

analysis
of a
general case history
(a superproject)

Obtaining a case history, either through interviewing or having the respondent fill out a questionnaire, is a common and useful clinical practice. An inspection of several published forms (Berry and Eisenson, 1956; Johnson, Darely, and Spriestersbach, 1963; Van Riper, 1963; Irwin, 1965; Rees, Herbert, and Coates, 1969; Milisen, 1971) reveals, as expected, a great deal of similarity in the major areas evaluated and even specific queries addressed to a client or parent. The creators of case-history forms undoubtedly select and frame each question to elicit certain relevant information about a client. It is instructive, however, for each clinician to analyze the form he intends to use. Every query should be scrutinized for its purpose: What is the rationale for including it? How pertinent is it in identifying the child's speech problem? Will the answer help the diagnostician to determine the etiology of the communication breakdown?

We have included below a general case-history form for children that was designed to be filled out by a parent and returned to the clinic before a child was seen for evaluation. By analyzing the responses to the various questions, a diagnostician presumably can prepare to assess the child and plan for a more detailed and specific parent interview. We suggest that you examine each item in this form—what purpose does it serve? In order to get you started, we have completed part of the first segment, Identification, and given several purposes for each item. Can you add any others? Instead of analyzing the

form below, you may prefer to study one used in your own clinical training program or a form designed to elicit information about a specific disorder.

I. IDENTIFICATION

A. *Client*

1. *Name*: Basic identifying information. Does the person's name reveal "ethnicity"? What relevance might this have for a speech or language disorder? What might an "unusual" name suggest (e.g., "Sue" for a male child)? Does the child have a nickname or a diminutive name?

2. *Date of birth*: Provides a basis for comparing the child's behavior to established age norms. How old were the parents when the child was born? What possible relationship might this information have to the speech or language disorder?

3. *Sex*: Norms differ for male and female children. Do parental expectations differ according to the sex of their children? Did the mother or father prefer a child of the opposite sex? Is the client the only boy (or girl) in a family of several female (male) children?

4. *Age*: May serve as a reliability check for Item No. 2.

5. *Address*: Provides data about socioeconomic status. Do the parents reside in an isolated rural area? What relationship is there between place of residence and speech or language disorders?

B. *Mother*

1. *Name*: See No. 1 above.

2. *Address*: Is the mother living with the family?

3. *Age*: See No. 2 above. Are birth injuries more frequent in very young (under eighteen) or older (over thirty-five) mothers? Is there any relationship between age of the mother and child-rearing practices?

4. *Occupation*: Does the mother work outside the home? Who cares for the child during her absence? Does her absence affect the child? Is there any conflict between the parents over the mother's employment?

5. *School*: Education level influences child-rearing practices. Is there any relationship between educational level and standards and expectations?

C. *Father*

1. *Name*: See above.

2. *Address*: Is the father living with the family?

3. *Age*: Is there marked difference in the ages of the parents?

4. *Occupation*: Provides basic data for socioeconomic status. Does the father have an occupation that may take him out of the home for prolonged intervals?

5. *Education*: Provides basic data for judgments of socioeconomic status. Is there a wide difference in educational levels between the parents? Could this create differing child-rearing beliefs or practices?

```
                              Date _____
                              Clinic No. _____

Person Completing this form _____
Relationship to the child _____

NOTE: It is important that you fill out this form as
      COMPLETELY as possible and have copies of all
      pertinent medical, educational and psychological
      information sent to us.  Feel free to explain your
      answers by writing on the margins or back of the
      sheet.

  I. IDENTIFICATION

     Name_____Date of Birth_____Sex___Age___

     Address_____Phone_____

     Mother's Name_____Address_____Age___

     Mother's Occupation_____

     Last Grade Completed in School_____

     Father's Name_____Address_____Age___

     Father's Occupation_____

     Last Grade Completed in School_____

     Brothers and Sisters:
```

Name	Age	Sex	Grade in School	Speech, Hearing, or Medical Problem

```
     Referred by_____
     Address_____

     Name of Family Doctor_____
     Address_____

 II. STATEMENT OF THE PROBLEM:

     Describe the problem (Use back if necessary)_____
     _____
     _____
     _____
```

FIGURE 14   Children's Case History.

313

When was the problem first noticed? _____

What is the child's reaction to the problem? _____

How do you and others in the family react to this
problem? _____

What do you think causes the problem? _____

What has been done about it? _____

III. GENERAL DEVELOPMENT

A. Pregnancy and Birth History

What illnesses and/or accidents occurred during
pregnancy? _____

Did mother have any miscarriages or stillbirths? ___

What was the length of labor? _____

Age of mother at child's birth? _____

Age of father at child's birth? _____

Were there any unusual problems at birth? (If so,
describe) _____

Were drugs used? ___ Instruments? ___ Were there any
bruises or abnormalities of the child's head? _____
Other abnormalities _____

Weight of child at birth _____

Did infant require oxygen? _____

Was child "blue" at birth? _____ Jaundiced? ____

Were there any health problems during first two
weeks of infant life? (Describe) _____

At what age did infant regain birth weight? _____

Describe how the infant was fed. (Breast, bottle?)

B. Developmental

At what age did the following occur:

Held head erect while lying on stomach _____
Sat alone unsupported _____ Crawled _____
Walked Unaided _____
Dressed and undressed himself _____
Fed self with spoon _____

FIGURE 14 (Continued)

314

Was completely toilet trained: waking ___ sleeping ___
Had first tooth ___ Had complete set of baby teeth ___

IV. MEDICAL HISTORY

At what ages did any of the following illnesses or
operations occur? Please indicate severity.

	Age	Severity		Age	Severity
Whooping cough			Earaches		
Mumps			Running ears		
Scarlet Fever			Chronic colds		
Measles			Head injuries		
Chicken Pox			Venereal Disease		
Pneumonia			Asthma		
Diptheria			Allergies		
Croup			Convulsions		
Influenza			Encephalitis		
Polio			High fevers		
Headaches			Typhoid		
Sinus			Tonsillitis		
Meningitis			Tonsillectomy		
Rickets			Adenoidectomy		
Rheumatic Fever			Mastoidectomy		
Pleurisy			Thyroid		
Tuberculosis			Heart trouble		
Smallpox			Enlarged glands		

Describe any other operations your child has had _____
_____

Where was he hospitalized? _____ When? _____

Name and address of attending doctor _____
_____

Describe any serious illnesses he has had _____
_____

Name and address of attending doctor _____
_____

What illnesses have been accompanied by an extremely high
fever? _____

Temperature _____ Duration of fever _____

Describe any other serious injuries, or deformities not
already mentioned. _____
_____

Have the child's ears been examined? _____ By whom? _____
Results _____

FIGURE 14   (Continued)

315

Is he now under the care of a doctor? _____

For what reason? _____

Is he presently taking any medication? _____

For what reason? _____

V. EDUCATIONAL HISTORY

School now attending _____ Address _____

Grade _____ Teacher _____

What are his average grades in the following subjects:

Reading _____ Spelling _____

Grades failed _____ Grades skipped _____

Did child attend nursery school? __ Kindergarten __ Age __

If so, where? _____

Is child frequently absent from school? _____ Why? _____

How does child feel about school and about his teachers?

_____

Has there been any previous speech or hearing therapy? ___

If so, where? _____ By whom? _____

VI. DAILY BEHAVIOR

Does your child sleep well? _____ Eat well? _____

Does he tend to play alone or with other children? _____

Age of playmates _____

How does he get along with other children? _____

With adults? _____

Is it difficult to discipline the child? (Explain as

fully as possible.) _____

_____

What types of discipline are used? _____

What types are most effective? _____

What types are least effective? _____

Would you describe your child as basically happy or

unhappy? _____

Does your child have difficulty in concentrating? _____

What are the child's favorite play activities? _____

_____

What is your most difficult problem with the child? _____

_____

FIGURE 14   (Continued)

VII. SPEECH AND HEARING HISTORY

Did infant babble and coo during first 6 months? _____

When did he speak his first word? _____

When did he begin to use two-word sentences? _____

What were child's first few words? _____

Does he use speech:
Frequently? _____ Occasionally? _____ Never? _____

Does he prefer to use speech or gestures? (Give
examples if possible.) _____

Which does the child prefer to use:
Complete sentences? _____ Phrases? _____
One or two words? _____ Sounds? _____

How well can he be understood by his parents? _____
By his brother and sisters and playmates? _____

Does he make sounds incorrectly? _____
If so, which ones? _____

Does he hesitate and/or repeat sounds or words? _____

Does he "get stuck" in attempting to say words? _____

Please answer the following with a "yes" or "no" for
each year:

	First Year	Second Year	After Second Year
Generally indifferent to sound			
Lack of response when spoken to			
Responded to noise and not voice			
Less than normal amount of crying			
Less than normal amount of laughter			
Meaningful speech (however limited)			
Yelling or screeching to attract attention or express annoyance			
Head-banging or foot-stamping			
Shuffles feet while walking			
Marked alertness to gesture, facial expression and movement			

Do you think your child hears adequately? _____
If not, what do you feel to be the cause? _____
_____

Does the child's hearing appear to be constant or does
it vary? _____

Is his hearing poorer when he has a cold? _____

FIGURE 14   (Continued)

VIII. HOME

Housing: House _____ Apartment _____
Other (Please describe) _____

How many rooms? _____

Members of household other than family _____
_____

Neighborhood: Check all that best describe your
neighborhood.
Residential _____ Business _____ Poor _____ Rural _____
Above Average _____ Crowded _____ Average _____ Run-
down _____ Excellent Condition _____ Suburban _____

FIGURE 14   (Continued)

BIBLIOGRAPHY

BERRY, M. and J. EISENSON (1956). *Speech Disorders.* New York: Appleton-Century-Crofts.

JOHNSON, W., F. DARLEY, and D. SPRIESTERSBACH (1963). *Diagnostic Methods in Speech Pathology.* New York: Harper & Row, Publishers.

IRWIN, R. (1965). *Speech and Hearing Therapy.* Pittsburgh: Stanwix.

MILISEN, R. (1971). "Methods of Evaluation and Diagnosis of Speech Disorders." In *Handbook of Speech Pathology and Audiology,* ed. L. Travis. New York: Appleton-Century-Crofts.

REES, M., E. HERBERT, and N. COATES (1969). "Development of a Standard Case Record Form." *Journal of Speech and Hearing Disorders,* 34: 68–81.

VAN RIPER, C. (1963). *Speech Correction: Principles and Methods,* 4th ed. Englewood Cliffs, N.J.: Prenitce-Hall, Inc.

index